International Sports Medicine Directory

International Federation of Sports Medicine
(Fédération Internationale de Médecine du Sport)

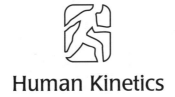

Human Kinetics

Library of Congress Cataloging-in-Publication Data

International Federation of Sports Medicine directory/International Federation of Sports Medicine.
    p. ; cm.
  ISBN 0-7360-3376-9
    1. International Federation of Sports Medicine--Directories. 2. Sports
medicine--Directories. I. International Federation of Sports Medicine.
   [DNLM: 1. Sports Medicine--Directory. 2. Physical Education and
Training--Directory. QT 22.1 I613 2001]
  RC1200 .I485 2001
  617.1'027'025--dc21

                  00-047234

ISBN: 0-7360-3376-9

Copyright © 2001 by Human Kinetics Publishers, Inc.

FIMS Coordinator: Edward Grogg
Sports Medicine Managing Editor: Julie Johnson
Special Projects Editor: Judy Park
Managing Editor: Laurie Stokoe
Assistant Editors: Wendy McLaughlin, Leigh Lahood
Copyeditors: Julie Marx, John Wentworth, Jan Feeney
Administrative Assistants: Connie Young, Sandra Shelton
Graphic Designer: Fred Starbird
Graphic Artist: Tara Welsch
Permissions Manager: Courtney Astle
Information Specialist: John Laskowski
Photo Manager: Gayle Garrison
Cover Designer: Nancy Rasmus
Photographers (interior): Photo on page 4 by Bruce Dill, Courtesy of Dr. Elsworth R. Buskirk and Dr. Charles M. Tipton; photo on page 7 by Bruce Dill, Courtesy of Dr. Jack Wilmore and Dr. David Costill; photo on page 8 Courtesy of Mankato State University; and photo on page 9 © Human Kinetics.
Printer: Versa

Printed in the United States of America   10 9 8 7 6 5 4 3 2 1

Human Kinetics
Web site: www.humankinetics.com

United States: Human Kinetics, P.O. Box 5076, Champaign, IL 61825-5076
800-747-4457
e-mail: humank@hkusa.com

Canada: Human Kinetics, 475 Devonshire Road Unit 100, Windsor, ON N8Y 2L5
800-465-7301 (in Canada only)
e-mail: hkcan@mnsi.net

Europe: Human Kinetics, P.O. Box IW14, Leeds LS16 6TR, United Kingdom
+44 (0) 113 278 1708
e-mail: humank@hkeurope.com

Australia: Human Kinetics, 57A Price Avenue, Lower Mitcham, South Australia 5062
08 8277 1555
e-mail: liahka@senet.com.au

New Zealand: Human Kinetics, P.O. Box 105-231, Auckland Central
09-309-1890
e-mail: hkp@ihug.co.nz

Contents

PART I

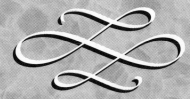

Sports Medicine Internationally

An Overview of Sports Medicine

Walter Frontera

The purpose of this chapter is to present an overview of the scientific and clinical discipline known as sports medicine. In a diverse world like ours, it is not surprising to see that there is no single definition of sports medicine that is accepted by all interested in the field. Different authors and professional groups throughout the world have their own conceptual and practical definitions of sports medicine. This intrinsic heterogeneity may explain why clinical sports medicine programs around the world vary in the nature and scope of their services. Also, educational and training programs in sports medicine do not have a common curriculum, and educational experiences vary from region to region. Finally, research in sports medicine covers a wide spectrum of topics. Some examples of research are the molecular mechanisms of force production in skeletal muscle, the surgical technique most appropriate for the reconstruction of the anterior cruciate ligament (ACL) of the knee, and the mental training that will enhance performance in specific athletic events such as archery. There

is little doubt that a consensus in sports medicine has not been achieved. Thus, for the purposes of this overview, it may be more relevant and fruitful to describe sports medicine as it is perceived and practiced around the world and to comment on the various approaches that have resulted from local or regional interests, needs, and beliefs.

Knowledge Base

All sports medicine practitioners benefit from the knowledge generated by research in many basic and applied sciences. Some of this knowledge is not unique to the field and serves as the foundation for the practice of many health-related professions and medical specialties including sports medicine. On the other hand, there is a body of knowledge that has accumulated over the last few decades that is unique to sports medicine. It has emerged from investigations designed to address specific questions related to the limits of human performance and the health care needs of the physically active population.

Many scientific disciplines contribute to the knowledge base in sports medicine—some more than others. Physiology and nutrition constitute the foundation that successful training programs are built on. In addition, an in-depth understanding of the physiological responses to acute and chronic exercise can guide the development of preventive exercise programs for the general population and rehabilitative interventions for patients with acute injuries and chronic diseases. Research on the psychological and biological bases of the human mind provides the framework for the mental preparation needed by the high-performance athlete and for the study of the benefits of physical activity and exercise on human behavior and mental health. Physics contributes to the basic understanding of the effects of therapeutic modalities such as cold and ultrasound in the rehabilitation of a sport-related injury. Chemistry and pharmacology explain the appropriate use and effectiveness of pharmacological agents in the treatment of pain and inflammation and serve to study the interaction between the metabolic changes associated with physical activity and drug metabolism. Knowledge of the anatomy and biomechanics of the musculoskeletal system is essential in the development of proper training and performance techniques for successful sport participation. This knowledge is also fundamental for the development of therapeutic and surgical techniques for injuries such as ligamentous tears and muscle-tendon sprains.

Practical and Operational Definitions

The content of study in sports medicine has evolved significantly during the last 50 years. In an editorial for the *Journal of Sports Medicine and Physical Fitness* published in 1977, Prof. Giuseppe La Cava, FIMS president from 1968 to 1976, described sports medicine as the application of medical knowledge to sport with the aim of preserving the health of the athlete while improving his or her performance. La Cava included sports biotypology, physiopathology, medical evaluation, traumatology, hygiene, and therapeutics as the main elements of sports medicine.

In 1988, Prof. Wildor Hollmann, FIMS president from 1986 to 1994, summarized the main aspects of sports medicine as follows: medical treatment of injuries and illnesses; medical examination before starting a sport to detect any damage that could be worsened by the sport; medical performance investigation to assess the performance capacity of heart, circulation, respiration, metabolism, and the skeletal musculature; performance diagnosis specific to the type of sport; medical advice on lifestyle and nutrition; medical assistance in developing optimal training methods; and scientifically based control of training.

More recently, many authors have expanded the nature of the clinical activities included in sports medicine. For example, according to Brukner and Khan (1993), clinical sports medicine includes management of medical problems

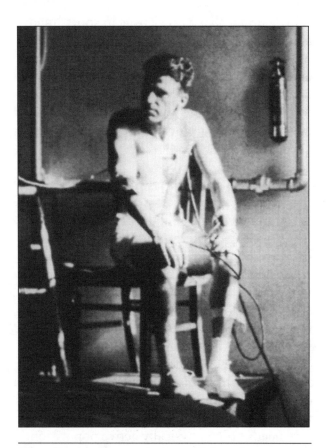

Glen Cunningham, sports medicine pioneer.

1954

Sports medicine, as defined by the ACSM, was a unique blend of physical education, medicine, and physiology, much as it was in ancient Greece.

Source: *Berryman, J. (1995) Out of Many, A History of the American College of Sports Medicine, p2.*

1958

Sports medicine embodies theoretical and practical medicine which examines the influence of exercise, training and sports, as well as lack of exercise, on healthy and unhealthy people of all ages to produce results that are conducive to prevention, therapy and rehabilitation as well as beneficial for the athlete himself.

Definition taken from the Foundation of the Institute for Circulatory Research and Sports Medicine in Cologne

Source: *Hollmann, W. & Hettinger, T. (1980) Sports medicine-foundations of work and training.*

1971

Sports medicine is the scientific study of the human organism:

1. Within the context of physical activity:
   a) Physical Activity: General
   b) Physical Activity: Sports, Games, and Exercise
2. As the organism (in physical activity) is influenced by or related to:
   a) Environment
   b) Emotions and intellect
   c) Growth, Development, and Aging
   d) Drugs
3. As physical activity is applied in:
   a) Prevention of Disease and Injury
   b) Special Application of Physical Activity in the Handicapped Individual
   c) Rehabilitation
4. As the organism is regulated (in physical activity) by:
   a) Safety and Protection

Source: *Encyclopedia of Sport Science and Medicine (1971).*

1976

The aspect of medicine concerned with the prevention and treatment of injuries related to or incurred during participation in sports.

Source: *Webster's Sports Dictionary (1976)*

1981

Sports medicine is the scientific and medical aspects of exercise and athletics. More specifically, sports medicine is the study of the physiological, biomechanical, psychosocial, and pathological phenomena associated with exercise and athletics and the clinical application of the knowledge gained from this study to the improvement and maintenance of functional capacities for physical labor, exercise, and athletics and to the prevention and treatment of disease and injuries related to exercise and athletics.

Definition taken from David Lamb's Sports Medicine Bulletin (1981)

Source: *Berryman, J. (1995) Out of Many, A History of the American College of Sports Medicine, p172.*

1984

An area of medicine that deals with the physiological, anatomical, psychological, and biomechanical effects of exercise; often includes other areas of concern such as training methods, injury prevention, injury treatment and rehabilitation, and nutrition.

Source: *The Facts on File Dictionary of Fitness (1984).*

1986

A subspecialty of clinical practice concerned with the injuries and disorders resulting from athletics and other sporting activities.

Source: *International Dictionary of Medicine and Biology, vII (1986).*

1989

The field of medicine concerned with injuries sustained in athletics, including their prevention, diagnosis, and treatment.

(continued)

Defining Sports Medicine (continued)

Source: *Dorland's Pocket Medical Dictionary 24th edition (1989)*.

1990

The field of medicine that uses a holistic, comprehensive, and multidisciplinary approach to health care for those engaged in a sporting or recreational activity.

Source: *Stedman's Medical Dictionary 25th edition (1990)*.

1993

Many authors have attempted to define sports medicine in relation to the management of sporting injuries. Sports medicine, however, has a much wider scope and should be defined as 'the medicine of exercise' or the 'total medical care of the exercising individual.' Clinical sports medicine includes injury prevention, diagnosis, treatment, and rehabilitation; performance enhancement through training, nutrition, and psychology; management of medical problems caused by exercise and the role of exercise in chronic disease states; the specific needs of exercising children, females, and older people; the medical care of sporting teams and events, as well as ethical issues such as the problem of drug abuse in sport.

Source: *Brukner & Khan, Clinical Sports Medicine (1993)*.

Field of medicine concerned with all aspects of physiology, pathology, and psychology as they apply to persons who participate in sports whether at the recreational, amateur, or professional level. An important facet of sports

medicine is the application of medical knowledge to the prevention of injuries in those who participate in sports.

Source: *Taber's Cyclopedia Medical Dictionary 17th edition (1993)*.

1998

A branch of medicine that specializes in the prevention and treatment of injuries resulting from training for and participating in athletic events.

Source: *Mosby's Medical, Nursing, and Allied Health Dictionary (1998)*.

A branch of medicine concerned with the welfare of athletes and deals with the science and medical treatment of those involved in sports and physical activities. The object of sports medicine includes the prevention, protection, and correction of injuries, and the preparation of an individual for physical activity in its full range of intensity. Sports medicine includes the study of effects of different levels of exercise, training, and sport on healthy and ill people in order to produce information useful in prevention, therapy, and rehabilitation of injuries and illness in athletes. The information is used to optimize performance in sports. Sports medicine originally dealt with medical aspects of sport, and its foremost objective was the welfare of the athlete. Recently, there has been an emphasis by some practitioners on the possible contribution of medical science to improve athletic performances, sometimes at the expense of morality and ethics.

Source: *Oxford Dictionary of Sports Science and Medicine 2nd edition (1998)*.

associated with physical activity and exercise; the role of exercise in the treatment and rehabilitation of chronic disease states; performance enhancement through various interventions such as physiological training, psychological training, and nutritional alterations; prevention, diagnosis, treatment, and rehabilitation of sports injuries; special and specific needs of the pediatric, female, and older populations of physically active people; health care needs of

the traveling sports team; and the use and abuse of substances prohibited in sports (doping).

A Personal View

It is clear that sports medicine includes a wide variety of themes and topics and that sports medicine practitioners must be familiar with many basic and applied sciences as well as with broadly diverse medical and clinical disciplines.

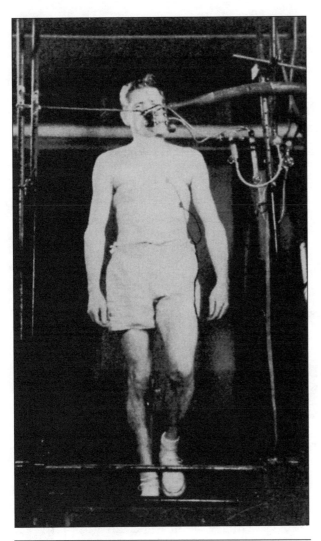

The Harvard Fatigue Laboratory (1938).

Sports medicine can be briefly and accurately defined as *the study of the interrelationship between physical activity and health*. In this context, physical activity includes daily and occupational activities, structured exercise training, and sport participation. This definition considers not only the presence of the stimulus of physical activity but also its absence since it is known that inactivity and deconditioning have deleterious effects on human health. Further, the possibility that excessive activity (and inappropriate training loads and techniques) and movements that test the limits of the musculoskeletal system lead to injury and disease is also recognized. Significant efforts and resources are dedicated to the diagnosis and treatment of these sport-related injuries.

Health must be defined (in accordance with the World Health Organization) as a state of physical, psychological, and social well-being, not only the absence of disease. Sports medicine is based on the reciprocal relationship between physical activity (in all its forms) and health. In other words, it is important to be healthy to participate in exercise and sport. Optimal performance is not possible without optimal health. The converse idea is equally important: a state of optimal health can be achieved by means of appropriate levels of physical activity, exercise, or sport participation. Physical activity, exercise, and sport participation contribute significantly to the prevention of chronic diseases and the enhancement of physical and psychological functional capacity. Thus, it is clear that the sports medicine practitioner must be an advocate for both health for sports and sports for health.

The Sports Medicine Team

Sports medicine is one of those professional disciplines in which the team approach is synonymous with the standard of care. The team is interdisciplinary in nature and the leader or coordinator of the team's efforts is a physician. The medical leader of the team can be a sports medicine specialist, an orthopedic surgeon, a physiatrist (specialist in physical medicine and rehabilitation), a specialist in internal medicine, a pediatrician, or a physician with experience working with physically active people and athletes. Frequently, the athlete interacts with any or all members of the health care team. Members of the sports medicine team may include, but are not limited to, athletic trainers, physiotherapists, nutritionists/dietitians, and psychologists.

The coach or manager should be included in the important decisions that are made about the ability of the athlete to train or compete with the team. The planning of sports medical services as well as the implementation of many medical clinical interventions require, with the consent of the patient/athlete, the active

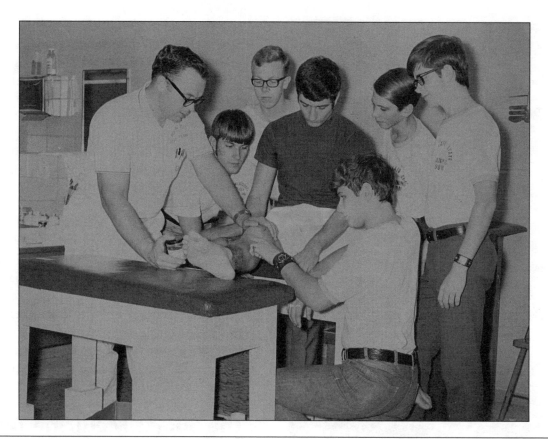

Graduates from Mankato State University's early undergraduate athletic training program (1950s).

participation of the coach. Further, the managers or administrators of sport teams or delegations sometimes must be aware of the nature of a health problem because their decisions directly affect the ability of the health care team to maintain the health status and enhance the performance of the athlete.

Sports Medicine Education in Different Countries

In some countries such as Brazil, Cuba, Italy, Germany, and Uruguay, sports medicine is a recognized specialty; formal postgraduate training has been instituted in various medical schools and universities. Education in sports medicine in these countries emphasizes the medical and physiological control of the athlete as well as many other nonorthopedic aspects of sports medicine. In other countries, such as Canada, Switzerland, and the United States, sports medicine is not recognized as a

specialty and training is available in the form of fellowships for physicians who have completed a primary medical specialty (for example, orthopedic surgery, physical medicine and rehabilitation, or family medicine). However, the scope of some of these fellowships is at times limited to a particular area of sports medicine such as the diagnosis and treatment of sport-related injuries. In many other countries where neither is available, physicians complete their professional training and acquire knowledge and expertise in sports medicine by participating in courses, attending seminars, and working with physically active people and competitive athletes.

Things That Make Sports Medicine Special

An interesting challenge in the practice of sports medicine is the nature of the patient and his or her environment. The underlying

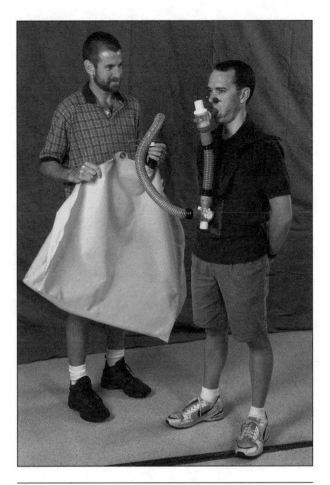

Early measurement of metabolic responses to exercise.

lete. Sports medicine has evolved from both the philosophical and clinical perspectives. The application of the sports medicine principles to the general population has become as important (some may say more important) as the use of sports medicine knowledge to maintain health and enhance performance in competitive athletics. Furthermore, the use of exercise and physical activity in the prevention, treatment, and rehabilitation of chronic diseases is now considered as effective as more traditional interventions such as the use of pharmacological agents. The importance of exercise and physical activity should be obvious if we consider that in many countries, chronic diseases are the most frequent causes of morbidity and mortality, the prevalence of disability resulting from such diseases is on the rise, and the aging population is experiencing functional loss and disability.

Walter Frontera was elected to the FIMS Executive Committee in 1994, and became the Secretary General in 1998. Dr. Frontera is the President of the Pan-American Confederation of Sports Medicine; the Earle P. and Ida S. Charlton Association Professor; the Department of Physical Medicine and Rehabilitation Chairman at Harvard Medical School; and the Physical Medicine and Rehabilitation Department Chief for both Spaulding Rehabilitation Hospital and Massachusetts General Hospital.

mechanism of injury or medical problem must be fully understood because the patient/athlete's objective is to return to the activity that caused the problem. Avoiding the activity associated with the injury, except in life-threatening situations, is not an option; the sports medicine team must do everything possible to correct the fundamental problem. Rehabilitation is needed to enhance the performance of the athlete not only in daily activities but most importantly in sport activities requiring the ultimate mastery of movement.

A Broadening Scope

It is important to highlight the fact that the current international perspective of sports medicine is no longer limited to the elite ath-

Bibliography

Brukner, P., and K. Khan. *Clinical Sports Medicine.* New York: McGraw Hill, 1993, pp. 3-7.

Darby, L., and K.D. Browder. Sports Medicine. In *Contemporary Sport Management.* J.H. Parks, B.R.K. Zanger, and J. Quarterman. Champaign, Il: Human Kinetics, 1998, pp. 197-213.

Holmann, W. The definition and scope of sports medicine. In *The Olympic Book of Sports Medicine.* A. Dirix, H.G. Knuttgen, and K. Tittel, eds. Oxford, UK: Blackwell Scientific Publications, 1988, pp. xi-xii.

La Cava, G. What is sports medicine: Definition and tasks. *J. Sports Med. Phys. Fitness.* 17:1-3, 1977.

2

International Federation of Sports Medicine

The International Federation of Sports Medicine (FIMS) was born in 1928, shortly after the birth of the modern Olympic Games. FIMS assists athletes in achieving their best performance based on their genetic potentials, health and nutrition, and medically supervised training. FIMS' strong association with the International Olympic Committee (IOC) is expressed in the five Olympic rings in the FIMS flag, which shows not only FIMS' origins but also the commitment to the basic principles of the Olympic movement.

FIMS promotes the study and development of sports medicine throughout the world. FIMS' missions are to preserve and improve the health of humankind through physical fitness and sport participation; to study the natural and pathological implications of physical training and sport participation; to organize and sponsor meetings, courses, congresses, and exhibits internationally in the field of sports medicine; to cooperate with national and international associations involved in sports medicine and related fields; to publish scientific information related to sports medicine; and to take all other steps either alone or in cooperation with any appropriate individuals or organizations to further FIMS' activities.

History of the Organization

When we look for the historical perspective of the International Federation of Sports Medicine, it is important to understand what was going on at the time it was founded and which forces and concerns moved our founders to bring together physicians from different countries to work toward a common goal.

The most important factor for establishing the specialization of sports medicine was the beginning of the modern Olympic Games in Athens, Greece, in 1896. At the beginning of the 20th century, advances in sport training required advances in medical care for world-class athletes' unique health concerns. The first sports medicine specialist, the first laboratory for the evaluation of athletes, the first scientific events, the first sports medicine journal, and the first association of sports medicine were established in Dresden, Germany, in 1913.

The international sport federations were founded at the time the Olympic Games were reestablished. In the late 19th century, there were only three associations: gymnastics (1881), rowing (1892), and cycling (1900). In the beginning of the 20th century, the associations for football (1904), weightlifting (1905),

> ### ∞ *What We Do* ∞
>
> Publications:
> - International Sports Medicine Directory
> - The World Of Sports Medicine, the quarterly newsletter
> - International Sports Medicine Journal, electronic journal at www.fims.org
>
> Education:
> - Offer distance education courses
> - Collaborate with Human Kinetics Publishers to create the electronic resource guide E-SportMed.com
> - Publish annual books on important Sports Medicine issues
>
> Networking:
> - Host regional and international Sports Medicine conferences
> - Network with Sports Medicine specialists worldwide

swimming (1908), and athletics (1912) were established.

While observing and being influenced by the organization of the sports, and considering the importance of promoting the ideas of sports medicine, the existing professionals in the field decided to move for the creation of an international association. The best opportunity for that was the Winter Olympic Games in Saint Moritz, Switzerland, in February 1928. At this time, 50 sports physicians from 11 nations founded the Association International Medico-Sportive (AIMS)—with a French name, as was the standard at that time. The purpose was to cooperate with the international sports federations and the International Olympic Committee to provide the best possible medical care for the athletes taking part in the Summer and Winter Olympic Games. The first executive board was formed by Prof. Knoll (Switzerland) as president, Dr. Mallwitz (Germany) as secretary, Prof. Latarjet (France), Prof. Buytendijk (Holland), and Dr. Dybowsky (Poland).

Prof. Buytendijk was asked to organize the 1st AIMS International Congress of Sports Medicine during the IX Summer Olympic Games in Amsterdam, Holland, in August 1928. The meeting was a great success, with the participation of 280 sports physicians from 20 countries. One important practical point of the event was the opportunity for a large group of professionals to analyze many of the athletes participating in the Games through a collection of anthropometric, cardiovascular, physiological, and metabolic information.

The name AIMS was changed to Fédération Internationale Medico-Sportive et Cientifique at the 2nd International Congress, held in September 1933 in Turin, Italy. In the next International Congress held in Chamonix, France, the association received the name that remains today: Fédération Internationale de Médecine Sportive (International Federation of Sports Medicine).

By 1960, the field of sports medicine experienced rapid growth and development in various parts of the world, partially due to the interest generated within individuals and nations and partially due to the projects and initiatives of FIMS. At a meeting held in Turin, Italy, in 1964, steps were taken to encourage the formation of multinational groups based on geographic and linguistic criteria.

To conclude, the development of FIMS can be divided into three periods. The first period was from 1928 to 1939, and its activities were essentially limited to Europe. During the second period, from 1946 to 1964, the International Olympic Committee and the World Health Organization recognized FIMS as the association responsible for bringing together the world's specialists in sports medicine. The third period, based on the internationalization of the specialization, started in 1964 and will probably conclude in 2002.

Dr. Eduardo Henrique De Rose is the 12th president of FIMS and the first president from a non-European country. Dr. De Rose is of Italian-Brazilian descent and was born in Porto Alegre. He completed his doctoral studies in Germany and Italy. Dr. De Rose has been a member of FIMS' executive committee since

Current Executive Committee

President

Eduardo De Rose, PhD
Rua Felipe Becker 95
Tres Figueiras
91330-250 Porto Alegre
RS-BRAZIL
BRAZIL
Telephone: (55 51) 381 2136
Fax: (55 51) 381 2205
E-mail: derose@vortex.ufrgs.br

Vice-Presidents

Constant Roux, MD
Chef de Service Chirurgie
Pediatrique
Chu de Yopougon
21 BP 632
Abidjan
(or)
01 BP v 166
Abidjan
Faculte de Medecine
Abidjan
IVORY COAST
Telephone: (225) 466 170/(225) 011 220/
    (225) 440 864
Fax: (225) 466 727/(225) 443 282
E-mail: roux.c@africaonline.co.ci

Kai-Ming Chan, MD
Hong Kong Centre of Sports
Medicine and Sports Science
Department of Orthopaedics &
Traumatology
Chinese University of Hong Kong
Prince Wales Hospital
Shatin
HONG KONG
Telephone: (852) 2632 2728
Fax: (852) 2637 7889
E-mail: kaimingchan@cuhk.hk
Home address: No. 152 Hong

Lok Road East
Hong Kong Yuen
Taipe, Hong
Telephone: (852) 2657 0822

Fabio Pigozzi, MD
University Institute of Motor Sciences
Pza. Lauro de Bosis 15
00196 Rome
ITALY
Telephone: (3906) 3609 5569/61/41
Fax: (3906) 3230 010
E-mail: medsporm@uni.net
Home address:
    Via Saluzzo—79
    00182 Rome
    ITALY
Telephone: (3906) 7011 576
Fax: (3906) 7011 576

Secretary General

Walter R. Frontera, MD, PhD
Department of Physical Medicine &
    Rehabilitation
Harvard Medical School
Spaulding Rehabilitation Hospital
Boston, MA 02114
UNITED STATES of AMERICA
Telephone: (617) 5737 180
Fax: (617) 5732 759
E-mail:
    frontera.walter@mgh.harvard.edu
Home address: 33 Summit Street
Concord, MA 01742
UNITED STATES of AMERICA
Telephone: (978) 3719 092

Treasurer

Costas Christodoulakis, MD
PO Box 5137
1307 Nicosia
CYPRUS

(continued on next page)

(Christodoulakis, continued)

Telephone: (357 2) 663 762
Fax: (357 2) 664 669
Home address: Indiras Gandhi 5, str.
Monparnasse Hill
2413, Engomi, Nicosi
CYPRUS
Telephone: (357 2) 350 931

Elected Members

Norbert Bachl, MD
Institute of Sports Science
Department of Sports & Exercise
   Physiology
University of Vienna
Auf der Schmelz 6A
1150 Vienna
AUSTRIA
Telephone: 431 4277 48870
Fax: 431 4277 48879
E-mail: norbert.bachl@univie.ac.at

Dusan Hamar, MD, PhD
Institute of Sports Sciences
Department of Sports Medicine
Comenuis University
Svobodovo nabr. 9
814 69 Bratislava
SLOVAKIA
Telephone: (421 7) 5441 1624
Fax: (421 7) 5441 4472
E-mail: hamar@fsport.uniba.sk
Home address:
   Vysehradska 5
   851 06 Bratislava
   SLOVAKIA
Telephone: (421 7) 6382 9290

Prof. Nishat Millack, MD
Hill Park General Hospital
Shaheet-e-Millat Hospital
Karachi
PAKISTAN
Telephone: (92 21) 4552 442

Fax: (92 21) 5060 343
E-mail: zsl@cyber.net.pk
Home address: 73-D, 29th Street
   DHA Phase V
   Karachi
   PAKISTAN
Telephone: (92 21) 5847 7567
Fax: (92 21) 5060 343

Lyle J. Micheli, MD
Children's Hospital
Department of Orthopaedic Surgery
319 Longwood Avenue
Boston, MA 02115
UNITED STATES of AMERICA
Telephone: (617) 355 6934/
   (617) 738 4314
Fax: (617) 730 0227

Anthony Parker, PhD
Queensland University of Technology
School of Human Movement Studies
Kelvin Grove Campus
Victoria Park Road, Kelvin Grove 4059
Queensland
AUSTRALIA
Telephone: (61 7) 3864 3512
Fax: (61 7) 3864 3980
E-mail: t.parker@qut.edu.au
Home address: 92/7 McQuarie Street
St. Lucia 4067
Brisbane, Queensland
AUSTRALIA
Telephone: (61 7) 3876 1941/
   0408 988 197

Patricia Sangenis, MD
Institute of Sports Medicine
Deporte y Salud Buenos Aires
Matienzo 1682 (C.F.)
(1426) Buenos Aires
ARGENTINA
Telephone: (541) 14 7774 949
Fax: (541) 14 7774 499
E-mail: Psangenis@datamarkets.com.ar

Martin P. Schwellnus, MD, MSc, PhD
Sports Science Institute of South Africa
The University of Cape Town
Boundary Road, Newlands 7700
SOUTH AFRICA
Telephone: (2721) 6867 330/
  (2721) 5314 615
Fax: (2721) 6867 530
E-mail: Mschwell@sports.uct.ac.az

John M. Wesseling, MD
AMALIASTRAAT 12
2514 JC Den Haag
THE NETHERLANDS
Telephone: 31.70.3521857
Fax: 31.70.3228313
E-mail: john.wesseling@wxs.nl
Home address:

Ypersestraat 4A
2587 AW Dan Haag
THE NETHERLANDS

Auditor
Mohammed H. Mufti, MD
PO Box 22486
Riyadh 11565
SAUDI ARABIA
Telephone: (966) 1 4776 448
Fax: (966) 1 4792 451
E-mail: 105362@compuserve.com
Home address:
  PO Box 60350
  Riyadh 11495
  SAUDI ARABIA
Telephone: (966) 1 4886 100
Fax: (966)1 4881 188

1976, and his main concerns are the regionalization of FIMS through the continental associations, an increase in individual membership, an emphasis on education including the full use of technology, and the use of professional administration. Dr. De Rose proposed to Human Kinetics an agreement that was signed in 1998 after the FIMS World Congress in Orlando, with a focus on individual membership (now administered by HK) and on education that uses new technologies.

As a member of the IOC Medical Commission, Dr. De Rose has strengthened the relationship with the IOC and also started exchanging information and activities with UNESCO, the World Health Organization, and the ICSSPER. Today, a great deal of FIMS' activities are done with the sport physician in mind, not only in high-level sport, but also in providing better health care to the general population through sport, exercise, and physical activities.

Statutes

CHAPTER I. Designation and Purpose of FIMS.

Article 01. FIMS-Fédération Internationale de Médécine Sportive is a non-profit organization founded at St. Moritz (Switzerland) in 1928.

Article 02. FIMS has a permanent legal status. Membership is not contingent on an individual's sex or race, or any political or philosophical belief or practice.

Article 03. The official address of FIMS shall be the address of the Secretary General.

Article 04. The aims of FIMS are:

a) To promote the study and development of Sports Medicine throughout the world.

b) To preserve and improve the health of mankind through physical fitness and sports participation.

c) To study scientifically the natural and pathological implications of physical training and sports participation.

d) To organize and/or sponsor scientific meetings, courses, congresses, and exhibits on an international basis in the field of Sports Medicine.

e) To cooperate with national and international organizations in Sports Medicine and related fields.

f) To publish scientific information in the field of Sports Medicine and related subjects.

g) To take all other such steps either alone or in cooperation with any appropriate individual or organization as shall from time to time be calculated to further the purposes above listed.

CHAPTER II. Composition of FIMS.

Article 05. The membership of FIMS shall include associations and individuals:

a) National Associations of Sports Medicine,

b) Multinational Groups in Sports Medicine,

c) Honorary members,

d) Individual members,

e) Associate members.

Article 06. National Associations.

06.01. The Council of Delegates shall admit to membership the National Association (not more than one from each country) which is recognized as representing the interests of Sports Medicine in each country.

06.02. Where two or more organizations in any country claim recognition as the National Association of that country, it shall be in the absolute discretion of the Council of Delegates to determine, after due consideration, which, if any, shall be recognized.

06.03. Applicant National Association must submit for consideration by the Executive the following documents before the petition can be presented to the Council of Delegates:

a) Application in writing signed by the President and the Secretary General of the National Association.

b) Copy of the Statutes of the Association.

c) List of Officers of the Association with their titles.

d) Total number of members in each category of membership.

e) Letter of recommendation attesting the fact that the applicant Association is the representative Sports Medicine organization in that country from one of the following bodies: National Medical Association, National Olympic Committee, or National Ministry of Health.

06.04. National Associations shall forward to the Secretariat of FIMS, in the event of changes, a revised copy of their institutional document, a current list of their officers, and the total numbers of their members in each category of membership.

06.05. National Associations shall forfeit their status as a member of FIMS:

a) As a result of a formal resignation in writing by the association being duly received by the Executive Committee.

b) As a result of non-payment of dues for four consecutive years. An application for re-instatement will be entertained by the Council of Delegates until the arrears are paid.

c) As a result of revocation of membership by a recommendation of the Executive Committee for that action.

Article 07. Multinational Groups in Sports Medicine.

a) Multinational groups of Sports Medicine shall represent continental or regional free groupings of National Associations of Sports Medicine, organized on a geographical or lingual basis.

b) The aims of Multinational Groups in Sports Medicine are to realize the purpose of FIMS as well as to organize specific activities in the field of Sports Medicine in the appropriate areas such as promotion of participation in FIMS, organization of regional conferences and courses, issuing of regional conferences and courses, issuing of regional journals, and ensuring a permanent exchange of information.

c) Activities of recognized Multinational Groups in Sports Medicine shall be promoted, sponsored, and coordinated by FIMS.

d) The creation of a recognized Multinational Group in Sports Medicine must be agreed to by the Council of Delegates upon request of the countries wishing to organize it and the approval of the FIMS Executive Committee.

Article 08. Honorary Member.

Individuals who have made exceptional contributions to the development of Sports Medicine may be elected to Honorary Membership. Nomination shall be made by the Member National Associations or other interested bodies to the Executive Committee who may then recommend the nominees to the Council of Delegates for election at the next regular meeting. Nominations which are not recommended by the Executive Committee or, having been recommended to the Council of Delegates fail election, may be made again after an interval of four years from the time that the original nomination was received.

The title will enable them:

a) to earn a diploma indicating honorary status.

b) to participate in the FIMS General Meeting.

c) to pay no dues to FIMS.

Article 09. Individual Member.

Granted by the Executive Committee on request to a person holding a degree in Medicine or a doctoral degree in related science who:

a) is member of the respective National Association where one exists.

b) has completed a FIMS Basic or Advance Course in Sports Medicine recognized by the Education Commission or has worked in the field at least for 5 years.

The title will enable the person:

a) to receive a FIMS certificate confirming the status of FIMS Individual Member.

b) to be elected for the Executive Committee, Standing or Special Commissions, and to represent his member National Association in the Council of Delegates.

c) to participate in the FIMS General Meeting.

d) to receive a reduction in the registration fee for FIMS sponsored congresses.

Article 10. Associate Member.

Granted by the Executive Committee on request to a non-medical professional who:

a) is a member of the respective National Association where one exists.

b) has completed a FIMS Basic or Advanced Course in Sports Medicine recognized by the Liaison Commission, or has worked in the field at least for 5 years.

The title will enable the person:

a) to receive a FIMS certificate confirming the status of FIMS Associate Member.

b) to participate in the FIMS General Meeting.

c) to receive a reduction in the registration fee for FIMS sponsored congresses.

Article 11. **Individuals shall lose their status as a Member of FIMS in the following situations:**

a) As a result of a formal resignation in writing by the individual being duly received by the Executive Committee.

b) As a result of failure to pay annual dues for more than 2 years in succession.

c) As a result of revocation of membership by a two-thirds majority of the Council of Delegates present and following a recommendation of the Executive Committee for that action.

CHAPTER III. Administrative Structure of FIMS.

Article 12. **The following bodies make up FIMS:**

a) The Council of Delegates,

b) The Executive Committee,

c) The Bureau,

d) The General Meeting.

Article 13. **The Council of Delegates.**

13.01. The Council of Delegates shall be constituted of one delegate from each of the Member National Associations. Each delegate has one vote.

13.02. Any Member National Association may appoint a delegate of another national body to represent it in the Council of Delegates. The proxy must be provided with a written power of attorney previously addressed to the Secretary General of FIMS. A delegate present in the meeting may not have more than one proxy.

13.03. The Members of the Executive Committee are entitled to debate in the Council of Delegates but may not vote unless they represent a Member National Association. The President, or his alternate, shall appoint one member of the Executive Committee to serve as Parliamentarian for the meeting of the Council.

13.04. The Council shall meet every 2 years at a location to be determined by the Executive Committee. All Member National Associations must be notified of the time, place, and agenda of the meeting 3 months in advance. In the year of the World Congress, it will meet at the time and place of the Congress. The host Member National Association is responsible for the local cost of the meeting and of the full board of the Executive members as well as the Chairperson of each Standing Commission.

13.05. Special meetings of the Council may be called at the initiative of the Executive Committee (by a vote of the majority of the members) or shall be called if there is a request by two-thirds of the Member National Associations to the General Secretary.

13.06. A quorum shall consist of one-third of the total number of Member National Associations in good standing. If there is no quorum, the National Associations must be notified within a month of the time of the meeting and the place of the next meeting must be decided by the Bureau. The new meeting must be held within 6 months of the cancelled one.

13.07. The Council of Delegates shall rule by a simple majority of delegates voting (including proxies), except when it is to amend the articles of the Statutes, or to dissolve the organization, or to expel one of its members, in which case a two-thirds majority is necessary of those voting.

13.08. The deliberations of the Council of Delegates shall be recorded in the form of minutes in a ledger kept for this purpose. These minutes shall be circulated to the Member National Associations and shall be published in "The World of Sports Medicine."

13.09. All matters of business which are not assigned to the Council of Delegates by the Statutes of FIMS shall fall within the jurisdiction of the Executive Committee. The Council of Delegates shall be the only body competent to conduct the following business:

a) Approve the biannual budget of FIMS.

b) Decide the affiliation of an applicant National Association as member based on a recommendation by the Executive Committee.

c) Recognize a Multinational Group of Sports

Medicine after approval by the Executive Committee.

d) Elect the officers, auditors, and other members of the Executive Committee (including substitutes from nominations).

e) Approve the awards of a FIMS Gold Medal and of a FIMS Citation of Honor based on recommendations of the Executive Committee.

f) Suspend or expel Member National Associations, Multinational Groups, Individual, or Associate Members.

g) Amend or alter the Statutes.

h) Receive and approve reports of the officers and chairpersons of the Standing Commissions.

i) Act on resolutions of the General Meeting.

j) Determine what other organizations shall be recognized by FIMS as having an active interest and/or involvement in Sports Medicine for the purpose of affiliation or other official contact.

k) Determine the site and date of the World Congress of Sports Medicine.

l) All other business which the Council shall from time to time reserve to itself.

Article 14. The Executive Committee.

14.01. The Executive Committee shall be composed of a President, a first, second, and third Vice-President, a Secretary General, a Treasurer, and eight members who have been elected from among FIMS Individual or Associate members after nomination by the Member National Associations.

14.02. Elections of the Executive Committee.

a) The Executive Committee shall be elected by the Council of Delegates for a period of four years.

b) The candidates shall be nominated only by their Member National Associations. No Association may nominate more than one candidate for officer or member of the Executive Committee.

c) Voting for each Officer shall take place by separate secret ballot. Those ballot slips which are not fully completed will be considered invalid.

d) Candidates for Officers who are not successful are entitled to be candidates for election as Members of the Executive Committee.

e1) If the result of any ballot for Officer results in a tie, additional ballots will take place until the tie is resolved. If the tie ballot pertains to the election of the Third Vice President, the ballot will involve only those candidates engaged in the tie.

e2) Following the ballot for the 8 elected Members of the Executive Committee, the 8 nominees with the highest number of votes shall be so named. If there is a tie among the final position(s), a new ballot will be held for these candidates only.

f) The two candidates who have the highest number of votes after those who are elected will be appointed Auditors and named substitutes. These substitutes shall replace elected Members of the Executive Committee if vacancies arise. If a vacancy occurs among the Officers, the Executive Committee shall elect one of its Members to the office for the balance of the unexpired term and that Member shall be replaced by the first substitute.

g) Officers and Members of the Executive Committee shall be eligible for immediate re-election in the same capacity only once.

h) To participate in a meeting of the Council of Delegates and have the right to vote, a Member National Association must have the membership dues for the current fiscal year and all previous years of membership paid in full on the occasion of the FIMS General Meeting which is held prior to the FIMS Council of Delegates meeting at which an election will take place.

i) A list of Member National Associations eligible to participate in and vote at a meeting of the Council of Delegates must be made available to each Delegate of a FIMS Member National Association prior to the meeting at which an election will be held.

j) Each Member National Association eligible to participate in and vote at a meeting of the Council of Delegates may designate one person to serve as its Delegate. To become accredited as the official Delegate of a Member National Association for a particular meeting of the Council of Delegates, that person must present typewritten authorization to the Secretary General of FIMS identifying the person as its Delegate. The authorization must be presented on the official letterhead stationery of the Member National Association and signed either by its President or other designated officer.

k) The designated Delegate of an eligible Member National Association is the only person permitted to vote on behalf of that Member National Association.

l) A Member National Association in good standing that is not able to send a Delegate to a meeting of the Council of Delegates may be represented by the accredited Delegate of another Member National Association. Both Member National Associations must be eligible to participate as regards completion of payment of annual dues.

m) To grant proxy, a Member National Association must submit to the Secretary General an official FIMS Proxy Form signed by its President. On the form, the specified Member National Association to receive the proxy must be identified. Only the accredited Delegate of the Member National Association receiving the proxy may use this proxy vote. A copy of the proxy form will be included with each announcement of a meeting of the Council of Delegates as distributed to all Member National Associations by the Secretary General. (As stated in the statutes, an accredited Delegate is entitled to use only one proxy vote in addition to the vote of the Delegate's own Member National Association.)

n) Preparation for FIMS election:

1. Nominations must be received from Member National Associations at least two months in advance of the meeting of the Council of Delegates at which the election will be held.

2. The ballot of the nominations must be circulated, together with biographical information on each candidate, at least one month in advance of the election.

o) Accreditation of Delegates:

Each sheet of the official ballot must be co-signed for validation in the voting procedure by the Secretary General and one Member of the Executive Committee, as appointed by the President.

p) Order of voting:

1. Separate elections will be held by roll call in the following order:

The President

The three Vice-Presidents

The Secretary General

The Treasurer

The eight Members of the Executive Committee

2. If a candidate is running unopposed for the office of President, Secretary General, or Treasurer, the election to that office may be accomplished by the Council's approval of a motion from the floor.

3. If there are only three nominations for the offices of the Vice Presidents, the election may be accomplished by approval of a motion from the floor after the determination of a method of designating the order of seniority as First Vice-President, Second Vice-President and Third-Vice President.

4. The ballot for the category of elected Members of the Executive Committee will list the candidates in alphabetical order by first letter of the family name.

q) Procedure for voting for each office:

1. Three Auditors will be elected from the Delegates of the Council of Delegates to receive and count the ballots. If more than three person are nominated, an election will be held.

2. When the agenda item for elections is reached during the meeting of the Council of Delegates, the President shall solicit ballots for the election of Officers and Executive Committee in the order prescribed above.

3. For the collection of ballots for each of the elected positions, the name of each Member National Association given the privilege of vot-

ing (both those with Delegates present and those represented by proxy) shall be read in alphabetical order, at which time the Delegate of the Member National Association or the Delegate carrying the proxy shall come forward and place the ballot in a closed ballot box.

4. The election Auditors will control that only one ballot at a time is placed in the ballot box and that the ballot carries the signature of the Secretary General and the appointed Member of the Executive Committee.

5. The votes for each of the elected positions will be tallied separately and publicly in front of the members of the Council of Delegates by the election Auditors.

6. A blackboard must be available for this purpose which can be viewed by all the members of the Council of Delegates.

14.03. The Executive Committee shall meet at least twice annually to transact the business of FIMS except for that reserved exclusively for the Council of Delegates, to receive and respond to reports from the officers and the chairpersons of the Standing Commissions, and to carry out programs and policies approved by the Council of Delegates. The date and place of such meetings will be decided by the Executive Committee and notices sent to all members at least 3 months in advance together with an agenda of business to be discussed. Any member who fails to attend three consecutive meetings shall forfeit the office or membership in the Executive Committee.

14.04. Between the meetings of the Council of Delegates, it is the responsibility of the Executive Committee:

a) To administer the affairs of FIMS.

b) To transact the business which is not reserved exclusively for the Council of Delegates.

c) To select and supervise the Standing Commissions, receiving and acting on their reports.

d) To decide the dates, venue, and agenda for the meeting of the Council of Delegates and the General Meeting as well as see that the necessary preparations are made.

e) To implement the decisions of the Council of Delegates.

f) To approve Individual and Associate Members of FIMS.

g) To examine the applications of National Associations and make recommendations regarding their acceptance or rejection to the Council of Delegates.

h) To approve the request of countries organized on a geographical or lingual basis to form a Multinational Group of Sports Medicine.

i) To recommend the appointments of Honorary Members and the awards of the FIMS Gold Medal and the FIMS Citation of Honor to the Council of Delegates.

j) To approve the contract with the National Association entrusted with the staging of the World Congress of Sports Medicine and to supervise regularly its preparation.

k) To act on the recommendation of the Scientific Commission regarding the scheduling, programs, and faculties for congresses and conferences to be sponsored by FIMS and to supervise the preparation and conduction of such events.

l) To review and take action on the minutes of the meeting of the Bureau.

m) Recommend to the Council of Delegates the award of the FIMS Gold Medal or the FIMS Citation of Honor following consideration of nominations by the Awards Committee and receipt of the Committee's endorsement.

14.05. The President shall be the representative of FIMS and responsible for the international relations of the organization. His special functions include:

a) Presiding over all the meetings of the Council of Delegates, General Meeting, Bureau, Executive Committee, and World Congress of Sports Medicine.

b) Maintaining contact between FIMS and other international organizations.

c) Signing together with the Secretary General any document which commits FIMS after its approval by the Executive Committee.

d) Referring to the Executive Committee a written report of FIMS activities to be submitted to the Council of Delegates.

e) Handing out the FIMS awards.

f) Fulfilling further tasks connected with FIMS activities according to the Statutes, By-Laws, and decisions of the Council of Delegates.

14.06. The 3 Vice-Presidents shall assume in the order of their precedence the place and duties of the President in his absence or if requested by him to do so.

14.07. The Secretary General is responsible for:

a) Preparing the agenda of the meetings of the Council of Delegates and the General Meeting, after decision of the Executive Committee, as well as the meetings of the Executive Committee and the Bureau, on request of the President, and circulating notice of these meetings in advance.

b) Preparing and circulating minutes of the meetings of the Council of Delegates, the General Meeting, the Executive Committee, and the Bureau of FIMS.

c) Maintaining official correspondence.

d) Preparing and circulating a Newsletter at least twice a year to all Member National Associations, the Executive Committee, and other appointed organizations and individuals.

14.08. The Treasurer is responsible for:

a) Keeping the financial accounts of FIMS in the official books together with all necessary supporting documents.

b) Preparing a detailed account and balance sheet for the preceding period which he shall submit to the Executive Committee and to the Auditors for each of their meetings.

c) Keeping a register of the Member National Associations, Multinational Groups, and Individual and Associate Members and to notify them at appropriate intervals of the dues which they must pay as well as to collect such income.

d) Preparing an annual budget for the Executive Committee and a biannual budget for the Council of Delegates.

14.09. The two auditors will review the financial account presented to them by the Treasurer and give a report of their review to the Executive Committee and the Council of Delegates.

Article 15.   The Bureau.

15.01. The Bureau is composed of the President, one of the Vice-Presidents, the Secretary General, and the Treasurer.

15.02. The Bureau shall meet at least once annually. The President shall preside at the meetings of the Bureau. If he is unable to do so, one of the Vice-Presidents shall take his place.

15.03. The minutes of the meetings of the Bureau are to be approved by the Executive Committee at the next subsequent meeting.

Article 16.   The General Meeting.

16.01. The General Meeting shall consist of:

a) The members of the Council of Delegates.

b) The members of the Executive Committee.

c) The representatives of the Multinational Groups of Sports Medicine recognized by FIMS.

d) The Honorary Members.

e) The Individual Members.

f) The Associate Members.

16.02. The General Meeting of FIMS meets every 4 years on the occasion of the World Congress of Sports Medicine. This meeting precedes the meeting of the Council of Delegates at that time.

16.03. The General Meeting shall discuss any question connected with the scientific and practical development of Sports Medicine throughout the world. Each person attending the General Meeting is entitled to one vote on any motion presented to the assembly. Motions that are carried shall be submitted to the Council of Delegates.

Article 17. The World Congress of Sports Medicine.

17.01. A World Congress of Sports Medicine will be held every 4 years. The Secretary General will inform the Member National Associations about the necessary conditions for staging this Congress and ask that proposals be submitted at least 3 years prior to the projected date of the next Congress.

The Executive Committee will review the received proposals and recommend to the Council of Delegates the site and date for their approval at their meeting at least 2 years before the designated date.

17.02. The Member National Association in the country selected shall assume full responsibility for the planning and financial support of all pertinent arrangements for the Congress.

17.03. The President of FIMS shall be the President ex-officio of the World Congress of Sports Medicine.

17.04. The secretariat of the Congress shall be established and maintained by the sponsoring Member National Association.

17.05. After the decision of the Council of Delegates as to where the next World Congress will be held, the President and the Secretary General of FIMS shall sign a contract with the representatives of the concerned Member National Association or the designated organizers.

Article 18. The Standing Commissions.

18.01. The Executive Committee is supported by Standing Commissions.

18.02. Each Standing Commission consists of FIMS Individual or Associate Members and is composed as:

a) A chairperson designated by the Executive Committee who directs the activities of the Commission and reports to the Executive Committee and Council of Delegates, with the right to attend both meetings.

b) Up to four Members designated by the Executive Committee from nominations submitted by Member National Associations after considering recommendations of the Commission chairperson.

c) Appointed Executive Committee members.

d) Corresponding members.

e) Observers nominated by appropriate international organizations.

f) Temporary members, co-opted ad hoc, for particular purposes.

18.03. The working period for a Standing Commission is 4 years.

18.04. A chairperson shall give rise to a record of meetings to be kept with the help of one Secretary and circulate it to the Commission membership, the FIMS President, and the Secretary General.

18.05. A Standing Commission

a) Reports directly to the Executive Committee which alone shall endorse policy.

b) Shall not have executive responsibility except where specific tasks are delegated to it by the Executive Committee.

18.06. The Standing Commissions are:

a) Scientific,

b) Interfederal,

c) Education,

d) Liaison.

18.07. The Scientific Commission.

The aims of the Scientific Commission are:

a) To promote scientific research in the field of Sports Medicine.

b) To prepare statements regarding specific problems in Sports Medicine proposed by the Executive Committee.

c) To cooperate with the organizers of the FIMS World Congress of Sports Medicine as well as with the organizers of other international scientific events sponsored by FIMS, especially as regards the choice of topics, invited lecturers, chairperson of sessions, and publication of proceedings.

d) To cooperate with the Editor of "The World

of Sports Medicine" to ensure the required scientific level of published contributions.

18.08. The Interfederal Medical Commission

The aims of the Interfederal Medical Commission are:

a) To study from a medical point of view practical problems related to sports activity submitted by the Executive Committee.

b) To disseminate scientific data regarding the medical aspects of sports activities in a form suitable to be understood by officers, physicians, paramedic staff, coaches and athletes.

c) To organize meetings of physicians attached to International Sports Federations and National Olympic Committees for the exchange of information on Sports Medicine.

18.09. The Education Commission.

The aim of the Education Commission is:

to provide advice and make recommendation to the Executive Committee on matters related to sports medicine education for medical and allied health professionals.

18.10. The Liaison Commission.

The aims of the Liaison Commission are:

to provide and make recommendations to the Executive Committee on matters related to communication, promotion, and membership.

In conjunction with the Secretary General the Liaison Commission will:

a) facilitate and enhance cooperation and collaboration with other international organizations related to sports medicine as defined by the Executive Committee.

b) assist in the maintenance of effective communication with national bodies, Individual Members, and associated organizations through acquisition and collation of materials for FIMS publications.

c) enlarge contacts with international organizations and institutions of non-medical professions related to the field of sports medicine.

In conjuction with the Treasurer, the Liaison Commission will:

a) raise the level of awareness and promote the benefits of individual membership of FIMS.

b) develop strategies for the maintenance and monitoring of effective membership services.

c) assist the Executive Committee in the implementation and conduct of procedures associated with the granting of Individual and Associate Membership.

d) identify countries with special needs with respect to sports medicine information and services and develop and implement mechanisms to expand the dissemination of information to these countries.

Article 19.   Financial Structure.

19.01. The capital of FIMS is derived from annual dues of the Member National Associations and Individual Members, administrative fees of Courses and Congresses, donations, legacies, and subsidies.

19.02. The Treasurer shall be in charge of financial operations and shall be supervised by two auditors appointed for 4-year terms by the Council of Delegates.

19.03. The Treasurer shall submit a report of the current status of the FIMS account at each meeting of the Executive Committee and a complete report to each meeting of the Council of Delegates. The report to the Council of Delegates should be certified by the Auditors.

19.04. Any transfer of budgetary credits or any expenditure must be approved by the Executive Committee.

19.05. FIMS is responsible for:

a) the administrative expenses of the Secretary General,

b) the expenses of the President in connection with his administrative functions,

c) the administrative expenses of the Treasurer and the Chairpersons of the Standing Commissions,

d) membership fees to international organizations to which FIMS belongs.

19.06. The expenses involved in attending

meetings of the Council of Delegates, Bureau, Executive Committee, Standing Commissions, and General Meeting are the responsibility of individual members or of the National Association to which each member belongs.

19.07. The financial year of FIMS begins on January 1st and terminates on December 31st of the same year.

19.08. In the event of dissolution of FIMS, the funds shall be allotted to one or more organizations in the field of Sports Medicine as designated by the Council of Delegates.

Article 20.   Annual Dues.

20.01. The annual dues shall be paid by each Member National Association, Multinational Group, as well as by each Individual or Associate Member in U.S. dollars according to the amount established by the Council of Delegates and specified in the By-Laws.

20.02. Waiting Member National Associations shall pay annually a service subscription established by the Council of Delegates and specified in the By-Laws.

20.03. Only members who have paid their dues and are not in arrears in relation to the previous fiscal year have voting privileges and may be elected or appointed for the Standing Commissions.

Article 21.   FIMS Awards.

21.01. A FIMS Gold Medal may be awarded to an individual who has demonstrated outstanding leadership which has resulted in advancement in sports medicine of international dimension and importance. A FIMS Citation of Honor may be awarded to an individual who has made outstanding contributions to sports medicine in one or more of the following categories: research in sports medicine and the sports sciences, scholarly activity and publication in sports medicine and the sports sciences, medical care of athletes, regional and/or national leadership, or service to FIMS.

21.02. Nominations for an award will be referred to the Awards Committee. Following review of credentials and discussion of the rationale for the nomination, the Awards Committee will make its recommendation to the Executive Committee which, by official action, will forward the nomination to the Council of Delegates which will have the power to approve the recommendation and make the award.

21.03. The FIMS Awards Committee shall consist of five members of the FIMS Executive Committee, one member of which will be a Vice-President and four will be elected members of the Executive Committee. The Vice-President will serve as the chairperson.

Article 22.   Liability.

22.01. FIMS shall recognize and acknowledge its responsibility towards third parties only by documents signed jointly by the President and the Secretary General.

22.02. The members of the Executive Committee, the Officers, the Member National Associations, the Honorary, Individual, and Associate Members, as well as the members of the Council of Delegates shall be exempt from any personal liability as far as the commitments undertaken by FIMS are concerned. Such commitments are guaranteed solely by the assets of FIMS.

Article 23.   Official Language.

23.01. The official administrative language of FIMS is English.

23.02. For the purpose of international meetings held under the patronage of FIMS, the French, Spanish, German, and Russian languages together with the language of the host country may be used in addition to English at the discretion of the organizing body.

By-Laws

The By-Laws of FIMS exist to facilitate the management of its affairs. They shall be approved and amended by the Council of Delegates by a simple majority of those present and voting.

CHAPTER I

Article 01. No by-law.

Article 02. No by-law.

Article 03. Address of FIMS.

03.01. Correspondence, except that intended especially for the President, shall be sent to the office of the Secretary General at the address indicated on his official stationery.

Article 04. No by-law.

CHAPTER II

Article 05. No by-law.

Article 06. Member National Associations.

06.01. Each applicant National Association shall, in the event of failure of the Executive Committee to recommend them for membership, have the absolute right to a personal hearing of its application before the Council of Delegates.

06.02. National Associations applying for membership in FIMS shall be admitted to waiting membership by the Executive Committee once they have satisfied the requirements specified in Chapter II, Article 06.03 of the Statutes, pending election by the Council of Delegates.

06.03. As waiting members, they may participate in the activities of FIMS and will receive all official communications to member nations but shall have no vote in the Council of Delegates.

06.04. Each Member National Association shall have only one representative entitled to vote on behalf of that Association in the Council of Delegates.

06.05. Before the commencement of each session of the Council, each Member National Association shall give notice in writing to the Secretary General of FIMS of the identity of its delegate.

Article 07. No by-law.

Article 08. No by-law.

Article 09. No by-law.

Article 10. No by-law.

Article 11. No by-law.

CHAPTER III

Article 12. No by-law.

Article 13. The Council of Delegates.

13.01. The business of the Council of Delegates shall be conducted under Roberts Rules of Order.

13.02. The President, or in his/her absence the Vice-President presiding, shall designate a Parliamentarian for the meeting.

Article 14. The Executive Committee.

14.01. Any voting member of the Executive Committee may propose a motion. If it is seconded by another voting member, a vote will be taken following discussion to accept or reject the motion. A simple majority will decide the result. If two-thirds or more of the voting members present agree to request it, the voting shall be by secret ballot.

14.02. The meetings of the Executive Committee are private. Other interested persons may be present as observers or consultants for a portion of these meetings with the approval of the Executive Committee and may participate in the discussions if invited to do so. They may be asked to withdraw if the majority of the Executive Committee votes that the subsequent proceedings shall be private.

14.03. The Executive Committee shall act as the Supervisory Board of the official FIMS publication, "The World of Sports Medicine."

14.04. No by-law.

14.05. No by-law.

14.06. No by-law.

14.07. No by-law.

14.08. The Treasurer will be empowered to act in any financial transactions for FIMS. An alternative person shall be appointed by the Executive to act as his substitute.

Article 15. The Bureau.

15.01. The rules of procedure for the Executive Committee apply to the meetings of the Bureau.

Article 16. No by-law.

Article 17. The World Congress of Sports Medicine.

17.01. Candidatures to organize the World Congress of Sports Medicine must be presented by a Member National Association whose membership is currently effective. Each must be accompanied by an official document from the National Government of the Member National Association ensuring the necessary co-operation for holding the Congress, including the issuance of any necessary visas for participants and a guarantee that prospective participants from all countries who wish to attend and are properly registered to do so will encounter no difficulties in being admitted to the event or in leaving the country after their attendance. They must also be accompanied by a detailed proposal concerning the physical and financial arrangements for the Congress and a declaration that the candidate National Association will respect the Statutes and By-Laws of FIMS.

17.02. If the Executive Committee considers it necessary to have an inspection of the proposed venue for the Congress in any candidature prior to the meeting of the Council of Delegates at which the decision on the site is to be made, the candidate Associations shall pay the costs of travel and full board for the inspecting FIMS representatives.

17.03. The Association organizing the Congress shall pay the travel cost and full board for the FIMS President and the Chairperson of the Scientific Commission to attend the meetings of the Organizing Committee of the Congress as it may be appropriate and necessary for them to do so.

17.04. The theme for the World Congress shall be proposed by the Organizing Committee and approved by the Executive Committee of FIMS upon recommendation of the Scientific Commission.

17.05. Invitations to take part in the World Congress must be dispatched by the Organizing Committee at least 18 months before the Congress. The text of the invitation must include the statement that free communication will be welcomed and provide information as to how and when the abstract forms may be obtained and the last date by which these abstracts must be received in order to decide whether or not presentation at the Congress will be accepted. Invitations must be addressed to:

a) Member National Associations and multi-national groups.

b) Honorary, Individual, and Associate Members.

c) International Associations which have an active interest and involvement of their members in Sports Medicine.

d) National Olympic Committees.

e) International Sports Federations.

17.06. The program of the World Congress shall include invited speakers and free communications. All speakers, whether invited or not, will be required to submit manuscripts to the Organizing Committee with appropriate tables, charts, and illustrations. The Organizing Committee shall establish an Editorial Committee to receive the manuscripts and, in conjunction with the Scientific Commission, to prepare them for publication. The cost of publication shall be assumed by the Organizing Committee.

17.07. The Organizing Committee of the World Congress shall pay the costs of travel and full board for the members of the Executive Committee, Chairpersons of the Standing Commissions, invited lecturers, and guests of honor during the time of the Congress.

17.08. The Organizing Committee of the World Congress shall provide meeting rooms, necessary staff, and equipment for the meeting of the Executive Committee, the General Meeting, and the Council of Delegates, as well as a temporary office for the Secretary General and the Treasurer of FIMS as close as possible to the Secretariat of the Congress.

17.09. At the World Congress, simultaneous translation of presentations shall be provided in English, and may be provided in French, Spanish, German, and Russian.

Article 18.   No by-law.

Article 19.   Financial Structure.

19.01. The Treasurer shall be empowered to reimburse each member of the Bureau and of the Executive Committee US$ 200.00 for attendance at each meeting for the purpose of helping to defray expenses.

Article 20.   Annual Dues.

20.01. Annual dues shall be established for each member National Organization according to the number of its members in the following amounts:

Up to 100 US$ 100.00

100 to 500 US$ 200.00

500 to 1000 US$ 300.00

1000 to 2000 US$ 400.00

2000 and over US$ 500.00

20.02. Waiting Member National Associations shall pay a service fee of US$ 100.00 annually.

20.03. Individual Members and Associate Members shall pay US$ 30.00 annually.

Article 21.   FIMS Awards.

21.01. Nomination for FIMS awards can be accomplished by means of one of two mechanisms:

a) by action of the highest executive body of a Member National Association of FIMS presented on that organization's official letterhead and signed by the organization's president or other authorized representative.

b) by action of three or more members of FIMS Executive Committee following consultation with the Member National Association of which the nominee is currently a member in good standing.

21.02. The procedure for nomination will involve the submission to the FIMS Executive Committee of the following:

a) a letter of nomination citing the specific rationale for the nomination and presenting background information about the nominee, and

b) a copy of the nominee's curriculum vitae. Following receipt of the nomination materials, a review will be conducted by the FIMS Awards Committee and, if there is a positive consensus, a recommendation will be forwarded to the FIMS Executive Committee for official action.

21.03. The Awards Committee shall be appointed by the President following the election of the Executive Committee by the Council of Delegates.

Article 22.   No by-law.

Article 23.   No by-law.

Future Plans of the Organization

In the dawn of the third millennium, FIMS is being adapted to reach a modern and dynamic concept of an important and active international association. Now that all continental associations are consolidated and have a solid representation in the FIMS executive board, the electoral system will be modified. Already in the FIMS World Congress of 2002, the council of delegates will elect only the president, the secretary general, and the treasurer. All other positions will be named by each continental group based on the number of countries in each continent.

The FIMS World Congress of Sports Medicine will be held every two years, increasing the budget and permitting a better promotion of sports medicine in different regions of the world. A new president will be elected every four years and FIMS will have a former president in its executive board, thereby bringing experience and guidance to the bureau.

Through the continental associations and multinational groups, major attention will be given to FIMS' national associations, assisting each one of them to grow strongly and steadily. The individual members will also receive spe-

∞ *Past and Current Presidents* ∞

Name:	Country of residence:	Terms of office:
Eduardo Henrique De Rose, MD, PhD	Brazil	1994-Current
Wildor Hollman	Germany	1986-1994
Ejnar Eriksson	Sweden	1980-1986
Ludrik Prokop	Austria	1976-1980
Giuseppe La Cava	Italy	1968-1976
Paul André Chailley-Bert	France	1964-1968
Paul Govaerts	Belgium	1946-1964
WWII 1940-1946		
Leonardi Conti	Germany	1937-1940
Raymond Latarjet	France	1933-1937
Fredrick Jacobus Johannes Buytendijk	Holland	1930-1933
W. Knoll	Switzerland	1928-1930

cial attention. Already this year there is an impressive amount of information and educational materials that are produced and circulated to our members. In this new century, the Internet will play a major role in FIMS' circulation, thanks to its agreement with Human Kinetics. Human Kinetics has an outstanding Web site, which is very dynamic and rich in information, and an educational electronic journal, a first in the area of sports medicine. And with the Traveling Fellows project, future leaders are crossing oceans and exploring cultures, preparing for their task in the future of FIMS.

The success of FIMS would not be possible without the commitment of each person involved. Each participant does his or her best to promote sports medicine among the regions and bring education, science, and technology to all areas of the world.

Affiliates

FIMS has an official working relationship with several international organizations. Each organization has a representative who is a part of the FIMS Executive Committee. The goal of this alliance with FIMS is to develop educational and research projects together. The following organizations work in accordance with FIMS:

ICSSPE (International Council of Sport Science and Physical Education)

Represented by: Anthony Parker, PhD (Australia—also an elected member of the FIMS Executive Committee)

C/O Queensland University of Technology

School of Human Movement Studies

Kelvin Grove Campus

Victoria Park Road, Kelvin Grove

Brisbane, Queensland

AUSTRALIA

Tel: (61.7) 3864 3512

Fax: (61.7) 3864 3980

E-mail: t.parker@qut.edu.au

IOC (International Olympic Committee)

Represented by: Patrick Schamasch, MD (Medical Doctor for IOC)

Chateau de Vidy

C.P. 356

(continued on next page)

(IOC, continued)

1007 Lausanne
SWITZERLAND
Tel: (41.21) 621.61.11
Fax: (41.21) 621.62.16
E-mail: patrick.schamasch@olympic.org

UNESCO (United Nations Educational, Scientific, and Cultural Organization)

Represented by: Michel Rieu, PhD (France)
7, Place de Fontenoy
75352 Paris
FRANCE
Tel: (33.1) 4569-1000
Fax: (33.1) 4567-1690
E-mail: rieu@cochin.univ-paris.fr

WHO (World Health Organization)

20 Avenue Appia
1211 Geneve 27
SWISSE
Tel: (41.22) 791-2111
Fax: (41.22) 791-0746

Scientific Commission

Aims:

- To promote scientific research in the field of Sports Medicine
- To prepare statements regarding specific problems in Sports Medicine proposed by Executive Committee.
- To cooperate with the organizers of the FIMS World Congress of Sports Medicine as well as with the organizers of other international scientific events sponsored by FIMS, especially as regards to the choice of topics, invited lecturers, chairperson of sessions, and publication of proceedings.
- To cooperate with the Editor of "The World of Sports Medicine" to ensure the required scientific level of published contributions.

Chairwoman

Éva Martos, MD
Vice Director
National Institute for Sports Medicine
Alkotás str. 48. Budapest 1123
HUNGARY
Tel: (361) 4886 189; (361) 4886 191
Fax: (361) 4886 196; (361) 3753 292
E-mail: Mar13880@Helka.IIF.HU

Members

André-Xavier Bigard, MD
Unité Bioénergétique et Environement du Centre de Recherches du Service de Santé des Armées
38702, La Tronche Cedex
FRANCE
Tel: 33 4 76 63 69 98
Fax: 33 4 76 63 69 45
E-mail: BigardXavier@Compuserve.com

Wayne Derman, MBChB, PhD
Sports Sciences Institute of South Africa
The University of Cape Town
Boundary Road Newlands 7700

SOUTH AFRICA
Tel: 27 21 686 7330
Fax: 27 21 686 7530
E-mail: wderman@sports.uct.ac.za

Toshihito Katsumura, MD, PhD
Department of Preventive Medicine and Public Health
Tokyo Medical University
6-1-1, Shinjuku, Shinjuku-ku
Tokyo 160-8402
JAPAN
Tel: 81 3 5379 4339
Fax: 81 3 3226 5277
E-mail: kats@tokyo-med.ac.jp

Luigi Di Luigi, MD
Endocrinology Department
University Institute of Motor Sciences
Pza L. De Bosis 15
00194, Rome
ITALY
Tel: 3906 487 3555 (home)
Tel: 3906 3609 5543 (office)
Fax: 3906 361 3065
E-mail: iusm.endocrinol@uni.net

Gideon Mann, MD
Department of Orthopaedic Surgery
Hadassah University Hospital
POB 24035
Mount Scopus, Jerusalem 91240
ISRAEL
Tel: 972 2 534 1217
Fax: 972 2 570 0367
E-mail: Howrob@Gezernet.Co.Il

Petra Platen, MD, PhD
International Adren
Institute of Cardiology and Sports Medicine
German Sports University
Carl-Diem-Weg 6

(continued on next page)

(Platen, continued)

50933 Cologne
GERMANY
Tel: 49 221 498 2522
Fax: 49 221 491 2906
E-mail: Platen@Hrz.Dshs-Koeln.De

James S. Skinner, PhD
Professor
Department of Kinesiology
Indiana University
11001 North 26th Street
Bloomington, IN 47408
UNITED STATES OF AMERICA
E-mail: jskinner@iupui.edu

Dah Cyrille Serge, MD
Faculte De Medecine
Departement De Physiologie
B. P. V 166 Abidjan
COTE d'IVOIRE
Tel: 225 44 53 33
Fax: 225 44 28 97

Willem van Mechelen, MD, PhD
Faculty of Medicine
Department of Social Medicine
Vrije Universiteit
Vander- Boechorststraat 7-9
NL- 1081 BT Amsterdam
THE NETHERLANDS
Tel: 31 20 444 8410
Fax: 31 20 444 8181
Home: 31 20 444 8387
E-mail:
    W.van_Mechelen.Emgo@med.vu.nl

Executive Committee Liaisons

Dušan Hamar, MD, PhD
Department of Sports Medicine
Institute of Sports Sciences
Comenius University
Svobodovo nabr. 9
814 69 Bratislava
SLOVAKIA
Tel: (421 7) 5441 1624
Fax: (421 7) 5441 4472
E-mail: hamar@fsport.uniba.sk

Anthony Parker, PhD
Queensland University of Technology
School of Human Movement Studies
Kelvin Grove Campus
Victoria Park Road
Kelvin Grove, 4059
Queensland
AUSTRALIA
Tel: (61 7) 3864 3512
Fax: (61 7) 3864 3980
E-mail: t.parker@qut.edu.au

Education Commission

Aim:
- To provide advice and make recommendation to the Executive Committee on matters related to sports medicine education for medical and allied health professionals.

Chairman

Andre Debruyne, MD
Kiewitstraat 141
3500 Hasselt
BELGIUM
Tel: 3211 265 100
Fax: 3211 265 101
E-mail: a.debruyne@debruyne.com

Members

Nicos Angelides, MD, PhD
Director
Department of Cardiovascular and Thoracic Surgery
Nicosia General Hospital
Nicosia 1450
CYPRUS
Tel: 357 2 801 502
Fax: 357 2 357 270

Antônio Claudio Lucas Da Nóbrega, PhD
Chairman, Department of Physiology
Instituto Biomédico-Unversidade Fed.
   Fluminense
Rua Hernani Meilo, 101 cep 2421-130
Niterói-RJ
BRAZIL
Tel: 5521 620-0623 X227
Fax: 5521 714-6821
E-mail: anobrega@web4u.com.br

David Michael Roberts, EdD
4/11 Gibbon Street, Mosman Park
Wetern Australia 6012
AUSTRALIA
Tel/Fax: 61 89 383-3364
E-mail: davmike67@yahoo.com

Angela Smith, MD
275 South Roberts Road
Bryn Mawr, PA 19010
UNITED STATES OF AMERICA
Tel: 610 909 0123
Fax: 610 519 0543
E-mail: asmithmd@aol.com

C. Thurairaja, MD
167 Rampart Road
Ethul Kotte
SRI LANKA
Tel: 941 863 656
Fax: 94 075 330 220

Temporary (ad-hoc) member

Gene Bayliss, MA, ATC
11718 Woodsong Court
Boca Raton, FL 33426
UNITED STATES OF AMERICA

Executive Committee Liaisons

Lyle J. Micheli, MD
Children's Hospital
Department of Orthopaedic Surgery
319 Longwood Avenue
Boston, MA 02115
UNITED STATES OF AMERICA
Tel: 1 617 355 6934
Home: 1 617 738 4314
Fax: 1 617 730 0227
E-mail: micheli_l@A1.tch.harvard.edu

Norbert Bachl, MD
Institute of Sports Science
Department of Sports and Exercise Physi-
   ology
University of Vienna
Auf de Schmelz 6A
1150 Vienna
AUSTRIA
Tel: 431 4277 48870
Fax: 431 4277 48879
E-mail: norbert.bachl@univie.ac.at

Interfederal Commission

Aims:

- To study from a medical point of view practical problems related to sports activity submitted by the Executive Committee.
- To disseminate scientific data regarding the medical aspects of sports activities in a form suitable to be understood by officers, physicians, paramedic staff, coaches, and athletes.
- To organize meetings of physicians attached to International Sports Federations and National Olympic Committees for the exchange of information on Sports Medicine.

Chairman

Ernst Raas, MD
University Hospital
Department of Sports Medicine
A-6020, Innsbruk
AUSTRIA
Tel: (+43 512) 504-3450
Fax: (+43 512) 504-3469
E-mail: trojan@oesv.at

(continued on next page)

(continued)

Members

Enrique Amy, DMD
P. O. Box 7402
Ponce, PR 00732
PUERTO RICO
Tel: 787 884-0125
Fax: 787 844-9019
Tel & Fax: 787-824-2669

Charoentasn Chintanaseri, MD
Sports Medicine Association of Thailand
2088 Ramkhamhaeny Road
Hua mark Bangkok 10240
THAILAND
Tel: 662 319 7435
Fax: 662 314 2596

Péter Jákó, MD
Director of National Institue for Sports
  Medicine
Alkotás str. 48
Budapest 1123
HUNGARY
Tel: 361-1753192
Fax: 361-1753292

Nicos Spanos, MD, PhD
Senior Specialist Neurosurgery
4, Skyros Str., Flat 24
1066, Nicosia
CYPRUS
Tel: +357-2-445974
Fax: +357-2-362029

Pierre Rochcongar, MD
Unité de Biologie et Médecine du Sport
CHR Pontchaillou 350033
RENNES CEDEX
FRANCE
Tel: 02-99-28-41-33
Fax: 02-99-28-41-86

Executive Committee Liaisons

Prof. Nishat Mallick, MD
Hill Park General Hospital
Shaheed-e Millat Road
Karachi – PAKISTAN
Tel: 92 21 455 2442
Fax: 92 21 506 0343
E-mail: zls@cyber.net.pk

John B. M. Wesseling, MD
AMALIASTRAAT 12
2514 JC Den Haag
THE NETHERLANDS
Tel: 31.70.352 1857
Fax: 31.70.322 8318
E-mail: john.wesseling@wxs.nl

Liaison Commission

Aims:
- To provide advice and make recommendations to the Executive Committee on matters related to communication, promotion, and membership.
- To work in conjunction with the Secretary General in maintaining and enhancing cooperation and contact with international organizations related to the field of Sports Medicine.
- To work in conjunction with the Treasurer to promote and expand awareness and membership to all countries.

Chairman

Wahid Al Kharusi, MD
P. O. Box 3007
Ruwi
Postal Code 112
SULTANATE OF OMAN
Tel: 968 560 937/968 560 939
Cel: 968 931 5212/968 938 3080
Fax: 968 603 485
E-mail: wahid@omantel.net.om

Members

Adnan Al-Edan, MD
Director
Physical Medicine and Rehabilitation
   Hospital
P. O. Box 4079
Safat 13041
KUWAIT
Tel: 965 487 0406
   965 487 5369
Fax: 965 487 4190

Simon John Bartold, FASMF
Sports Medicine Australia
32 Payneham Road, Stepney
South Australia 5069
AUSTRALIA
Tel: 61 8 8362 8111
Fax: 61 2 6253 1489
E-mail: sbartold@sportsmed.com.au

Peter Baumgartl, MD
Krankenhaus St. Johann
Bahnhofstr. 10
6380 St. Johann in Tirol
AUSTRIA
Tel: +43 5352 606514
Fax: +43 5352 606270
E-mail: baumgartl@khsj.net

Rose P. Macdonald, SRP
Consultant in Sports Physiotherapy
Hillside
Fountain Drive
London – SE191UP

UNITED KINGDOM
Tel: 208 670 3055
Fax: 208 670 3055
E-mail: Rosian@cwcom.net

Danish Zaheer, MBBS
Head, Sports Medicine and Research
   Centre
Suite No. 26-B, Block-2
Mabohai Apartments
SPG-10, Jalan Jawatan, Dalam,
BRUNEI
Tel: 673 2 221503
Fax: 673 2 380754
E-mail: smrcdan@byunet.bn

Executive Committee Liaisons

Patricia Sangenis, MD
Institute of Sports Medicine
Deporte y Salud Buenos Aires
Matienzo 1682 (C.F.)
(1426) Buenos Aires
ARGENTINA
Tel: 541 14 777 4949
Fax: 541 14 777 4499
E-mail: psangenis@datamarkets.com.ar

Costas Christodoulakis, MD
P. O. Box 5137
1307 Nicosia
CYPRUS
Tel: 357 2 663 762
Fax: 357 2 664 669
E-mail: sportsmedicine@cytanet.com.cy

International Federation of Sports Medicine (FIMS) Business Office

Contact Human Kinetics for any of the following information, education, and business services for FIMS.

- ❑ Information for the International Sports Medicine Directory
- ❑ Information about FIMS activities
- ❑ Information about cooperative programs between FIMS and National Associations of Sports Medicine
- ❑ Forthcoming conferences
- ❑ FIMS courses
- ❑ Submission of articles to newsletter and journal
- ❑ Receipt of publications
- ❑ New membership or renewal (including payment or certificate questions)

Sports Medicine Coordinator: Edward Grogg

Sports Medicine Managing Editor: Julie Johnson

Sports Medicine Administrative Assistant: Connie Young

Human Kinetics
P.O. Box 5076
Champaign, IL 61825-5076
United States of America
Tel: (217) 351-5076, in the U.S. call (800) 747-4457
Fax: (217) 351-2474
E-mail: fims@hkusa.com
www.humankinetics.com
www.fims.org

PART II

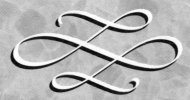

Association Directory

CHAPTER 3

Multinational Sports Medicine Associations

Arab Federation of Sports Medicine

AFSM

P.O. Box 29191

Riffa

BAHRAIN

Telephone: +973 682612

Fax: +973 684108

Name of Contact Person: Dr. Ali Al Khalifa

Countries belonging to group: Algeria, Egypt, Bahrain, Saudi Arabia, Syria, Mauritania, Morocco, Tunisia, and the Arab Emirates.

Founding Date: 1982

Asian Federation of Sports Medicine

AFSM

To foster the development of sports medicine in Asia for sporting excellence and health for all.

Prof. Dr. Nishat Mallick

Hill Park General Hospital

Shaheed-e-Millat Road

Karachi

PAKISTAN

Telephone: 92 21 455 2442

Fax: 92 21 506 0343

E-mail: mallick@cyber.net.pk

Web site: www.afsm.com.hk

Name of Contact Person: Dr. Wahid Al-Kharusi

Title of Contact Person: Secretary General

Contact Address: Post Box: 3007

Ruwi, Postal Code 112

OMAN

Telephone: 968 601 600

Fax: 968 603 485

E-mail: wahid@omantel.net.com

Countries belonging to group: 27 National and Regional Associations from all of Asia: Bangladesh, Chinese Taipei, DPR Korea, Hong Kong, India, Indonesia, Iran, Japan, Korea, Malaysia, Macau, Mongolia, Nepal, Oman, Pakistan, PR of China, Philippines, Saudi Arabia, Singapore, Sri Lanka, Syria, Thailand, and United Arab Emirates

(continued on next page)

(AFSM, continued)

Founding Date: 1990

Publications: Quarterly Newsletter; AFSM Newsletter

Association of Sports Medicine of the Balkans

Name of Contact Person: Prof. John Dragan

Title of Contact Person: President

Contact Address: Bd. Basarabiel

District 2

Bucharest

ROMANIA

Telephone: (+401) 322 0097

Fax: (+401) 323 1570

Countries belonging to group: Albania, Bulgaria, Croatia, Cyprus, Greece, Romania, Slovenia, Turkey, and Yugoslavia

Founding Date: 1967

Caribbean Association of Sports Medicine

Name of Contact Person: Dr. Adrian Lorde

Title of Contact Person: President

Contact Address: 20 Edghill Heights 2

St. Thomas

BARBADOS

Telephone: (246) 424 8236, (246) 436 9360, (246) 425 4025

Fax: (246) 425 3323

Countries belonging to group: Aruba, Barbados, Jamaica, the Netherlands Antilles, Puerto Rico, Trinidad and Tobago, and Haiti.

Founding Date: 1986

Confederacion Centroamericano de Medicina del Deporte (Central American Federation of Sports Medicine)

Promotes the advancement of Sports Medicine in Central America.

Apartado Postal 172

Heredia 3000

COSTA RICA

Telephone: 506 2378956

Fax: 506 2378956

Name of Contact Person: Dr. Rafeal Brenes Rojas

Title of Contact Person: President

Contact Address: Apartado Postal 172

Heredia 3000

506 2378956

COSTA RICA

Telephone: 506 2378956

Fax: 506 2378956

Countries belonging to group: Costa Rica, El Salvador, Guatemala, Honduras, Nicaragua, and Panama.

Founding Date: 1986

Confederacion Panamerican de Medicina del Deporte–COPAMEDE

Name of Contact Person: Walter R. Frontera, MD, PhD

Title of Contact Person: President

Contact Address: Dept. of Physical Medicine and Rehabilitation

Spaulding Rehabilitation Hospital

125 Nashua Street

Boston, Massachusetts

02114

UNITED STATES OF AMERICA

Telephone: (617) 573-7180

Fax: (617) 573-2759

Countries belonging to group: Antilles, Argentina, Aruba, Bolivia, Barbados, Brazil, Canada, Chile, Colombia, Costa Rica, Cuba, Dominican Republic, Ecuador, El Salvador, Guatemala, Haiti, Honduras, Jamaica, Mexico, the Netherlands, Nicaragua, Panama, Paraguay, Peru, Puerto Rico, Trinidad and Tobago, United States of America, Uruguay, and Venezuela

Founding Date: 1975

Confederacion Sudamericana de Medicine del Deporte

This group coordinates sports medicine regulations for national associations in Sur America

Atlantico 1605

Montevideo C.P. 11400

URUGUAY

Name of Contact Person: Dr. Italo Moneti

Title of Contact Person: President

Contact Address: Atlantico 1605

Montevideo C.P. 11400

URUGUAY

Telephone: 598 2 6199 526

Fax: 598 2 9023 175

Founding Date: 1986

Publications: *Medicina del Ejercicio*

European Federation of Sports Medicine

Name of Contact Person: Dr. Norbert Bachl

Title of Contact Person: President

Contact Address: Head of Department of Sports Physiology

Auf de Schmetz 6

AUSTRIA

Telephone: (+43-1) 982 2661 174

Fax: (+43-1) 982 2661 247

Countries belonging to group: Andorra, Austria, Belgium, Bosnia, Bulgaria, Croatia, Cyprus, Czech Republic, Denmark, Estonia, Finland, France, Germany, Great Britain, Greece, Hungary, Ireland, Italy, Kazakhstan, Letonia, Lithuania, Luxembourg, Malta, the Netherlands, Norway, Poland, Portugal, Romania, Russia, Slovakia, Slovenia, Sweden, Switzerland, Turkey, Yugoslavia

Founding Date: 1997

Fédération Internationale de Médecine du Sport (International Federation of Sports Medicine)

FIMS

To promote the study and development of sports medicine throughout the world; preserve and improve the health of mankind through physical fitness and sports participation; study scientifically the natural and pathological implications of physical training and sports participation; organize or sponsor scientific meetings, courses, congresses, and exhibits on an international basis in the field of sports medicine; cooperate with national and international organizations in sports medicine and related fields; and publish scientific information in the field of sports medicine and in related subjects.

Dept. of Physical Medicine and Rehabilitation

Harvard Medical School

Spaulding Rehabilitation Hospital

125 Nashua St.

Boston, MA

02114

UNITED STATES OF AMERICA

Web site: www.fims.org

Name of Contact Person: Walter R. Frontera

Title of Contact Person: Secretary-General

Telephone: (617) 573-7180

Fax: (617) 573-2759

E-mail: frontera.walter@mgh.harvard.edu

Founding Date: 1928

Publications: *International SportMed Journal* (bimonthly); *The World of Sports Medicine* (quarterly newsletter); *International Sports Medicine Directory* (expanded directory).

Federation Magrebine de Medecine du Sport (Moroccan Federation of Sports Medicine)

Name of Contact Person: Dr. Abdelmalek Sentissi

Title of Contact Person: President

Contact Address: 206, Av. Mers Sultan

Casablanca

MOROCCO

Telephone: (+212.2) 2-27-4434

Fax: (+212.2) 2-20-2172

Countries belonging to group: Algeria, Libya, Mauritania, Morocco, and Tunisia

Founding Date: 1990

Groupement Latin et Mediterranean de Medecine du Sport (Latin and Mediterranean Group for Sport Medicine)

GLMMS (LMGSM)

Objectives are to further sports medicine and to conduct studies on medical problems related to amateur and professional sports and physical activity in general. Offers continuing education classes to members. Operates speakers' bureau.

23 Blvd.

Carabacel

F-06000 Nice

FRANCE

Name of Contact Person: Dr. Francisque Cammandre

Title of Contact Person: Secretary General

Contact Address: 23 Blvd.

Carabacel

F-06000 Nice

FRANCE

Telephone: 33 93 853377

Fax: 33 93 130762

Countries belonging to group: Andorra, Belgium, France, Greece, Israel, Italy, Luxembourg, Monaco, Portugal, Romania, Spain, Algeria, Cyprus, Malta, Morocco, Switzerland, Tunisia, and Turkey

Number of Members: 2,000

Founding Date: 1956

Publications: *Apunto* (in Spanish—periodic); *Archivos de Medicina del Deporte* (in Spanish—quarterly); *Cinesiologie* (in French—bimonthly); *Medecine du Sport* (in English, French, Italian, and Portuguese—bimonthly); *Medecine du Sud-Est* (in French—quarterly).

North European Chapter of Sports Medicine

Snarestad 8

S-271 93 YSTAD

SWEDEN

Telephone: 46 411 70007

Fax: 46 411 70007

Name of Contact Person: Dr. Sven-Anders Sölveborn

Title of Contact Person: Secretary General

Founding Date: 1998

Union Africaine de Medecine du Sport (African Union of Sports Medicine)

Name of Contact Person: Prof. Dr. Constant Roux

Title of Contact Person: President

Contact Address: Abidjan 01

IVORY COAST

Telephone: (+225) 440 864

Fax: (+225) 443 282

Founding Date: 1982

National Associations of Sports Medicine

ALGERIA

Group Algerien de Medecine et de Traumatologie du Sport

BR 61
El Biar
ALGERIA
Telephone: (213.2) 921810

ANDORRA

Federacion Andorrana Medicina de l'esport (Sports Medicine Federation of Andorra)

Edifici Credit Centre
Carrer Bonaventura
Armengol
6/8 Andorra la Vella
ANDORRA
Telephone: (376) 866585
Fax: (376) 868308

ARGENTINA

Federacion Argentina de Medicina del Deporte (Sports Medicine Federation of Argentina)

FAMEDEP
The scientific promotion of sports medicine, medical doctors, meetings of specialty, institutional associations, and physical activity in the community
Casilla del Correo 994
Castros Barros 75-C 1000 WAJ
Ciudad de Buenos Aires
ARGENTINA
Telephone: 54 11 4981 2965
Fax: 54 221 425 9324
E-mail: famedep@redcadeco.com.ar
Name of Contact Person: Dr. Alberto Omar Ricart
Title of Contact Person: President
Contact Address: 508 N. 2831
1900 La Plata

(continued on next page)

(FAMEDEP, continued)

Prov de Buenos Aires
ARGENTINA
Telephone: 54 221 471 0589
Fax: 54 221 425 9324
E-mail: aricart@redcadeco.com.ar
10 regional associations
Membership: 300
Publications: *ERGUM,* official magazine of
FAMEDEP

ARUBA

Instituto di Medicina Pa Deporte di Aruba (Sports Medicine Institute of Aruba)

Bernhardstraat 75
San Nicolaas
ARUBA
Telephone: (297.8) 57290 / 48832
Fax: (297.8) 52994

AUSTRALIA

Sports Medicine Australia

PO Box 897
Belconnen ACT 2616
AUSTRALIA
Telephone: (02) 6251 6944
Fax: (02) 6253 1489
E-mail: smanat@ozE-mail.com.au
Web site: www.ausport.gov.au/sma
Publications: *The Sportsmed News* is a quarterly publication of SMA Queensland Branch.

AUSTRIA

Austrian Society of Sports Medicine

Auf der Schmelz 6
A-1150 Wien
AUSTRIA
Telephone: (43.1) 9822661/174
Fax: (43.1) 9822661/198

B.S.B. BRUNEI DARUSSALAM

Brunei Association of Sports Medicine

BASM
To promote research and clinical advancement in the field of sports medicine in the ASEAN and BRUNEI.
c/o Dr. Hj. Danish Zaheer
Ste. 26-B, Block II
Mabohai Apt. 5pg-10
Jalan Jawatan Dalam
B.S.B. BRUNEI DARUSSALAM
Telephone: +673-8-870369
Name of Contact Person: Dr. Hj. Danish Zaheer
Title of Contact Person: President
Telephone: +673-2-221503
Fax: +673-2-380754
E-mail: smrcdan@brunet.bn
Membership: 246
Publications: *AFSM Newsletter* (quarterly in English); *Sports Medicine Watch* (monthly in English)

BAHRAIN

Bahrain Sports Medicine Association

PO Box 29191
Riffa
BAHRAIN
Telephone: (973) 682612
Fax: (973) 684108
Founding Date: 1984

BANGLADESH

Bangladesh Association of Sports Medicine

Bangabandhu National Stadium
VIP Gate 3, Second Floor
BANGLADESH
Telephone: 880 2 9660025, 894291
Fax: 880 2 9561567
Name of Contact Person: Prof. Rashiduddin Ahmed
Title of Contact Person: President

BARBADOS

Barbados Sport Medicine Association

PO Box 89
Welches Rd.
St. Michael
BARBADOS
Telephone: (1.246) 429-8269
Fax: (1.246) 228-5251
Name of Contact Person: Adrian Lorde
Title of Contact Person: Chair
E-mail: doclorde@caribsurf.com
Founding Date: 1985/1988

BELGIUM

Belgische Vereniging Sport—Geneeskunde & Sportwetenschappen (Sports Medicine Association of Belgium)

Flok Ku-Leuven
Prof. P. Hespel
Tervuursevest 101
B-3001 Leuven
BELGIUM
Telephone: (32) 16329091
Fax: (32) 16329196

BOLIVIA

Federacion Boliviana de Medicina Deportiva (Sports Medicine Federation of Bolivia)

Avenida Busch 1539
La Paz
BOLIVIA
Telephone: (5912) 220086
Fax: (5912) 377709

BOSNIA

Bosnia and Herzegovina Sports Medicine Association

c/o Dr. Zlatan M. Hrelja
Titova 9A
71000 Sarajevo
BOSNIA & HERZEGOVINA
Telephone: (387.71) 663514
Fax: (387.71) 663362
Name of Contact Person: Dr. Zlatan M. Hrelja
Title of Contact Person: Secretary-General

BRAZIL

Sociedade Brasileira de Medicina de Esporte (Brazil Sports Medicine Society)

Av. Ipiranja, 5311

Porto Alegre-RS

90610-001

BRAZIL

Telephone: (55.51) 3392899

Fax: (55.51) 3392998

E-mail: DEROSE@VORTEX.UFRGS.br

BULGARIA

Bulgarian Society of Sport Medicine and Kinestherapy

The society fosters research in sports medicine and kinestherapy.

Gurguliat 1

BG-1000 Sofia

BULGARIA

Telephone: 359 2 894145

Fax: 359 2 894145

Name of Contact Person: Prof. Maria Totera, MD

Title of Contact Person: President

Membership: 200

Founding Date: 1953

BURKINA FAZO

Association Burkinabe de la Medecina du Sport

08 BP 11061 Ouagadougou

BURKINA FAZO

Telephone: (226) 314995

Fax: (226) 303330

CANADA

Canadian Academy of Sport Medicine

CASM

The CASM is an organization of physicians committed to excellence in the practice of medicine as it applies to all aspects of physical activity. Its mission is to be a leader in advancing the art and science of sports medicine, including health promotion and disease prevention, for the benefit of all Canadians through programs of education, research, and service. The CASM promotes development and application of improved sports medicine techniques, facilitates professional advancement of members, serves as a clearinghouse on sports medicine, conducts educational programs, and participates in charitable activities.

1010 Polytex St. #14

Gloucester ON K1B 5N4

KIJ 9H9

CANADA

Telephone: (613) 748-5851

Fax: (613) 748-5792

E-mail: jburke@casm-acms.org

Web site: www.casm-acms.org

Name of Contact Person: Jacqueline Burke

Title of Contact Person: Executive Director

Membership: 500

Founding Date: 1970

Publications: *Clinical Journal of Sport Medicine* (quarterly)

Canadian Athletic Therapists Association

CATA

The CATA is a national nonprofit organization dedicated to the promotion and delivery of the highest quality care to active individuals through injury prevention, emergency services, and rehabilitative techniques.

National Office

Ste. 312, 902 - 11th Ave. SW

Calgary AB T2R 0E7

CANADA

Telephone: 403-509-CATA (2282)

Fax: 403-509-2280

E-mail: cata12@telusplanet.net

Web site: www.mtroyal.ab.ca/CATA

Name of Contact Person: Maggie Kayes

Title of Contact Person: President

Membership: 1,000

Founding Date: 1965

Publications: *Athletic Therapy Update* (periodic newsletter); *Canadian Athletic Therapists Association* (quarterly newsletter); *Directory* (periodic)

Canadian Sport Massage Therapists Association

CSMTA

The CSMTA enhances the health care needs of Canadian athletes through its National Sport Massage Certification Program and the effective application of sport massage during all phases of their training, performance, and competition. The CSMTA promotes a professional climate for the growth of sport massage therapy in Canada.

CSMTA National Office

Box 1330

Unity SK S0K 4L0

CANADA

Telephone: (306) 228-2808

Fax: (306) 228-2808

E-mail: headoffice@csmta.ca

Web site: www.csmta.ca

E-mail: gerrygee@sk.sympatico.ca

Founding Date: 1987

CHILE

Sociedad Chilena de Medicina del Deporte (Chile Sports Medicine Society)

Esmeralda 678, Of. 307

Santiago de Chile

CHILE

Telephone: (56.2) 6396171

Fax: (56.2) 6391085

Web site: www.sochmedep.cl

CHINA

Chinese Association of Sports Medicine

11 Tiyuguan Rd.

100061 Beijing

CHINA

Telephone: (86.1) 7120293

Fax: (86.1) 7146035

COLUMBIA

Asociacion de Medicina del Deporte de Colombia (Association of Sports Medicine of Colombia)

Tr. 9A BIS No. 133-25

El. Milton Arguello, 3er Piso

Santafe de Bogota, D.C

COLOMBIA

Telephone: (57.1) 626 9117

Fax: (57.1) 626 8924

E-mail: amedco@mixmail.com

Web site: www.encolombia.com/amedcom.htm

CONGO REPUBLIC

Conseil Nationale de Medecine du Sport du Congo (Sports Medicine National Council of the Congo)

BP 2290

Brazzaville

CONGO REPUBLIC

Telephone: (242) 823 710

COSTA RICA

Asociacion Costaricense de Medicina Deportiva (Sports Medicine Association of Costa Rica)

Apartado Postal 172

3000 Heredia

COSTA RICA

Telephone: (506) 2371835

Fax: (506) 2378956

E-mail: cinco@medscope.com

CROATIA

Croatian Sports Medicine Society

The Croatian Sports Medicine Society regulates national associations, collaborates in postgraduate courses of sports medicine, and organizes seminars and workshops in fields related to sports medicine.

Faculty of Physical Education

Horvacanski zavoj 15

HR-10 000 Zagreb

CROATIA

Telephone: 00385 1 3658 630

Fax: 00385 1 3634 146

E-mail: hdsm@ffk.hr

Name of Contact Person: Prof. Stjepan Heimer, PhD

E-mail: hdsm@ffk.hr

Membership: 120

Publications: *Croatian Sports Medicine Journal* (biquarterly)

CUBA

Federacion Cubana de Medicina Deportiva (Sports Medicine Federation of Cuba)

Calle 10 E 100 y 14

Reparto Embil, Municipio Boyeros

Codigo Postal 10800

Cuidad Habana, Apartado Postal 8003

CUBA

Telephone: (537) 447257

Fax: (537) 335310

E-mail: cinid@ceniai.cu

CYPRUS

Cyprus Association of Sports Medicine

CASM

The CASM is locally active for the implementation of the medical certification of athletes, medical coverage of athletic events, the antidoping campaign, and all medical problems related to athletes.

PO Box 25137

1307 Nicosia

CYPRUS

Telephone: (357.2) 663762

Fax: (357.2) 664669

E-mail: sportsmedicine@cytanet.co.cy

Web site: www.cydem.com/page7.html

Name of Contact Person: Dr. Costas Christodoulakis, MD

Title of Contact Person: President

Telephone: (357.2) 677022

Fax: (357.2) 664669

E-mail: sportsmedicine@cytanet.com.cy

Membership: 85

Founding Date: 1977

Publications: Newsletter (biannually in Greek)

CZECH REPUBLIC

Czech Society of Sports Medicine

c/o Fakultni nemocnise motol

V Uvalu 85

CZ-150 18 Praha 5

CZECH REPUBLIC

Telephone: (420) 2244.35500

Fax: (420) 2244.35820

DENMARK

Danish Association of Sports Medicine

To promote the interest for and knowledge of sports medicine and work to put sports medicine to practical use.

c/o Danmaks Idraets-Forbund

Idraettens Hus

Brondby Stadium 20

DK-2605 Brondby

DENMARK

Telephone: (45) 4326 2001

Fax: (45) 4326 2991

E-mail: birthe@jochumsen.dk

Web site: www.sportsmedicin.dk

Name of Contact Person: Mrs. Birth Jochumsen

Membership: 640

Publications: *Dansk Sportsmedicin* (quarterly journal in Danish)

DOMINICAN REPUBLIC

Sociedad Dominicana de Medicina del Deporte (Dominican Society of Sports Medicine

c/o Aruba 82 Ens. Ozama

Santo Domingo

DOMINICAN REPUBLIC

Telephone: (1. 809) 594-6892

Fax: (1.809) 591-3444

Name of Contact Person: Dr. Milton Pinedo

Title of Contact Person: President

ECUADOR

Federacion Ecuatoriana de Medicina Deportiva (Sports Medicine Federation of Ecuadorian)

FEMED

Training and continual education

Name of Contact Person: Dr. Bolivar Gonzalex Delgado

Title of Contact Person: General Secretary

Contact Address: Amazonas 607 y Carrion

Roca 538 y Juan Leon Mera Quito

ECUADOR

Telephone: (5932) 491069/545501

Fax: (5932) 567664

E-mail: gonzacuero@hotmail.com

Membership: 20

EGYPT

Egypt Sports Medicine Association

Gabalaya Str.

Elguezira

Cairo

EGYPT

EL SALVADOR

Sociedad Salvadorena de Medicina Deportiva (El Salvador Sports Medicine Society)

45 Av. Sur 632 Colonia
Flor Blanca, San Salvador
EL SALVADOR
Name of Contact Person: Dr. Edgar Alberto

ESTONIA

Estonian Sports Medicine Federation

Dept. of Sports Medicine & Rehabilitation
University of Tartu
1A Puusepa St.
EE2400 Tartu
ESTONIA
Telephone: (372.7) 449221
Fax: (372.7) 449402
E-mail: yllar@cut.ee

ETHIOPIA

Sports Medical Committee of Ethiopia

Ministry of Physical Culture of Sport
(National Sport Medical Centre)
Addis Ababa
ETHIOPIA
Telephone: (251.1) 159152 / 515363
Fax: (251.1) 513345

FINLAND

Finnish Association of Sports Medicine

Likes Research Center
Rautpohjankatu 10
FIN-40700, Jyvalkyla
FINLAND
Telephone: (358.14) 2601576
Fax: (358.14) 2601571
E-mail: jmdsa@jyu.fi

FRANCE

International Society for Ski Traumatology and Medicine of Winter Sports

Encourages an international exchange of medical experiences and ideas on the treatment of injuries resulting from mountaineering and other winter sports.

Name of Contact Person: Dr. M. Binet
Contact Address: Centre Medical
F-74110 Avoriaz
FRANCE
Telephone: 33 4 50740542
Fax: 33 4 50740758
Founding Date: 1956
Publications: *Congress Reports* (biennial)

Societe Francaise de Medecine du Sport (French Sports Medicine Society)

C. M. S.
200, rue du Pere Soulas
Montpellier
FRANCE
Telephone: (33.4) 6754.5102
Fax: (33.4) 6752.1316
Web site: www.sfms.asso.fr

GABON

Association Gabonaisede Medicine du Sport

BP 13050
Libreville
GABON
Telephone: (241) 736253
Fax: (241) 731629

GERMANY

Geschäftsstelle des Deutscher Sportärztebund (German Federation of Sports Medicine and Prevention)

DGSP Hugstetter
Strabe 55
79106 Freiburg
GERMANY
Telephone: 761-2707456
Fax: 761-2024881
E-mail: german.sportmed@msm1.ukl.uni-
    freiburg.de

GHANA

Ghana Association of Sports Medicine

PO Box 10540
Accra North
GHANA
Telephone: (23321) 664282

GREECE

Greece Sports Medicine Association of Northern Greece

26 Agiar Sofias Street
54622
Thessaloniki
GREECE
Telephone: 003031 (992181)
Fax: 003031 (992183)
E-mail: stregios@med.auth.gr
Name of Contact Person: Prof. A. Deligiannis

GRENADA

Grenada Sports Medicine Association

c/o Olympic Committee
P.O. Box 370
Scott Street
St. George's
GRENADA-WEST INDIES
Name of Contact Person: Dr. David Lambert
Title of Contact Person: President

GUATEMALA

Asociacion Guatemalteca de Medicina Deportiva

17 Avenida <<A>> 6-05
Zona 15, Colonia El Maestro
Ciudad Guatemala
GUATEMALA
Fax: (5022) 324469
Name of Contact Person: Dr. Rafael Robles

HONDURAS

Asociacion Hondurena de Medicina del Deporte

Apartado Postal 3143
Est. Nacional, Tegucigulpa
HONDURAS

HONG KONG

Hong Kong Association of Sports Medicine & Sports Science

The association's aims and objectives are to promote and advance the practice, education, and research of medicine and science in relation to sport and exercise, including the basic physiological, biomechanical, structural, and behavioral mechanisms; the maintenance and enhancement of physical and mental fitness for daily living; the evaluation of and conditioning for sport performance; and the prevention, treatment, and rehabilitation of disease and injury related to sport and exercise. The association promotes and establishes friendly relationships with other medical and scientific associations and organizations both in Hong Kong and abroad; promotes, supports, or opposes legislative or other measures affecting the interest and affairs of the association; and appoints or nominates for appointment by the Hong Kong government persons to sit on any government or statutory body or the like.

Sports Science Department
Hong Kong Sports Development Board
Sports Institute, Shatin
HONG KONG
Telephone: (852) 2681.6368
Fax: (852) 2681.6330
E-mail: raymonds@hksdb.org.hk

Web site: http://medicine.org.hk/hkasmss (or) http://home4u.hongkong.com/health/fitness/hkasmandss
Name of Contact Person: Dr. Lobo Lonie
Title of Contact Person: Secretary
Contact Address: c/o Department of Physical Education
Hong Kong Baptist University
Kowloon Tong
HONG KONG
Telephone: 852-23395631
Fax: 852-23395757
E-mail: 562591@hkbu.edu.hk
Membership: 50
Founding Date: 1988
Publications: *Hong Kong Journal of Sports Medicine & Sports Science* (biannual)

HUNGARY

Hungarian Society of Sports Medicine

The society organizes the activity of sport physicians, prepares guidelines in the field of sports medicine, and organizes scientific activity, conferences, courses, etc.

1123
Alkotás str. 48 Budapest
H-1123
HUNGARY
Telephone: (361) 4886111
Fax: (361) 13753292
Name of Contact Person: Dr. Eva Martos
Title of Contact Person: Secretary
E-mail: Mar13880@Helka.IIF.hu
Membership: 226
Publications: *Hungarian Review of Sports Medicine* (bilingual quarterly journal)

INDIA

Indian Association of Sports Medicine

IASM
1, Adishwar Flats
P.O. RoocdKhokhara
Mayinagdr (E) 380008
New Delhi
INDIA
Telephone: 911-79-2161675
Fax: 911-79-5530034
E-mail: spspomed@ad1.vsul.net.in
Name of Contact Person: Dr. P.S.M. Chandran
Title of Contact Person: President
Telephone: 011-4368320/011-6493016/
011-6492016
Fax: 011-4369653
E-mail: dvpsmc@del3.vsnl.net.in
Founding Date: 1971
Publications: *Indian Journal of Sports Traumatology and Sport Science* (biannual)

INDONESIA

Indonesian Association for Sports Health

Gate III Senayan Main Stadium
Jakarta, 10270
INDONESIA
Telephone: (62.21) 579181
Name of Contact Person: Dr. Hario Tilarso
Contact Address: PPKORI
Pintu III Stadion Utama Senayan
Jakarta
INDONESIA
Telephone: (62.21) 5719191
Fax: (62.21) 5711140
E-mail: dangsina@rad.net.id

IRAN

Sports Medicine Federation of Iran

Shiroudi Sports Complex
Varzandah St. Shehid
Mofatteh Ave.
Tehran, I.R.
IRAN
Telephone: (98.21) 8825937
Fax: (98.21) 8840100

IRELAND

Irish Sports Medicine Association

c/o Anatomy Department
Human Performance Laboratory
Trinity College
Dublin 2
IRELAND
Telephone: (353.1) 6081182
Fax: (353.1) 6790119

ISRAEL

Israel Society of Sports Medicine

Department of Orthopaedics
Hadassah University Hospital
Mount Scopus
il-91240 Jerusalem
ISRAEL
Telephone: (972.2) 5341217
Fax: (972.2) 5619686

ITALY

Italian Sports Medicine Federation

Viale Tiziano 70
I-00196 Rome
ITALY
Telephone: (36.6) 3233774
Fax: (39.6) 3858206

IVORY COAST

Asociacion Ivorienne de Medicine Sportive

s/c Prof. Constant Roux
Faculte de Medicine
01 BP V 166
Abidjan
COTE D'IVOIRE
Telephone: (225) 440864
Fax: (225) 443282
Name of Contact Person: Prof. Constant Roux

JAMAICA

Jamaican Association of Sports Medicine

Institute of Sports
Nacional Areana
Kingston
JAMAICA

JAPAN

Japan Athletic Trainers Organization

JATO's objectives are to educate the community about the value of NATA standards and to promote the athletic training profession in Japan, to provide continuous education opportunities for the membership, to exchange opinions among the membership about the current sports medicine environment, to communicate with other organizations to promote higher standards of care for athletes, and to share knowledge and experience with other health care providers in Japan.

JAPAN
Telephone: +81-3-3448-2806
Fax: +81-3-3448-2849
E-mail: jato@tokyoonline.co.jp
Web site: www.tokyoonline.co.jp/jato
Membership: Solely NATA members. Currently, the majority of ATCs in Japan are members of the JATO. There are three categories of membership: regular, associate, and student. NATA certification is required to become a regular member, while any associate member of the NATA can become an associate member of the JATO.
Founding Date: 1996
Publications: *JATO Newsletter* (quarterly)

Japanese Federation of Physical Fitness and Sports Medicine

To promote the progress and development of research on physical fitness, sports medicine, and science by facilitating and collaborating research, and to strive for practical applications from the research outcomes.

Business Center for Academic Societies Japan
16-9, 5-Chome
Hon-Komagome, Bunkyo-ku
Tokyo 113-8622
JAPAN
Telephone: (81.3) 5814.5801
Fax: (81.3) 5814.5820
Name of Contact Person: Toshito Katsumura, MD, PhD
Title of Contact Person: Professor

Contact Address: Department of Preventive Medicine and Public Health, Tokyo Medical University

1-1, 6-Chome

Shinjuku, Shinjuku-Ku

Tokyo 160-8402

JAPAN

Telephone: (81.3) 5379.4339

Fax: (81.3) 3226.5277

E-mail: kats@tokyo-med.ac.jp

Membership: 4900

Publications: *Japanese Journal of Physical Fitness and Sports Medicine*

KAZAKHSTAN

Kazakhistanian Association of Sports Medicine

4800 Goldenfish

Almati

Abai St. 48

KAZAKHSTAN

E-mail: m-iveyd-k@hotmail.com

KOREA

Popular Democratic Republic of Korea: The Sport Medical Association

Munsin- Dong 2

Dongdaewon District

Pyongyang

PEOPLE'S REPUBLIC OF KOREA

Korean Society of Sports Medicine

50 Ilwon Dong

Kangnam Ku

Seoul 135-230

KOREA

Telephone: (82.2) 3410-3840

Fax: (82.2) 3410-0054

E-mail: W.H.Park@SMC.SAM.SUNG

KUWAIT

Kuwait Sports Medicine Association

c/o Dr. Adnan Al-Edan, MD

PO Box 4079 Safat

13041

KUWAIT

Telephone: (+965) 4870406 / (+965) 4875369

Fax: (+965) 4874190

Name of Contact Person: Dr. Adnan Al-Edan, MD

LATVIA

Latvia Sports Medicine Association

Bruninieku str. 813

Riga, LV-1010

LATVIA

Telephone: (371) 2279163

Fax: (371) 2274114

LITHUANIA

Lithuanian Sports Medicine Association

Roziu A1 2/5

2009 Vilnius

LITHUANIA

Telephone: (370.2) 612455

LUXEMBOURG

Societe Luxembourgeoise de Medecine du Sport (Luxembourg Sports Medicine Society)

Institut Nacional des Sports
BP 180
L-2011 Luxembourg
LUXEMBOURG

MACAU

Macau Sports Medicine Association

PO Box 1954
MACAU
Telephone: (853) 700139
Fax: (853) 355539

MACEDONIA

Association of Physicians of Sports Medicine Macedonian Medical Association

ul. Dame Gruev br. 3
PO Box 174
MK-91000 Skopje
MACEDONIA
Telephone: (389.91) 232577

MALAYSIA

Malaysian Association of Sports Medicine

MASM
c/o Olympic Council of Malaysia
Mezzanine Floor, Wisma OCM
Hang Jebat Rd.
50150 Kuala Lumpur

MALAYSIA
Telephone: (603) 7761469
Fax: (603) 7750687
Name of Contact Person: Dr. Ramlan Abd. Aziz
Title of Contact Person: President
Contact Address: Institut Sukan Negara (National Sports Institute of Malaysia)
Bukit Jalil, SRI Petaling
PO Box 10440
50714, Kuala Lumpur
MALAYSIA
Telephone: (603) 9579735
Fax: (603) 9587244
E-mail: ramlan@nsc.gov.my
Publications: *MASM Bulletin* (quarterly)

MALTA

Sports Medical Commission of Malta

Warq U. Zahar, Triq ID-Dawwara, Attard BZNI3
MALTA
Telephone: 00356 414736
Fax: 00356 414736
E-mail: nocmalta@waldonet.net.mt
Name of Contact Person: Dr. Kirill Micallef Starface

MAURITANIA

Association Mauritaninne de Medecine du Sport

c/o Dr. B.A. Mohamed Lemine
BP 30
Nouakchott
MAURITANIA
Telephone: (2222) 50498
Fax: (2222) 52915

MEXICO

Federacion Mexicana de Medicina del Deporte (Sports Medicine Federation of Mexico)

Av. Rio Churusco Puerta 9
Ciudad Deportiva
Magdalena Mixhuca
Delegacion Iztacalco
08010 Mexico DF
Telephone: (52.2) 519-0991
Fax: (52.2) 519-1213
Web site: www.codeme.org.mx/mexicana

MONGOLIA

Mongolian Association of Sports Medicine

c/o Dr. D. Dagrasuren
Baga Toiruu-55
Ulaanbaatar 210648
MONGOLIA
Telephone: (212.2) 274434
Fax: (212.2) 202173

MOROCCO

Association Marocaine de Medecine du Sport

Polyclinique Notre Dame
206 Avenue Mers Sultan
Casablanca
MOROCCO
Telephone: (212.2) 274434
Fax: (212.2) 202172

NETHERLANDS ANTILLES

Netherlands Antilles Foundation of Sports Medicine

Sta. Rosa Sports Medicine Institute
Sta. Rosaweg 353
Curacao
NETHERLANDS ANTILLES
Telephone: (5999) 7676666
Fax: (5999) 7674139
Name of Contact Person: Wallid Elhage, MD

NEW ZEALAND

Sports Medicine New Zealand Inc.

PO Box 6398
Dunedin
NEW ZEALAND
Telephone: (64.3) 477-7887
Fax: (64.3) 477-7882
E-mail: smnznat@xtra.com.nz

New Zealand Sports Medicine

NEW ZEALAND
E-mail: website@sportsmedicine.co.nz
Web site: www.sportsmedicine.co.nz

NICARAGUA

Associacion Nicaraguense de Medicina del Deporte

De Radio Mundial Z
Cuadras Arriba
Managua
NICARAGUA
Telephone: (505.2) 224772
Fax: (505.2) 662576

NIGERIA

Nigerian Association of Sports Medicine

c/o Nigeria Olympic Committee
PO Box 3156
Marina, Lagos
NIGERIA
Telephone: (234.1) 5450105
Fax: (234.1) 5450104 / 2693304

NORWAY

Norwegian Sports Medicine Association

Teaching through doctors and physical therapists of both athletes and nonathletes of health benefits related to physical activities as well as treatment and prevention of injuries.

c/o NyComed
Pharma As
P.O. Box 4220
Torshov N-0401
Oslo
NORWAY
Telephone: +4773998000
Fax: +4773998722
Name of Contact Person: Anders Walloe
Title of Contact Person: Consultant
Contact Address: Dept. of Ort. Surgery Ulleval Hospital 0407
Oslo
NORWAY
Telephone: +4722119500 or +4722060932
Fax: +4722119558
E-mail: anders.walloe@ulleval.no
Membership: 535
Publications: *Norwegian Sports Medisin*

OMAN

Oman Sports Medicine Committee

PO Box 2842
Ruwi
Postal Code 112
OMAN
Telephone: (968) 799891 / 892
Fax: (968) 799890

PAKISTAN

Sports Medicine Association of Pakistan

Hill Park General Hospital
Shaheed Millat Rd.
Karachi
PAKISTAN
Telephone: (92.21) 4552442
Fax: (92.21) 5060343
E-mail: zsl@cyber.net.pk
Name of Contact Person: Prof. Nish Mallick
Title of Contact Person: President
E-mail: mallick@cybernet.pk
Membership: 137
Founding Date: 1989

PANAMA

Federacion de Medicina Deportiva de Panama (Sports Medicine Federation of Panama)

Residencial San Fernando #4
PO Box 6A-8772
El Dorado
PANAMA
Fax: (507) 694345
Name of Contact Person: Dr. Daniel Herrera

PARAGUAY

Sociedad Paraguaya de Medicina del Deporte (Paraguayan Sports Medicine Society)

c/o Dr. Jorge Acosta
Jose Marti, 5352
Casilla postal 1420
Asuncion
PARAGUAY
Telephone: (595.21) 603718
Fax: (595.21) 603968
Name of Contact Person: Dr. Jorge Acosta

PERU

Sociedad Peruana de Medicina y Ciencias Aplicadas al Deporte

Aplicadas al Deporte
c/o Dr. Pedro Riega
Recuay 122-203
Brena, Lima
PERU
Telephone: (51.14) 257180
Fax: (51.12) 654956
Name of Contact Person: Dr. Pedro Riega

PHILIPPINES

Sports Medicine Association of Philippeans

Rizal Memorial Complex
Adriatico St.
Manila
PHILIPPINES
Telephone: (632) 521-9123
Fax: (632) 522-2374
E-mail: bebet@mnl.seqnel.net

POLAND

Poland Sports Medicine Association

ul. Wawelska 5
PL-02-034 Warszawa
POLAND
Telephone: (4822) 256738
Fax: (4822) 257385

PORTUGAL

Sociedade Portuguesa de Medicina Desportiva (Portugal Sports Medicine Society)

Av. Almirante Gago
Coutinho 151
P-1700 Lisboa
PORTUGAL
Telephone: (3511) 8470654
Fax: (3511) 8471215

PUERTO RICO

Federacion de Medicina Deportiva de Puerto Rico (Sports Medicine Federation of Puerto Rico)

Casa Olimpica
Box 8
San Juan 00902
PUERTO RICO
Telephone: (787) 722-2826 or (787) 723-3890
Fax: (787) 723-3898
E-mail: enramy@coqui.net
Name of Contact Person: Dr. William Mecheo
Title of Contact Person: President
Telephone: (787) 751-9625/(787) 740-2270
Membership: 60

REPUBLIC OF GEORGIA

Georgian Association of Sports Medicine

12, Chitadze str. 380008
Tbilisi
REPUBLIC OF GEORGIA
Telephone: 995 32 99 81 44; 995 32 98 84 59
Fax: 995 32 92 23 32; 995 32 98 75 01
E-mail: pdmed@access.sanet.ge

REPUBLIC OF MOLDOVA

Moldova Federation of Sports Medicine & Medical Rehabilitation of the Republic of Moldova

27 Testemitanu str.
2025 MD Chilsnau
REPUBLIC OF MOLDOVA
Telephone: 3732 733 784 or 3732 733 819
Fax: 3732 494 989
E-mail: sportmed@mail.md

ROMANIA

Societatea Romana de Medicina Sportiva (Romania Sports Medicine Society)

Boul. Basarabiei No. 37-39
District 2, Code 73401
Bucharest
ROMANIA
Telephone: (401) 3248375
Fax: (401) 3248376

RUSSIA

United All-Russia Federation of Sports Medicine

107120, Moscow
Zemlianoi val, 53
RUSSIA
Telephone: (7095) 928-2992
Fax: (7095) 928-2992

SAUDI ARABIA

Saudi Arabian Sports Medicine Association

SASMA
The SASMA contributes to scientific and academic efforts aiming at enhancing athletes' performance, disseminates health awareness and preventive guidance among youth and athletes, assists in qualifying and polishing the expertise of technical cadres working in the various aspects of sports medicine, and offers specialized consultations on sports medicine services.

PO Box 22486
Riyadh 11495
SAUDI ARABIA
Telephone: (9661) 482-6142
Fax: (9661) 482-0750
Name of Contact Person: Dr. Mohammad H. Mufti
Title of Contact Person: President
E-mail: info@smc.com.sa
Membership: 530
Publications: *The Saudi Journal of Sports Medicine* (biannual), *Sports Medicine Message* (quarterly newsletter). Over the past 15 years, the Association has published 19 reference books on the various aspects of sports medicine, 4 directories, 8 documentary books, and 17 handouts.

SLOVAKIA

Slovak Society of Sports Medicine

The society promotes sports medicine as a branch of medical sciences and a clinical specialization.

Svobodovo nabr. 9

SK-814 69 Bratislava

SLOVAKIA

Telephone: 4217 5441 4472

Fax: 4217 5441 4472

Name of Contact Person: Prof. Dasan Hamar, MD, PhD

Title of Contact Person: President

E-mail: hamar@fsport.uniba.sk

Membership: 150

Publications: *Medicina Sportiva Bohemica at Slovaca* (quarterly journal done jointly with the Czech Society of Sports Medicine)

SLOVENIA

Slovenia Sports Medicine Society

Celovska 25

SI-1000 Ljubljana

SLOVENIA

Telephone: (38661) 315184

Fax: (38661) 315184

E-mail: vanja.vuga@animos.mf.uni.lj.sl

SOUTH AFRICA

South Africa Sports Medicine Association

PO Box 2598

Claremch

7440

SOUTH AFRICA

Telephone: (2721) 686-7330

Fax: (2721) 686-7530

E-mail: Tnoakes@sports.uct.ac.za

SPAIN

Federacion Espanola de Medicina del Deporte (Sports Medicine Federation of Spain)

FEMEDE

Apartado 1207

31080 Pamplona

Navarra

SPAIN

Telephone: 0034 948 267706

Fax: 0034 948 174325

E-mail: femede@arrakis.es

Web site: www.femede.es

SRI LANKA

Sri Lanka Sports Medicine Association

Dte of Army Medical Services

Military Hospital

Colombo 3

SRI LANKA

Telephone: (941) 431693

Fax: (941) 531011

E-mail: thurai@sri.lanka.net

SWEDEN

Swedish Society of Sports Medicine, The

The society's purpose is to promote sports medicine education, and to hold annual meetings and courses.

(continued on next page)

(Swedish Society of Sports Medicine, continued)

Klockarvagen 104

SE-151 61 Sodertalje

SWEDEN

Telephone: (468) 550-102-00

Fax: (468) 550-104-09

E-mail: IMF.kansli@mailbox.calypso.net

Web site: www.IMF.a.se

Name of Contact Person: Prof. Jon Karlsson

Title of Contact Person: Chair

Contact Address: Department of Orthopaedic

Sahlgrenska University Hospital

OSTRA

SE-416 85 Goteborg Sverige

SWEDEN

Telephone: +46 31 343 4090

Fax: +46 31 343 4092

E-mail: jon.karlsson@telia.com

Membership: 1,200

Publications: PSvensk Idrottsmedicin, quarterly newsletter

Society for Tennis Medicine and Science

STMS

STMS aims to serve as an international forum for the generation and dissemination of knowledge of tennis medicine and science.

Web site: www.stms.nl

Name of Contact Person: Per A.F.H. Renström

Title of Contact Person: President

Contact Address: Karolinska Institute

Stockholm

SWEDEN

E-mail: President@STMS.nl

Publications: Sports Medicine and Science in Tennis, quarterly newsletter

SWITZERLAND

International Olympic Association for Medico-Sport Research

IOAMSR

Seeks to advance sports medical research and practice. Conducts research programs; serves as a clearinghouse on sports medicine.*

Name of Contact Person: Juan Antonio Samaranch

Contact Address: c/o COI

Chateau de Vidy

CH-1007 Lanne

SWITZERLAND

Telephone: 41 21 6216111

Fax: 41 21 6216116

Societe Swisse de Medecine du Sport (Switzerland Sports Medicine Society)

PO Box 408

CH-3000 Bern 25

SWITZERLAND

Telephone: (4131) 333-0254

Fax: (4131) 332-9879

SYRIA

Syrian Association of Sports Medicine

PO Box 5473

Damascus

SYRIA

TAIWAN

Chinese Tapei Sports Medicine Association

5, Fu-Hsig St.
Kweishan, Taoyuan
TAIWAN
Telephone: (886.3) 3281200
Fax: (886.3) 3284564

TCHAD

Association Tchadienne de Medecine du Sport (Tchad Association of Sports Medicine)

BP 2203 N Djamcna
TCHAD
Telephone: (235) 517174
Fax: (235) 521498

THAILAND

Sports Medicine Association of Thailand

2088 Ramkhamhaeng Rd.
Hua Mark
Bangkok
10240
THAILAND
Telephone: (662) 319-7435
Fax: (662) 314-2596

THE NETHERLANDS

Netherlands Association of Sports Medicine

Postbus 52
3720 AB Bilthoven
THE NETHERLANDS
Telephone: (31.30) 225 2290
Fax: (31.30) 225 2498
E-mail: vsg@sportgeneeskunde.com
Web site: www.sportgeneeskunde.com
Name of Contact Person: Prof. Bronkhorotlaan
Title of Contact Person: A.M.G.Y. Bruinsma
Contact Address: P.O. Box 52
3723 MB Bilthoven
THE NETHERLANDS
Membership: 600
Publications: *Geneeskunde en Sport*

TUNISIA

Societe Tunisien de Medecine du Sport (Tunisia Sports Medicine Society)

c/o Prof. Bey Abid Moncef
Clinique Avicenne
El Manar
1004 Tunis
TUNISIA
Fax: (2161) 231180

TURKEY

Turkish Association of Sports Medicine

P.K. 24
Bornova
TR-35040
Izmir
TURKEY
Telephone: (90) 232.3881097
Fax: (90) 232.3422142
E-mail: Meaterg@united states of america.net
Web site: www.ege.edu.com.tr

UGANDA

Uganda Games and Sports Medicine Association

PO Box 9194

Kampala

UGANDA

Telephone: (256.41) 233879

Fax: (256.41) 222093

UNITED ARAB EMIRATES

United Arab Emirates Sports Medicine Committee

PO Box 4350

Dubai

UNITED ARAB EMIRATES

Telephone: (9714) 687333

Fax: (9714) 698886

UNITED KINGDOM

Association of Chartered Physiotherapists in Sports Medicine

ACPSM

The ACPSM seeks to improve techniques and facilities for the prevention and treatment of sport injuries, offers sport physiotherapy courses, and produces an educational journal.

14 Mayfield Ct.

Moseley, Birmingham

B13 9YD

UNITED KINGDOM

Telephone: 44 115 9627681

Fax: 44 115 9606993

Web site: www.wlv.ac.uk/leisure/carss.html

Name of Contact Person: Nicola Phillips

Title of Contact Person: Hon. Sec.

Contact Address: 81 Heol W. Plas Coity

Budgend

CF35 6BA

UNITED KINGDOM

Membership: 954

Founding Date: 1975

Publications: *Directory* (biennial), *Physiotherapy in Sport* (newsletter, 3 per year, in English)

British Association of Sport and Medicine

The British Association of Sport and Medicine seeks to promote public health and fitness as well as to conduct research into the treatment of medical problems aligned with sport and exercise. The organization is also concerned with the postgraduate education of medical professionals with regard to sports medicine.

c/o The Anatomy Building

Medical School of St. Bartholomews Hospital Charterhouse Sq.

London EC1M 6BQ

UNITED KINGDOM

Telephone: 44 171 2533244

Fax: 44 171 2510774

Name of Contact Person: Donald Angus David Macleod

Title of Contact Person: President

Contact Address: The Haining

Woodland Park

Livingston EH54 8AT

UNITED KINGDOM

Membership: 1,400

Founding Date: 1953

Publications: *British Journal of Sport Medicine* (bimonthly)

National Sports Medicine Institute of the United Kingdom

NSMI

The NSMI works to improve the quality of sports and exercise medicine and sport sciences in the United Kingdom. The institute will endeavor to earn the respect of the sporting, medical, and scientific communities by enabling the continuing education and development of all those involved in the delivery of support services to those participating in sport and exercise at all levels.

c/o Medical College of St. Bartholomew's Hospital

Charterhouse Square

London

EC1M 6BQ

UNITED KINGDOM

Telephone: +44 (0)20 7251 0583

Fax: +44 (0)20 7251 0774

E-mail: enquiry@nsmi.org.uk

Web site: www.nsmi.org.uk

Founding Date: 1992

UNITED STATES OF AMERICA

Academy for Sports Dentistry

ASD

The ASD fosters research, development, and education in all sciences related to sports dentistry and its relationship to the body as a whole. The ASD encourages utilization of this knowledge in promoting better approaches to the prevention and treatment of athletic injuries and oral disease and facilitates the exchange of ideas and experience among members.

c/o Mailcode 555

University of Illinois College of Dentistry

801 S. Paulina St.

Chicago, IL 60612

UNITED STATES OF AMERICA

Telephone: (217) 824-6819 / (800) 273-1788

Fax: (312) 996-3535

E-mail: sportdds@uic.edu

Web site: www.sportsdentistry.com/academy.htm

Name of Contact Person: Susan D. Ferry

Title of Contact Person: Executive Director

Contact Address: Academy of Sports Dentistry

875 N. Michigan Ave., Ste. 4040

Chicago, IL 60611-1901

UNITED STATES OF AMERICA

Telephone: (217) 824-4990

Membership: 750

Founding Date: 1983

Publications: *ASD Newsletter* (2 to 3 per year, in English)

American Academy of Pediatrics: Sports Medicine Committee

AAP

The Committee on Sports Medicine and Fitness develops policy to educate pediatricians about all aspects of exercise, sports medicine, and physical fitness for children and adolescents.

141 Northwest Point Blvd.

Elk Grove Village, IL 60009-0927

UNITED STATES OF AMERICA

Telephone: 847-228-5005

Fax: 847-228-5097

E-mail: kidsdoc@aap.org

Web site: www.aap.org

Name of Contact Person: Joe M. Sanders, Jr., MD

Title of Contact Person: Executive Director

Membership: 66 State groups; 55,000

Founding Date: 1930

Publications: *Sports Medicine: Health Care for Young Athletes* (manual); *AAP News*

(continued on next page)

(AAP, continued)

(monthly); *Pedatrics* (monthly scientific journal); *Pediatrics in Review* (continuing education journal); *Healthy Kids* (magazine); *Guide to Your Child's Symptoms* (book); *Guide to Your Child's Nutrition* (book); *Guide to Your Child's Sleep* (book)

American Academy of Podiatric Sports Medicine

AAPSM

The AAPSM promotes professional participation and research in sports medicine and has a series of major objectives:

1. To provide and stimulate programs for research and education

2. To promote and encourage publication of research findings and other literature pertaining to podiatric sports medicine

3. To provide a consultative service for those persons engaged in sports medicine

4. To increase awareness of the medical profession, sport population, and general public to the profession of podiatric sports medicine and modalities available to those who participate in sports

5. To coordinate student chapters and to acquaint the podiatric medical student with the needs and demands placed upon athletes

1729 Glastonberry Rd.

Potomac, MD 20854

UNITED STATES OF AMERICA

Telephone: (301) 424-7440

Web site: www.aapsm.org

Name of Contact Person: Larry I. Shane

Title of Contact Person: Executive Director

Founding Date: 1970

Publications: *AAPSM Newsletter* (quarterly)

American Academy of Sports Physicians

AASP

The AASP's objectives are to educate and inform physicians whose practices comprise mainly sports medicine and to register and recognize physicians who have expertise in sports medicine. The AASP also sponsors seminars.

17445 Oak Creek Ct.

Encino, CA 91316

UNITED STATES OF AMERICA

Telephone: (818) 501-4433

Fax: (818) 501-8855

Name of Contact Person: Janie Zimmer

Title of Contact Person: Coordinator

Membership: 150

Founding Date: 1979

Publications: Newsletter (quarterly)

American Association of Cardiovascular and Pulmonary Rehabilitation

AACVPR

The AACVPR's mission is to reduce morbidity, mortality, and disability from cardiovascular and pulmonary diseases through education, prevention, rehabilitation, and aggressive disease management. Central to this mission is the improvement of the quality of life for patients and their families.

7600 Terrace Ave., ste.203

Middleton, WI 53562

UNITED STATES OF AMERICA

Telephone: (608) 831-6989

Fax: (608) 831-5122

E-mail: aacvpr@tmahq.com

Web site: www.aacvpr.org

Name of Contact Person: Susan M. Rees, MS

Title of Contact Person: Executive Director

Membership: 3,000

Founding Date: 1985

Publications: Publications related to pulmonary and cardiac rehabilitation. *Journal of Cardiopulmonary Rehabilitation* (bimonthly); *News and Views of AACVPR* (quarterly newsletter); *Media Resource Guide; Outcome Tools Resource Guide Recovering From Heart Problems Through Cardiac Rehabilitation: Consumer Guidelines*

American Chiropractic Association Council on Sports Injuries and Physical Fitness

The council's mission is to advance chiropractic principles and education with practical applications of chiropractic sports medicine and exercise science to enhance athletic performance and promote physical fitness.

ACA Sports Council

2444 Solomons Island Rd., #218

Annapolis, MD 21401

UNITED STATES OF AMERICA

Telephone: (410) 266-8285 / (800) 593-3222

Web site: www.cais.net

Name of Contact Person: Francis M. Czajka

Title of Contact Person: Executive Director

American College of Sports Medicine

The ACSM's mission is to promote and integrate scientific research, education, and practical applications of sports medicine and exercise science to maintain and enhance physical performance, fitness, health, and quality of life. The ACSM certifies fitness leaders, fitness instructors, exercise test technologists, exercise specialists, health/fitness program directors, and U.S. military fitness personnel and grants continuing medical education (CME) and continuing education credits (CEC).

ACSM

PO Box 1440

Indianapolis, IN 46206-1440

UNITED STATES OF AMERICA

Telephone: (317) 637-9200

Fax: (317) 634-7817

Web site: www.acsm.org

Name of Contact Person: James R. Whitehead

Title of Contact Person: Executive Vice President

Membership: 17,500

Founding Date: 1954

Publications: *ACSM Fitness Book; ACSM's Guidelines for Exercise Testing and Prescription; ACSM's Health/Fitness Facility Standards and Guidelines; ACSM's Resource Manual for Guidelines for Exercise Testing and Prescription; American College of Sports Medicine Directory of Graduate Programs in Sports Medicine and Exercise Science* (annual); *American College of Sports Medicine Guidelines for the Team Physician Exercise and Sport Sciences Reviews* (annual); *Medicine and Science in Sports and Exercise* (monthly journal); *Medicine and Science in Sports and Exercise Cumulative Index Sports Medicine Bulletin* (quarterly magazine)

American Kinesiotherapy Association

The AKTA's mission is to promote kinesiotherapy by improving recognition of the profession through the pursuit of legislation and public relations. The AKTA will serve the interest of its members and will represent the profession to the public as well as work to enhance the standard of care provided by kinesiotherapists through educational opportunities.

AKTA

1 IBM Plaza, Ste. 2500

Chicago, IL 60611-7617

(continued on next page)

(AKTA, continued)

UNITED STATES OF AMERICA

Telephone: 800-296-AKTA

Web site: www.akta.org

Name of Contact Person: Lisa V. Hedrick

Title of Contact Person: Admin. Officer

E-mail: lhedrick@aapmr.org

Membership: 450

Founding Date: 1946

Publications: *Career in Kinesiology, Clinical Kinesiology* (quarterly journal); *Mobility* (quarterly newsletter)

American Medical Athletic Association (previously known as the American Medical Joggers Association)

AMAA/AMJA

To educate and motivate fellow physicians to disseminate information about exercise and nutrition to their patients, thereby enhancing the quality of life.

4405 East West Hwy., Ste. 405

Bethesda, MD 20814

UNITED STATES OF AMERICA

Telephone: (301) 913-9517 / (800)-776-2732

Fax: (301) 913-9520

E-mail: amaasportsmed@aol.com

Web site: www.americanrunning.org/

Name of Contact Person: Susan Kalish

Title of Contact Person: Executive Director

Membership: 2,000

Founding Date: 1969

Publications: *AMAA Newsletter* (quarterly)

American Medical Equestrian Association

AMEA

The AMEA is dedicated to the philosophy, principles, and application of safety of people in equestrian activities. This purpose is achieved through education, research, and resource:

- Education of health care professionals, organizational representatives and individuals, including an emphasis on public awareness
- Research to better define injury patterns and risks, efficacy of safety measures and equipment, and assistance in equipment design
- A resource of experience and expertise to be shared and utilized for the benefit of equestrian safety

103 Surrey Rd.

Waynesville, NC 28786

UNITED STATES OF AMERICA

Telephone: 800-399-0138

Fax: 903-509-2474

E-mail: ammedeqassn@bigfoot.com

Web site: www.law.utexas.edu/dawson

Name of Contact Person: LaJuan Skiver

Title of Contact Person: Executive Director

Contact Address: 5318 Old Bullard Road

Tyler, TX 75708-3612

UNITED STATES OF AMERICA

Membership: 100

Founding Date: 1990

Publications: *AMEA News* (quarterly newsletter); *Planning Event Coverage* (booklet); *When Can My Child Ride a Horse?* (brochure)

American Medical Soccer Association

AMSA

350 Cheshire Dr.

Birmingham, AL 35242-3100

UNITED STATES OF AMERICA

Telephone: (205) 991-6054

Name of Contact Person: Robert M. Cosby, MD

Title of Contact Person: President

American Medical Society for Sports Medicine

AMSSM

The AMSSM's purpose is to foster a collegial relationship among dedicated and competent primary care sports medicine physicians and to provide a quality educational resource for AMSSM members, other sports medicine professionals, and the general public.

11639 Earnshaw

Overland Park, KS 66210

UNITED STATES OF AMERICA

Telephone: 913-327-1415

Fax: 913-327-1415

E-mail: amssm@swbell.net

Web site: www.sportsmed.upmc.edu/~amssm/index.html

Founding Date: 1991

American Medical Tennis Association

AMTA

The AMTA is a nonprofit educational organization whose purpose is to provide Continuing Medical Education (CME) programs for physicians. A nonelimination tennis tournament for physicians and spouses complements the scientific program.

7736 Wynlakes Blvd

Montgomery, Alabama 36117

UNITED STATES OF AMERICA

Telephone: (800) 326-2682 / (334) 273-7983

Fax: (770) 479-3382

E-mail: tatread@mdtennis.org

Web site: www.mdtennis.org

Name of Contact Person: Sheryl Treadwell

Title of Contact Person: Executive Director

Contact Address: 7736 Wynlakes Blvd.

Montgomery, AL 36117

UNITED STATES OF AMERICA

Telephone: (800) 326-2682

Fax: (334) 273-7983

Membership: 3,000

Founding Date: 1967

Publications: *AMTA Newsletter* (quarterly); Official directory (annual)

American Orthopedic Rugby Football Association, The

AORFA

The AORFA's mission is to create an awareness of the orthopedic and medical aspects of rugby and promote competitive rugby in North America. AORFA wants to make rugby safer without changing the spirit of the game and believes that this can be accomplished through research, education, and medical coverage and resources for individuals and teams.

PO Box 539

Washington Crossing, PA 18977

UNITED STATES OF AMERICA

Telephone: (215) 493-0743

E-mail: infoAORFA@aol.com

Web site: www.sechrest.com/ortho/aorfa

Name of Contact Person: Merrick J. Wetzler, MD

Title of Contact Person: President

E-mail: MJWETZ@aol.com

American Orthopaedic Society for Sports Medicine, The

AOSSM

The objectives of the AOSSM are the following:

- To provide orthopaedic surgeons with special training in sport-related medical and surgical techniques
- To offer education and research programs that benefit athletes and persons concerned with physical fitness

(continued on next page)

(AOSSM, continued)

- To support scientific research in sports medicine
- To develop methods for safer, more productive, and enjoyable fitness programs
- To publish educational materials for medical professionals as well as for professional and amateur athletes
- To promote education and research in the prevention, recognition, treatment, and rehabilitation of sport injuries.

6300 N. River Rd., Ste. 200

Rosemont, IL 60018

UNITED STATES OF AMERICA

Telephone: (847) 292-4900 / (877) 321-3500

Fax: (847) 292-4905

E-mail: aossm@aossm.org

Web site: www.sportsmed.org

Name of Contact Person: Krista Blazek Hogarth

Title of Contact Person: Director of Communications

Membership: 1,500

Founding Date: 1972

Publications: *American Journal of Sports Medicine* (bimonthly); *Sports Medicine Update*

American Osteopathic Academy of Sports Medicine

AOASM

The AOASM's objectives are to promote education, development of high ethical standards, communication, and research in the field of sports medicine. The AOASM conducts study programs, lectures, forums, and seminars; encourages publication of articles and dissertations in scientific and professional journals; sponsors student academy organizations at osteopathic education institutions; and maintains a speakers' bureau. The AOASM is a specialty affiliate of the American Osteopathic Association (AOA), which is organized to advance the philosophy and practice of osteopathic medicine by promoting excellence in education, research, and the delivery of quality, cost-effective health care in a distinct, unified profession.

7611 Elmwood Ave., Ste. 201

Middleton, WI 53562

UNITED STATES OF AMERICA

Telephone: (608) 831-4400

Fax: (608) 831-5122

E-mail: aoasm@tmahq.com

Web site: www.am-osteo-assn.org

Name of Contact Person: Sheila Endicott

Title of Contact Person: Executive Director

Membership: 700

Founding Date: 1975

Publications: *Sport Medicine Today* (quarterly newsletter)

American Osteopathic Orthopedic Society for Sports Medicine

AOOSSM

RD 3

Clarion, PA 16214

UNITED STATES OF AMERICA

Web site: www.doitsports.com/epc/exersci/orgs.html

Name of Contact Person: Robert Armstrong

Association for Equine Sports Medicine

AESM

The AESM works to improve the health of horses competing in athletic events; disseminates information on current research in equine medicine, physiology, and biomechanics; and offers wet lab training.

3579 E. Foothill Blvd., No. 288

Pasadena, CA 91107

UNITED STATES OF AMERICA

Telephone: (909) 869-4859

Fax: (909) 869-6788

E-mail: aesm@relaypoint.net

Web site: www.aesm.org

Name of Contact Person: Holly M. Greene, MS

Title of Contact Person: Executive Director

Membership: 260

Founding Date: 1982

Publications: *Quarterly Issues of the World Equine Veterinary Review Proceedings of Annual Conference*

Association of Major League Baseball Team Physicians

To improve the medical and surgical care of baseball players and to promote the health and welfare of baseball personnel.

E-mail: straw@probaseballteamdoctors.com

Web site: www.probaseballteamdoctors.com

Name of Contact Person: William E. Straw, MD

Contact Address: 370 Distel Circle

Los Altos, CA 94022

UNITED STATES OF AMERICA

Telephone: 650-254-5225

E-mail: wes@straws.com

Association of Professional Baseball Physicians

APBP

The APBP's aim is to provide the best possible medical care to all players and associated personnel.

c/o L.J. Michienzi, MD, PhD

1661 St. Anthony Ave.

St. Paul, MN 55104

UNITED STATES OF AMERICA

Telephone: (651) 646-0491

Fax: (651) 646-0205

Membership: 36

Founding Date: 1970

Association of Volleyball Medical Doctors

AVMD

PO Box 4990

Chicago, IL 60680

UNITED STATES OF AMERICA

Telephone: (708) 210-3112

E-mail: avmd1@aol.com

Web site: www.avmd.org

Name of Contact Person: T. Eric Yokoo, MD, MM

Title of Contact Person: President

Telephone: (310) 318-6500

Publications: Newsletter (periodic)

Association of Volleyball Physicians

1229 N. North Branch, Ste. 122

Chicago, IL 60622

UNITED STATES OF AMERICA

Telephone: (708) 210-3112

International Society for Sport Psychiatry

ISSP

316 North Milwaukee Street

Suite 318

Milwaukee, Wisconsin 53202

UNITED STATES OF AMERICA

Telephone: (414) 271-2900

Name of Contact Person: Daniel Begel, M.D.

Title of Contact Person: President

International Society of Arthroscopy, Knee Surgery, and Orthopedic Sports Medicine

145 Town and Country Drive, Suite 106

Danville, CA 94526-3963

UNITED STATES OF AMERICA

Telephone: (925) 314-7920

(continued on next page)

(International Society of Arthroscopy, Knee Surgery, and Orthopedic Sports Medicine, continued)

Fax: (925) 314-7922

E-mail: isakos@isakos.com

Web site: www.isakoas.com

Name of Contact Person: Cathryn Grady

Title of Contact Person: Society Manager

Contact Address: 6300 River Rd.

Suite 727

Rosemont, IL 60018-1632

UNITED STATES OF AMERICA

Telephone: (847) 698-1632

Fax: (847) 823-0536

Founding Date: 1978

Publications: *The Journal of Arthroscopic and Related Surgery*

National Athletic Trainers Association

The NATA's mission is to enhance the quality of health care for athletes and those engaged in physical activity and to advance the profession of athletic training through education and research in the prevention, evaluation, management, and rehabilitation of injuries.

2952 Stemmons Fwy., Ste. 200

Dallas, TX 75247-6196

UNITED STATES OF AMERICA

Telephone: (214) 637-6282 / (800) 879-6282

Fax: (214) 637-2206

E-mail: webdude@nata.org

Web site: www.nata.org

Name of Contact Person: Eve Becker-Doyle, CAE

Title of Contact Person: Executive Director

E-mail: ebd@nata.org

Membership: 26,000

Founding Date: 1950

Publications: *Journal of Athletic Training* (quarterly); *Minimizing the Risk of Injury in High School Athletes; What is an Athletic Trainer; Code of Ethics; About the NATA; NATA News* (monthly)

North American Society for Pediatric Exercise Medicine

NASPEM

NASPEM's mission is to promote exercise science, physical activity, and fitness in the health and medical care of children and adolescents.

Web site: www.naspem.org

Name of Contact Person: Stephen Paridon, MD

Title of Contact Person: President

Contact Address: Cardiology Division

Children's Hospital of Philadelphia

34th. St. & Civic Center Blvd.

Philadelphia, PA 19104

UNITED STATES OF AMERICA

Telephone: 215-590-2226

Fax: 215-590-1411

E-mail: paridon@E-mail.CHOP.edu

Publications: Pediatric Exercise Science

URUGUAY

Sociedad Uruguaya de Medicina del Deporte (Uruguay Sports Medicine Society)

Achives 1432

A.P. 603, CP 11300

URUGUAY

Telephone: (5982) 7075976

Fax: (5982) 2039764

VENEZUELA

Sociedad Venezolana de Medicina Deportiva (Venezuela Sports Medicine Society)

Lagoven, Apartado 889
Caracas 1010-A
VENEZUELA
Telephone: (582) 606-8203
Fax: (582) 606-8204 / 606-8253

WEST INDIES

St. Vincent and the Grenadines Sports Medicine Association

c/o Dr. Perry De Freitas
Kingston General Hospital
St. Vincent and the Grenadines
WEST INDIES
Telephone: (1809) 456-1185

Trinidad and Tobago Sports Medicine Association

6 Albion St.
Port of Spain
Trinidad and Tobago
WEST INDIES
Telephone: (1868) 623-8864
E-mail: t&ali@carib.link.net

YUGOSLAVIA

Yugoslav Association of Sports Medicine

29, M. Gregoran
YU-11000 Belgrade
YUGOSLAVIA
Telephone: (38111) 648443
Fax: (38111) 753900

ZIMBABWE

Zimbabwe Sports Medicine Association

c/o Zimbabwe Olympic Committee
PO Box 4718
Harare
ZIMBABWE
Telephone: (263.4) 700746
Fax: (263.4) 795796
E-mail: tags@msasa.samara.co.zw

5

International Sports Federations

Archery

International Archery Federation

FITA

Medical Committee, Chair: Mr. Karol Hibner

Avenue de cour 135

CH-1007 Lausanne

SWITZERLAND

Telephone: (41) 21 61 43 050

Fax: (41) 21 61 43 055

E-mail: fita@worldcom.ch

Web site: www.worldsport.com

Name of Contact Person: James Easton

Title of Contact Person: President, 1997-2001

E-mail: jeaston@esimail.eastonsports.com

Membership: 124 affiliated national federations

Founding Date: 1931

Athletics (Track and Field)

International Amateur Athletic Federation

IAAF

Medical Committee, Chair: Prof. Arne Ljungqvist

17, rue Princesse Florestine

BP 359

MC-98007 Monte-Carlo

PRINCIPALITY OF MONACO

Telephone: (377) 93 10 88 88

Fax: (377) 93 15 95 15

Web site: www.iaaf.org

Name of Contact Person: Diack Lamine

Title of Contact Person: President

Founding Date: 1912

International Biathlon Union

IBU

Medical Committee, Chair: Dr. Jurgen Haberstroh

Airport Center

Postfach 1

Kasernenstrasse 1

A-5073 Wals Himmelreich

AUSTRIA

Telephone: (43.662) 85 50 50

Fax: (43.662) 85 50 508

E-mail: biathlon@ibu.at

Web site: www.ibu.at

Name of Contact Person: Mr. Anders Besseberg

Title of Contact Person: President

Bessebergveien

N-3320 Vestfossen

NORWAY

Telephone: +00 47 32 75 81 34

Fax: +00 47 +32 75 83 83

E-mail: an-bes@online.no

Membership: 59 affiliated national federations

Founding Date: 1993

International Triathlon Union

ITU

Doping Control Commission, Chair: Dr. Mark Sisson

1154 West 24th St.

North Vancouver BC V7P 2J2

CANADA

Telephone: (1.604) 926 72 50

Fax: (1.604) 608 31 95

E-mail: ituhdq@home.com

Web site: www.worldsport.com

Name of Contact Person: Les McDonald

Title of Contact Person: President

1154 West 24th St.

North Vancouver BC V7P 2J2

CANADA

Telephone: (1.604) 926 72 50

Fax: (1.604) 926 72 60

E-mail: ituhdq@home.com

Membership: 123 affiliated national federations

Founding Date: 1989

Union Internationale de Pentathlon Moderne

Stade Louis II-Entrée E

13, Avenue des Castelans

MC-98000 Monaco

MONACO

Telephone: +377 9777 8555

Fax: +377 9777 8550

Web site: www.pentathlon.org

Name of Contact Person: Schormann Klaus

Title of Contact Person: President

Membership: 94 affiliated national federations

Founding Date: 1948

Badminton

International Badminton Federation

IBF

Medical Commission

4, Manor Park Place

Rutherford Way

Cheltenham

GL51 9TU

ENGLAND

Telephone: (44.1242) 23 49 04

Fax: (44.1242) 22 10 30

E-mail: info@intbadfed.org

Web site: www.intbadfed.org (or) www.worldsport.com

Name of Contact Person: Neil Cameron

Title of Contact Person: Executive Director

9 Tiyukuan Rd.

100763 Beijing

CHINA

Telephone: +86 10 6842 0395

Fax: +86 10 6842 5960

E-mail: lshr@public3.bta.bet.cn

Membership: 145 member associations

Founding Date: 1934

Publications: *World Badminton Magazine* (online); *Physical Training for Badminton IBF Statute Book* (annually); *Drug Testing Information* (video)

Baseball

International Baseball Federation

IBAF

Medical Commission, Chair: Gianfranco Beltrami

The International Baseball Federation is the International Governing Body for the Olympic Sport of Baseball which is in charge of all Baseball activities in their various categories in all the countries of the world which accept it statutes, rules, and regulations.

Avenue de Mon-Repos 24

CP 131

CH-1000 Lausanne 5

SWITZERLAND

Telephone: (41.21) 318 82 40

Fax: (41.21) 318 82 41

E-mail: iba@baseball.ch

Web site: www.baseball.ch

Name of Contact Person: Mr. Miquel Ortin

Title of Contact Person: Executive Director

E-mail: Press.ibaf@baseball.ch

Membership: 109 affiliated national federations

Founding Date: 1938

Publications: *I.B.A.F World Baseball Magazine; I.B.A.F News*

Basketball

International Basketball Federation

FIBA

To promote basketball worldwide.

Medical Council, President: Dr. Jacques Huguet

Boschetsrieder Str. 67

81379 Munich

GERMANY

Telephone: (49.89) 74 81 58 0

Fax: (49.89) 74 81 58 33

E-mail: secretariat@office.fiba.com

Web site: www.fiba.com

Name of Contact Person: Borislav Stankovic

Title of Contact Person: Secretary General

PO Box 700607

81306 Munich

GERMANY

Membership: 208 affiliated national federations

Founding Date: 1932

Publications: *Official Basketball Rules and Referee's Manual; General By-Laws; European Regulations, FIBA Bulletin, FIBA World Directory, European Directory, Basketball for Everyone; FIBA Media Guide; The Basketball World; FIBA Basketball Results (1932-1993); From Minibasket to Basketball; 100 Years of Basketball; 60 Years of Basketball Rules; Guide to Basketball Facilities; Guide to Small Basketball Facilities; A Concise Dictionary of American Basketball*

Billiards

World Confederation of Billiards Sports

WCBS

Meidoorn 133 6226 WH Maastricht

NETHERLANDS

Telephone: 31 43 362 6011 / 362 6380

Fax: 31 43 362 7095

E-mail: jean.graus@worldonline.nl

Web site: www.worldsport.com

Name of Contact Person: Sindhu Pulsirivong

Title of Contact Person: President

SPC-Building

1 Soi Chaemchan

Sukhumvit 55

Bangkok 10110

THAILAND

Telephone: 66-2-3817223 / 4682398

Fax: 66-2-3810850 / 3810857

Membership: 97 affiliated national federations

Founding Date: 1992

Bobsleigh

International Bobsleigh and Tobogganing Federation

FIBT

Medical Committee, President: Giorgio Santjlli

Via Piranesi 44B

I-20137 Milan MI

ITALY

Telephone: (39.0) + 02-757 3319

Fax: (39.02) 757 33 84

E-mail: egarde@tin.it

Web site: www.bobsleigh.com

Name of Contact Person: Robert H. Storey

Title of Contact Person: President, 1998-2002

1941 Castlewood

Ottawa ON K2A 2Z6

CANADA

Telephone: (+1.613) 722-7847

Fax: (+1.613) 722-7160

E-mail: storeyco@magi.com

Membership: 54 affiliated national federations

Founding Date: 1923

Body Building

International Federation of Body Builders

IFBB

Medical Commission, Chair: Dr. Bob Goldman

The IFBB's objectives are the following:

1. To develop, promote, and control the sport of bodybuilding and fitness on an international scale
2. To promote an interest in and a dedication to better health and fitness through physical culture, proper nutrition, and weight training
3. To develop and strengthen friendship and cooperation among the members of the IFBB
4. To supervise the activities of the national federations
5. To legislate rules for the sport of bodybuilding and fitness
6. To sanction, regulate, and control all international bodybuilding and fitness competitions, including both amateur and professional events
7. To implement doping control programs at designated IFBB-sanctioned

competitions and to ensure that such programs are carried out by the national federations

8. To conduct research into the benefits of bodybuilding and fitness as it relates to physical conditioning, both as a basis towards reaching peak athletic performance in sport and to improve the general health of the population at large

9. To conduct training programs for athletes, coaches, judges, and other officials

10. To distribute research information on physical culture, nutrition, and weight training to its members and other interested individuals and organizations

11. To act as the official international representative of the sport of bodybuilding and fitness at all international sports federation meetings and events

12. To collaborate with the International Olympic Committee, the General Association of International Sports Federations, and other organizations having as their purpose the promotion of sport on an international scale

13. To qualify judges in both international amateur and professional divisions

2875 Bates Rd.

Montreal PQ H3S 1B7

CANADA

Telephone: (514) 731-3783

Fax: (514) 731-7082

E-mail: ifbb@weider.ca

Web site: www.ifbb.commain.html

Name of Contact Person: Ben Weider

Title of Contact Person: President

E-mail: bweider@ifbb.com

Membership: 169 affiliated national federations

Founding Date: 1946

Publications: *Congress Report* (annual); *Flex* (monthly magazine); *Scientific Athlete Reports* (periodic)

International Powerlifting Federation

IPF

Medical Committee, Chair: Richard Herrick

Amselweg 3

D-64572 Klein Gerau

GERMANY

Telephone: 43-13699981

Fax: 43-13173136

Web site: www.worldsport.com

Name of Contact Person: Norbert Wallauch

Title of Contact Person: President

Krottenbachstrasse 16

A-1190 Wien

AUSTRIA

Telephone: +43-13699981

Fax: 0043-13173136

Membership: 95 member federations

Publications: *IPF Newsletter* (published as needed)

International Weightlifting Federation

IWF

Medical Committee, President: Dr. Juan Marcos Becerro

Budapest

Hold U. 1

Pf. 614

H-1374

HUNGARY

Telephone: (36.1) 353 05 30

Fax: (36.1) 353 01 99

E-mail: iwf@iwf.net

Web site: www.iwf.net

Name of Contact Person: Tamas Ajan

(continued on next page)

(IWF, continued)

Title of Contact Person: General Secretary

E-mail: g.schoedl@online.edvg.cb.at

Membership: 167 affiliated national federations

Founding Date: 1905

Publications: *IWF Handbook; Medals and World Records in Weightlifting; The Lost Past; Weightlifting—Fitness for All Sports; IWF Coaching-Refereeing-Medical Symposium; 1989, 1993, 1997, From Alexeev to Zubricky: 100 Years' Weightlifting Medals 1891-1991; Guidebook for Weightlifting Referees; IWF Medical Handbook*

Boules

Confédération Mondiale des Sports de Boules

Boules is a French ball game, similar to bowls or boccie.

CSMB

The CSMB is essentially an umbrella organization that unites the three international federations governing the sport of boules: the International Boules Federation, the International Federation of Pétanque and le Jeu Provençal, and the International Confederation of Boules Players.

Club Bouliste du Rocher

Avenue des Pins

MC-98000 Monaco

PRINCIPALITY OF MONACO

Telephone: 33/(0) 4 92 52 43 01

Fax: 33/(0) 4 92 52 43 02

E-mail: cmsb@alpes-net.fr

Web site: www.worldsport.com

Name of Contact Person: Alphonse Lagier-Bruno

Title of Contact Person: President

Celle Du President, Square

Aritide Briand, 05000

Gap

FRANCE

Membership: 73 affiliated national federations

Founding Date: 1985

Bowling

Fédération Internationale des Quilleurs (International Bowling Federation)

FIQ

1631 Mesa Ave., Ste. A

Colorado Springs, CO 80906

UNITED STATES OF AMERICA

Telephone: (719) 636-2695

Fax: (719) 636-3300

E-mail: bowling@fiq.org

Web site: www.fig.org

Name of Contact Person: Gerald L. Koenig

Title of Contact Person: President

Membership: 120 affiliated national federations

Founding Date: 1952

Boxing

International Amateur Boxing Association

AIBA

Medical Commission, Chair: Dr. Peter Jaco

PO Box 76343

Atlanta, GA 30358

UNITED STATES OF AMERICA

Telephone: (770) 455-8350

Fax: (770) 454-6467

Web site: www.aiba.net

Name of Contact Person: Loring Baker

Title of Contact Person: General Secretary

E-mail: lbaker27@mindspring.com

Membership: 190 affiliated national federations

Founding Date: 1946

Canoeing

International Canoe Federation

ICF

Medical Committee, Chair: Jan Verstuyft

Budapest

Dózsa György út. 1-3

H-1143

HUNGARY

Telephone: (36.1) 363 48 32

Fax: (36.1) 221 41 30

Web site: www.worldsport.com

Name of Contact Person: Ulrich Feldhoff

Title of Contact Person: President

Bertaallee 8

D-47055 Duisburg

GERMANY

Telephone: +49 203 7200 197

Fax: +49 203 7200 205

E-mail: service@kanu.de

Membership: 108 affiliated national federations

Founding Date: 1924

Casting

International Casting Federation

ICF

The ICF is dedicated to the promotion of the sport of casting. The federation sanctions world championships and international competitions in bait, fly, and surf casting; promotes the standardization of rules and methods of casting, scoring, and judging; and compiles statistics on national and world records.

c/o Secretary General Mr. Ulf Persson

Rinnbovägen 19

S-244 33 Kävlinge

SWEDEN

Telephone: 46 46 735645

Fax: 46 46 735645

E-mail: upersson@casting.worldsport.org

Web site: www.worldsport.com/worldsport/sports/casting/home.html

Name of Contact Person: Ulf Janson

Title of Contact Person: President

GrevTuregatan 78nb

S-114 38 Stockholm

SWEDEN

Telephone: 46 8 662 31 06

Fax: 46 8 662 31 06

E-mail: ujanson@casting.worldsport.org

Membership: 35 affiliated federations

Founding Date: 1957

Publications: Newsletter

Curling

World Curling Federation

WCF

74 Tay St.

Perth PHZ 8NN

SCOTLAND

Telephone: (44 173) 8 451630

Fax: (44 173) 8 451641

E-mail: Wcf@dial.pipex.net

Web site: www.worldsport.com

Name of Contact Person: Mike Thomson

Title of Contact Person: Secretary

c/o Waltham Group

(continued on next page)

(WCF, continued)

Rosenheimer Strasse 143a

D-81671 Munich

GERMANY

Membership: 35 affiliated national federations

Founding Date: 1966

Cycling

International Cycling Union

ICU

The UCI's mission is to develop and promote all aspects of cycling without discrimination of any kind, in close cooperation with national federations and major associates.

Rte de Chavannes 37

CH-1007 Lausanne

SWITZERLAND

Telephone: (41.21) 622 05 80

Fax: (41.21) 622 05 88

Web site: www.uci.ch

Name of Contact Person: Hein Verbruggen

Title of Contact Person: President

Founding Date: 1900

Dance

International Dance Sport Federation

IDSF

The IDSF's aims are to promote DanceSport internationally and to work for further acceptance by the IOC; to enhance the sporting appearance of DanceSport and make it attractive to a worldwide television audience; to protect and develop our cooperation with IMG, our joint-venture marketing partner; to provide standardized rules to which all international competitions organized by its members are subject; and to advise and assist its members with their work in their own countries.

Avenue Mon-Repos 24

CP 83

CH-1000 Lausanne 5

SWITZERLAND

Telephone: (41.21) 310 47 47

Fax: (41.21) 310 47 60

E-mail: chfenn@t-online.de

Web site: www.idfs.net

Name of Contact Person: Rudolf Baumann

Title of Contact Person: President

Im Hungerbuel 22

CH-8614 Bertschikon

SWITZERLAND

Telephone: (:.41) 1-935 19 73

Fax: (..41) 1-936 19 73

E-mail: rudolfbaumann@compuserve.com

Membership: 76

Founding Date: 1957

Publications: *The International News* (magazine)

Equestrian

International Equestrian Federation

FEI

The FEI's primary mission is to advance the orderly growth of equestrian sport worldwide by promoting, regulating, and administering humane and sportsmanlike international competition in the traditional equestrian discipline and by helping them to evolve in ways that enhance their attractiveness both for the participants and the public, while respecting and furthering the ideals and principles of horsemanship.

Medical Committee, Chair: Dr. Roland Devolz

Avenue Mon-Repos 24

CP 157

CH-1000 Lausanne 5

SWITZERLAND

Telephone: (41.21) 312 56 56

Fax: (41.21) 312 86 77

E-mail: info@horsesport.org

Web site: www.horsesport.org

Name of Contact Person: Bo Helander

Title of Contact Person: General Secretary

Membership: 125 affiliated national federations

Founding Date: 1921

Publications: *The FEI Bulletin* (9 to 10 per year, in English and French)

Federation of International Polo

FIP

FIP is the leading international polo federation that organizes international tournaments worldwide for professionals, amateurs, and children while actively promoting the sport of polo throughout the world.

9663 Santa Monica Blvd.

PMB 848

Beverly Hills, CA 90210

UNITED STATES OF AMERICA

Telephone: (310) 472-4312

Fax: (310) 472-5220

E-mail: info@fippolo.com

Web site: www.fippolo.com

Name of Contact Person: Glen Holden

Title of Contact Person: President

9663 Santa Monica Blvd.

PMB 848

Beverly Hills, CA 90210

UNITED STATES OF AMERICA

Telephone: (310) 472-4312

Fax: (310) 472-5220

E-mail: fippolo@aol.com

Membership: 41 affiliated national federations

Founding Date: 1985

Publications: Newsletter

Faustball

International Faustball-Verband

IFV

Heltorfer Mark 134

D-40489 Dusseldorf

GERMANY

Telephone: 00 49 02 03 74 19 57

Fax: 00 49 02 11 61 88 131

E-mail: wjapp@vdi-nachrichten.com

Web site: www.worldsport.com

Name of Contact Person: Ernesto Dohnalek

Title of Contact Person: President

Wiedstr.12

D-41540 Dormagen

GERMANY

Telephone: 02133 / 62254

Fax: 02133 / 60584

Membership: 14 affiliated national federations

Fencing

Federation Internationale d'Escrime

FIE

Avenue Mon-Repos 24

CP 128

CH-1000 Lausanne 5

SWITZERLAND

Telephone: +41 21 320 31 15

Fax: +41 21 320 31 16

(continued on next page)

(FIE, continued)

E-mail: contact@fie.ch

Web site: www.fie.ch

Name of Contact Person: Rene Rock

Title of Contact Person: President

Membership: 99 affiliated national federations

Founding Date: 1913

Flying Disc

World Flying Disc Federation

WFDF

200 Linden

Fort Collins, CO 80524

UNITED STATES OF AMERICA

Web site: www.wfdf.org (or) www.worldsport.com

Name of Contact Person: Bill Wright

Title of Contact Person: President

Telephone: (970) 484-6932

Fax: (970) 490-2714

E-mail: bwright@wrightlife.com

Football (Soccer)

Fédération Internationale de Football Association (International Federation of Association Football)

FIFA

Sports Medicine Society, Dr. Michael D'Hooghe

Hitzigweg 11

CP 85

CH-8030 Zurich

SWITZERLAND

Telephone: (41.1) 384 95 95

Fax: (41.1) 384 96 96

Web site: www.fifa2.com

Name of Contact Person: Joseph Blatter

Title of Contact Person: President, 1998-2002

Membership: 203 affiliated national federations

Founding Date: 1904

Publications: *FIFA News* (monthly); *FIFA Magazine* (bimonthly, in English, French, Spanish and German); *FIFA Handbook* (yearly)

Golf

World Amateur Golf Council

To encourage the International development of golf and to foster friendship and sportsmanship among the peoples of the world through the conduct biennially of Amateur Team Championships for the Eisenhower Trophy and the Espirito Santo Trophy. To promote golf as an Olympic sport and to act as the Federation for golf in the Olympic Games.

Golf House

PO Box 708

Far Hills, NJ 07931-0708

UNITED STATES OF AMERICA

Telephone: (908) 234-2300

Fax: (908) 234-2178

E-mail: sparel@usga.org

Web site: www.wagc.org

Name of Contact Person: David B. Fay

Title of Contact Person: Co-Secretary

Membership: 77 affiliated national federations

Founding Date: 1958

Gymnastics

Fédération Internationale de Trampoline (International Trampoline Federation)

FIT
Medical Commission
Rue des Oeuches 10
CP 359
CH-2740 Moutier 1
SWITZERLAND
Telephone: 41 32 494 64 15
Fax: 41 32 494 64 19
E-mail: figymps@bluewin.ch
Name of Contact Person: Ronald Froehlich
Title of Contact Person: President
Membership: 46 affiliated national federations
Founding Date: 1964

International Federation of Sports Acrobatics

IFSA
75, Blvd. Vassil Levski
BG-1040, Sofia
BULGARIA
Telephone: 359 2 86 54 83
Fax: 359 2 980 09 13
Web site: www.worldsport.comworldsport/sports/sports_acrobatics/home.html
Name of Contact Person: Lily Dimitrova
Title of Contact Person: Administrative Secretary
Founding Date: 1973

International Gymnastics Federation

FIG
Rue des Oeuches 10
CP 359
2740 Moutier 1
SWITZERLAND
Telephone: (41.32) 494 6410
Fax: (41.32) 494 6419
E-mail: gymnastics@fig.worldsport.org
Web site: www. worldsport.com
Name of Contact Person: M. Bruno Grandi
Title of Contact Person: President
Viale Tiziano 74
I-00196 Roma
ITALY
Telephone: 39.06.3685.81.79
Fax: 39.06.36.85.82.92
E-mail: fig.president@flashnet.it
Membership: 122 affiliated national federations
Founding Date: 1881
Publications: *World of Gymnastics* (magazine); *FIG Bulletin* (annually); *FIG Flash*

Handball

International Handball Federation

IHF
PO Box 302
CH-4052 Bâle
SWITZERLAND
Telephone: 41 61 2721300
Fax: 41 61 2721344
E-mail: ihf@ihf.ch
Web site: www. worldsport.com
Name of Contact Person: Frank Birkefeld
Title of Contact Person: Managing Director
Feldkellergasse 70
A-1130 Wien
AUSTRIA
Telephone: 43-1-804 99 65 or 43-1-504 64 37
Fax: 43-1-505 32 36

(continued on next page)

(IHF, continued)

E-mail: iip@aon.at

Membership: 142 affiliated national federations

Founding Date: 1946

Publication: *WHM—World Handball Magazine*

Federation Intervacional de Pelota Vasca (International Federation of Pelota Vasca)

Pelota Vasca developed from a form of handball.

FIPV

Medical Commission

Poblado Vasco de Urdanibia

Palacio de Urdanibia

Apdo. de Correos 468

E-20300 Irún

SPAIN

Telephone: 34 943 61 00 06

Fax: 34 943 61 00 44

E-mail: fipv@facilnet.es

Web site: www.worldsport.com

Name of Contact Person: Enrique Gaytán de Ayala

Title of Contact Person: President

Membership: 25 affiliated national federations

Founding Date: 1929

Hockey

International Bandy Federation

Bandy is a game similar to ice hockey, played on a larger rink.

IBF

Minstr Ditleffsr. 23

N-0862

Oslo

NORWAY

Telephone: 47 2 2232290

Fax: 47 2 2232616

E-mail: bandy@bandy.worldsport.org

Web site: www.worldsport.com

Name of Contact Person: Anki Pettersson

Title of Contact Person: Assistant Secretary-General

c/o The Swedish Bandy Federation

Box 78

S-641 21 Katrineholm

SWEDEN

Telephone: -46-150-722 03

Fax: -46-150-722 01

Membership: 9 affiliated national federations

International Hockey Federation

FIH

Medical Committee, Chair: Dr. Kathleen Watson

Avenue des Arts 1

BP 5

B-1210 Bruxelles

BELGIUM

Telephone: (32.2) 219 45 37

Fax: (32.2) 219 27 61

E-mail: FIH@FIHockey.org

Web site: www.hockey.worldsport.com

Name of Contact Person: Juan Angel Calzado

Title of Contact Person: President

Membership: 120 affiliated national federations

Founding Date: 1924

International Ice Hockey Federation

IIHF

Medical Committee, Chair: Murray Costello

Parkring 11

CH-8002 Zürich

SWITZERLAND

Telephone: (+41.1) 289 86 00

Fax: (+41.1) 289 86 22

E-mail: iihf@iihf.com

Web site: www.iihf.com

Name of Contact Person: Jan –Ake Dvinsson

Title of Contact Person: General Secretary

Parkring 11

CH-8002 Zürich

SWITZERLAND

Telephone: +41 1 289 86 00

Fax: +41 1 289 86 20

Membership: 55 affiliated national federations

Founding Date: 1908

Ice Skating

International Skating Union

ISU

Medical Advisors Committee, Chair: Dr. Jane M. Moran

Chemin de Primerose 2

CH-1007 Lausanne

SWITZERLAND

Telephone: (41.21) 612 66 66

Fax: (41.21) 612 66 67

E-mail: info@isu.ch

Web site: www.isu.org (or) www.worldsport.com

Name of Contact Person: Fredi Schmid

Title of Contact Person: Secretary General

Via Cerva 30

I-20122 Milano MI

ITALY

Telephone: (+39) 02 760 244 36

Fax: (+39) 02 760 246 93

Membership: 72 affiliated national federations

Founding Date: 1892

Korfball

International Korfball Federation

IKF

Medical Committee, Chair: Mr. Leo Heere

PO Box 1000

3980 DA Bunnik

THE NETHERLANDS

Telephone: 31 30 656 63 54

Fax: 31 30 657 04 68

E-mail: office@ikf.worldsport.org (or) ikf.office@kss.nl

Web site: www.worldsport.com

Name of Contact Person: Bob de Die

Title of Contact Person: President

Laagveld 24

5707 GS Helmond

THE NETHERLANDS

Telephone: +31 492 599340

Fax: +31 492 599341

E-mail: bobdedie.korfball@worldsport.org

Membership: 34 affiliated national federations

Founding Date: 1933

Publications: *Updated History of the IKF and the World Championships; Updated History of the IKF and the World Games*

Luge

International Luge Federation

FIL

Rathausplatz 9

D-83471 Berchtesgaden

GERMANY

Telephone: (49.8652) 669 60

Fax: (49.8652) 669 69

E-mail: office@fil-luge.org

(continued on next page)

(FIL, continued)

Web site: www.fil-luge.org
Name of Contact Person: Josef Fendt
Title of Contact Person: President
Kirchplatz Gern 2
D-83471 Berchtesgaden
GERMANY
Membership: 41 affiliated national federations
Founding Date: 1957

Martial Arts

International Aikido Federation

IAF
c/o Aikikai Foundation
17-18 Wakamatsu-cho
Shinjuku-ku
Tokyo 162
JAPAN
Telephone: 81-3-3203-9236
Fax: 81-3-3204-8145
E-mail: aikido@aikikai.or.jp
Web site: www.aikido-international.org
Name of Contact Person: Dr. Peter A. Goldsbury
Title of Contact Person: IAF
3-29 Ushita Honmachi 4-chome Higashi-ku
Hiroshima 732-0066
JAPAN
Telephone: + 81-82-211-1271
Fax: + 81-82-211-1955
E-mail: chairman@aikido-international.org
Membership: The IAF consists of 42 national organizations for aikido around the world.
Founding Date: 1976

International Judo Federation

IJF
33rd FL Doosan Tower
18-12, Ulchi-Ro, 6-Ka
Chung-Ku
Seoul 100-730
KOREA
Telephone: (82.2) 3398 10 17
Fax: (82.2) 3398 10 20
E-mail: yspark@ifj.org
Web site: www.ijf.org
Name of Contact Person: Yong Sung Park
Title of Contact Person: President
Membership: 182 affiliated national federations
Founding Date: 1951

International Wushu Federation

3, Anding Rd.
Chaoyang District
100101 Beijing
CHINA
Telephone: (86.10) 649 121 53 / 649 122 33 ext. 413
Fax: (86.10) 649 121 51
E-mail: iwuf@wushu.com.cn
Web site: www.wushu.com
Name of Contact Person: Wu Shaozu
Title of Contact Person: President
Membership: 77 affiliated national federations
Founding Date: 1990

Ju-Jitsu International Federation

JJIF
Vesterbrogade 173, Frederikberg
C DK-1800
DENMARK
Telephone: +45 33 23 13 13
Fax: +45 33 24 01 13
Web site: www.worldsport.com

Name of Contact Person: Rinaldo Orlandi

Title of Contact Person: President

Via Bellini 40

Monza

I-20052 Milano MI

ITALY

Telephone: +39 039 23 00 381

Fax: +39 093 23 00 381

Membership: 63 affiliated national federations

World Karate Federation

WKF

Medical Committee

WKF Headquarters

149 Vizantiou St

GR-142 35 Athens

GREECE

Telephone: 30 1 2717564

Fax: 30 1 2717563

E-mail: karate@ath.forthnet.gr (or) espinos@wkf.net

Web site: www.wkf.net

Name of Contact Person: George Yerolimpos

Title of Contact Person: General Secretary

Membership: 150 affliated national federations

Founding Date: 1992

Publications: Newsletter

World Karate Federation

WKF

Medical Committee, Dr. Rafael Arriaza

c/o Spanish Karate Federation

Princesa 22.4° Izqda

E-28008 Madrid

SPAIN

Telephone: 34 91 542 4625

Fax: 34 91 542 9163

Web site: www.worldsport.com

Name of Contact Person: Antonio Espinós

Title of Contact Person: President

E-mail: w.k.f@arrakis.es

Membership: 160 affiliated national federations

World Taekwondo Federation

WTF

Medical Committee

635 Yuksam-Dong

Kangnam-ku

Seoul 135-080

KOREA

Telephone: (82.2) 566 25 05 / 557 54 46

Fax: (82.2) 553 47 28

E-mail: office@wtf.worldsport.org

Web site: www.worldsport.com

Name of Contact Person: Dr. Kim Un Yong

Title of Contact Person: President

Membership: 157 affiliated national federations

Founding Date: 1973

Motor Sports

Fédération Aéronautique Internationale

FAI

International Commission of Medicine and Physiology

Avenue Mon Repos 24

CH-1005 Lausanne

SWITZERLAND

Telephone: (41.21) 345 10 70

Fax: (41.21) 345 10 77

E-mail: info@fai.org

Web site: www.fai.org

Name of Contact Person: Eilif Ness

Title of Contact Person: President

E-mail: president@fai.org

Membership: 95 affiliated national federations

Founding Date: 1905

Fédération Internationale de l'Automobile (International Automobile Federation)

FIA

FIA member clubs provide vital assistance and rescue services for roadside breakdowns or emergencies as well as touring information, insurance, and travel bookings. They carry out research and consumer testing, promote road safety and driver education, and publish maps, technical guides, and hotel ratings. They try at all times to protect the mobility of their members and the interest of the ordinary motorist. FIA member clubs also organize motor sport events in their own countries.

Medical Commission

Chemin de Blandonnet, 2

CH-1215 Genève 15

SWITZERLAND

Telephone: (41.22) 544 44 00

Fax: (41.22) 544 44 50 (Sport) / (41.22) 544 45 50 (Tourisme et Automobile)

Web site: www.fia.com

Name of Contact Person: Max Mosley

Title of Contact Person: President

Membership: 117 affiliated national federations

Founding Date: 1904

Fédération Internationale Motorcycliste

FIM

The purpose of the FIM is to develop, promote, coordinate, supervise, and govern motorcycling activities throughout the world.

Medical Commission

11 Route Suisse

CH-1295 Mies

SWITZERLAND

Telephone: (41.22) 950 9500

Fax: (41.22) 950 9501

E-mail: info@fim.ch

Web site: www.fim.ch

Name of Contact Person: Mr. MaitreGuy

Membership: 80 affiliated national federations and 6 continental unions

Founding Date: 1904

Union Internationale Motonautique

UIM

International Medical and Safety Commission, President: Bob Wartinger

1, Avenue des Castelans

Stade Louis II Entrés H

MC-98000 Monaco

MONACO

Telephone: (377) 92 05 25 22

Fax: (377) 92 05 04 60

E-mail: uim@powerboating.org

Web site: www.powerboating.org (or) www.worldsport.com

Name of Contact Person: Ralf Fröhling

Title of Contact Person: President

Rommersceider Str.

72

D-51465 Bergisch

Gladbach

GERMANY

Telephone: +49 2202 300 02

Fax: +49 2202 300 03

Membership: 60 affiliated national federations

Founding Date: 1922

Netball

International Federation of Netball Associations

IFNA

The IFNA is dedicated to promoting and

developing netball as a desirable sport in all countries of the world and to raise awareness and appreciation of the game.

Birmingham Sports Centre

201 Balsall Heath Rd.

Highgate, Birmingham

B12 9DL

UNITED KINGDOM

Telephone: 44 121 446 44 51

Fax: 44 121 446 5857

E-mail: ifna@btinternet.com

Web site: www.netball.org (or) www.worldsport.com

Name of Contact Person: Anne Steele

Title of Contact Person: Executive Officer

Founding Date: 1960

Publications: *Book of Administration; Rules Book; The Organization of World Netball Championships; The Organization of World Youth Netball Championships; Dope Control&Information and Regulations; Netball in the 1998 Commonwealth Games; IFNA News*

Orienteering

International Mountaineering and Climbing Federation

UIAA

The UIAA gathers together leading experts from all over the world into working commissions that study and help to resolve issues and problems that mountaineers encounter wherever they climb.

Monbijoustrasse 61

CH-3007 Bern

SWITZERLAND

Telephone: 41 31 370 18 28

Fax: 41 31 370 18 38

E-mail: uiaa@compuserve.com

Web site: www.worldsport.com

Name of Contact Person: Ian McNaught-Davis

Title of Contact Person: President

80, Abingdon Rd.

Kensington

London

W8 6QT

UNITED KINGDOM

Telephone: +44.171 / 937 6559

Fax: +44.171 / 937 7664

E-mail: MACDAVIS@compuserve.com

Membership: 82 affiliated national federations

Founding Date: 1932

International Orienteering Federation

IOF

Radiokatu 20

FIN-00093 Slu

FINLAND

Telephone: 358 9 3481 3112

Fax: 358 9 3481 3113

E-mail: iof@orienteering.org

Web site: www.orienteering.org (or) www.worldsport.com

Name of Contact Person: Sue Harvey

Title of Contact Person: President

Mile End, Main St., Doune

Perthshire FK16 6BJ

SCOTLAND

Telephone: +44 1786 841202

Fax: +44 1786 841098

E-mail: iof@harveymaps.co.uk

Membership: 55 affiliated national federations

Founding Date: 1961

Publications: *Orienteering World; Scientific Journal of Orienteering; IOF Headlines*

Racquetball

International Racquetball Federation

1685 W. Uintah

Colorado Springs, CO 80904

UNITED STATES OF AMERICA

Telephone: (719) 635-5396

Fax: (719) 635-0685

E-mail: usrapr@webaccess.net

Web site: www.worldsport.com

Name of Contact Person: Han van der Heijden

Title of Contact Person: President

Heulweg 10

2641 KR Pijnacker

THE NETHERLANDS

Telephone: 00-31-15-369-7643

Fax: 00-31-15-369-7745

E-mail: info@h-vd-heijden-import.nl

Membership: 90 affiliated national federations

Founding Date: 1968

Publications: *Racquetball Magazine*

Roller Skating

International Roller Skating Federation

FIRS

Rambla Catalunya 121

Piso 6, Puerta 7

E-08008 Barcelona

SPAIN

Telephone: (34.93) 237 7055

Fax: (34.93) 237 2733

E-mail: bilo@compuserve.com

Web site: www.worldsport.com

Name of Contact Person: Isidro Oliveras

Title of Contact Person: President

E-mail: firs@idgrup.ibernet.com

Membership: 107 affiliated national federations

Founding Date: 1924

Rowing

International Rowing Federation

FISA

Avenue de Cour 135

CH-1007 Lausanne

SWITZERLAND

Telephone: (41.21) 617 83 73

Fax: (41.21) 617 83 75

E-mail: info@fisa.org

Web site: www.worldsport.com

Name of Contact Person: Dénis Oswald

Title of Contact Person: President

CP 352

CH-2001 Neuchatel

SWITZERLAND

Telephone: -41-32-7257121

Fax: -41-32-7259118

E-mail: etudeoswald@swissonline.ch

Membership: 106 affiliated national federations

Founding Date: 1892

Rugby

International Rugby Board

IRB

Huguenot House

35/38 St. Stephen's Green

Dublin 2

IRELAND

Telephone: (353.1) 240 92 00

Fax: (353.1) 240 92 01

Web site: www.irfb.com (or) www.worldsport.com

Name of Contact Person: Vernon Pugh

Title of Contact Person: Chair

First Floor, Huguenot House

35/38 St. Stephens Green

Dublin 2

IRELAND

Membership: 91 affiliated national federations

Founding Date: 1886

Sailing

International Sailing Federation

ISAF

Ariadne House

Town Quay

Southampton

SE1 9PL

UNITED KINGDOM

Telephone: (44.1703) 635111

Fax: (44.1703) 635789

E-mail: SAIL@isaf.co.uk

Web site: www.sailing.org (or) www.worldsport.com

Name of Contact Person: Paul Henderson

Title of Contact Person: President

100 Thorncliffe Park Dr.

PO Box 128

Toronto ON M4H 1G9

CANADA

Membership: 121 affiliated national federations

Founding Date: 1907

Scuba Diving

World Underwater Federation

CMAS

Viale Tiziano 74

00196 Rome

ITALY

Telephone: 39.0 + 06 36 85 84 80

Fax: 39.0 + 06 36 85 84 90

E-mail: cmasmond@tin.it

Web site: www.cmas/orgindex.htm

Name of Contact Person: Pierre Dernier

Title of Contact Person: Secretary General

Membership: 94 affiliated national federations

Founding Date: 1959

Sepaktakraw

International Sepaktakraw Federation

Sepaktakraw is a skill ball game originating from Asia.

ISTAF

The ISTAF's mission is to control, manage, and develop sepaktakraw worldwide through planning, organizing, marketing, and promotional activities aimed at developing sepaktakraw as a major world sport.

220 Ban Ampawan

Pitsanulok Rd.

Bangkok

10300

THAILAND

Telephone: +662 2811 038

Fax: +662 2803 758

E-mail: info@sepaktakraw.com

Web site: http://sepaktakraw.com (or) www.worldsport.com

Name of Contact Person: Senator Maj. Gen. Charouck Arirachakaran

Title of Contact Person: President, 1996-2000

Membership: 25 affiliated national federations

Shooting

International Shooting Sport Federation

ISSF

Medical Committee

Bavariaring 21

D-80336 Munich

GERMANY

Telephone: (49.89) 5443550

Fax: (49.89) 54435544

E-mail: issfmunich@Compuserve.com

Web site: www.issf-shooting.org (or)
    www.worldsport.com

Name of Contact Person: Horst Schreiber

Title of Contact Person: Secretary General

Avenida Universidad 2014, 4th Floor

Colonia Copilco Universidad

04360 Mexico City DF

MEXICO

Telephone: 52-5-6582850

Fax: 52-5-5549191

E-mail: 74751.1514@Compuserve.com

Membership: 151 affiliated national federations

Founding Date: 1907

Skibob (Skibike)

Fédération Internationale de Skibob

FISB

 Doctor and Medical Advisors

Peberinger Str 3

A-5301 Eugendorf

AUSTRIA

Telephone: (0043) 0662 66 25 31

Fax: (0043) 0662 66 25 32

Web site: www.skibob.org

Name of Contact Person: Richard Aistleitner

Title of Contact Person: President

Membership: 10 affiliated national federations

Skiing

International Ski Federation

FIS

The FIS's objectives are to promote the sport of skiing and to supervise and direct the development of all skiing activities; to establish and maintain friendly relations with and between member associations; to support within its possibilities the objectives of member associations; to promote the cooperation and mutual understanding between athletes from all countries; to organize World Ski Championships and World and Continental Cups, as well as other competitions that are approved by the Congress or the Council; to establish rules for all ski competitions approved by the FIS; to recognize only those international competitions that comply with the statutes and rules of the FIS and to ensure that those statutes and rules are observed at such competitions; to draft and impose sanctions; to prepare rules and make recommendations for recreational skiing; to serve as the highest court of appeal for protests and other legal questions concerning international ski competitions and for all questions concerning FIS rules; to generally promote skiing as a recreational and leisure sport in the interest of all skiers, especially as an activity for children and youth; to take all possible steps to avoid accidents; and to take into consideration the protection of the environment and to take care of external relations.

 Medical Committee, Chair: Ernst Raas

Blochstrasse 2

CH-3653 Oberhofen/Thunersee

SWITZERLAND

Telephone: (41.33) 44 61 61

Fax: (41.33) 43 53 53

E-mail: Lewis@fisski.ch

Web site: www.fis-ski.com

Name of Contact Person: Kasper Gian Franco

Title of Contact Person: President

Membership: 100 affiliated national federations

Founding Date: 1924

Sleddog Sports

International Federation of Sleddog Sports

IFSS

881 County Rd. 14

Grand Marais, MN 55604

UNITED STATES OF AMERICA

Telephone: (218) 387-2712

Web site: www.worldsport.com

Name of Contact Person: Sally Blair

Title of Contact Person: Secretary-General

16406 257th Ave.

Big Lake, MN 55309

UNITED STATES OF AMERICA

Telephone: (612) 263-2818

Fax: (612) 263-8471

E-mail: sbair@sherbtel.net

Membership: 30 affiliated national federations

Founding Date: 1984

Softball

International Softball Federation

ISF

Medical Commission, Chair: Dr. Fernando Jorge Aren

1900 S. Park Rd

Plant City, FL 33566-8113

UNITED STATES OF AMERICA

Telephone: (813) 707-7204

Fax: (813) 707-7209

E-mail: isfsoftball@ci.plant-city.fl.us

Web site: www.worldsport.com

Name of Contact Person: Don E. Porter

Title of Contact Person: President

4141 NW Expressway, Ste. 340

Oklahoma City, OK 73116-1675

UNITED STATES OF AMERICA

Telephone: (405) 879-2004

Fax: (405) 879-9801

E-mail: dporter@accessacg.net

Membership: 112 affiliated national federations

Founding Date: 1952

Squash

World Squash Federation

WSF

Medical Committee

6, Havelock Rd.

Hastings

East Sussex

TN34 1BP

UNITED KINGDOM

Telephone: (44 1424) 42 92 45

Fax: (44 1424) 42 92 50

E-mail: squash@wsf.cablenet.co.uk

Web site: www.worldsport.com

Name of Contact Person: Edward J. Wallbutton

27a Portland Rd.

Remuera

Auckland 5

(continued on next page)

(Squash, continued)

NEW ZEALAND
Telephone: (64) 9 524 9360
Fax: (64) 9 529 0674
E-mail: simcock@voyager.co.nz
Membership: 115 affiliated national federations
Founding Date: 1967

Surfing

International Surfing Association

ISA
Medical Committee, Chair: Mark Bracker
5580 La Jolla Blvd.
PMB 145
La Jolla, CA 92037
UNITED STATES OF AMERICA
Telephone: (858) 551-5292
Fax: (858) 551-5290
E-mail: surf@isasurf.org
Web site: www.worldsport.com
Name of Contact Person: Fernando Aguerre
Title of Contact Person: President
Membership: 43 affiliated national federations
Founding Date: 1976

Swimming

Fédération Internationale de Natation Amateur (International Amateur Swimming Federation)

FINA
Medical Committee
Av. de Beaumont 9
Rez-de-Chaussée
CH-1012 Lausanne
SWITZERLAND
Telephone: (41.21) 310 47 10
Fax: (41.21) 312 66 10
Web site: www.fina.org
Name of Contact Person: Mustapha Larfaoui
Title of Contact Person: President
26 rue Larbi Ben M'Hidi
16000 Algiers
ALGERIA
Telephone: (213-2) 92 41 27 or 92 37 28
Fax: (213-2) 740 096 or Telex: 55224 FINA DZ
Membership: 171 affiliated national federations
Founding Date: 1908

Table Tennis

International Table Tennis Federation

ITTF
53, London Rd.
St. Leonards-on-Sea
East Sussex
TN37 6AY
UNITED KINGDOM
Telephone: (44.1424) 72 14 14
Fax: (44.1424) 43 18 71
E-mail: hg@ittf.cablenet.co.uk
Web site: www.ittf.com (or)
    www.worldsport.com
Name of Contact Person: Adham Sharara
Title of Contact Person: President
1125 Colonel By Dr., Ste. 2900
Ottawa ON K1S 5R1
CANADA
Membership: 185 affiliated national federations
Founding Date: 1926
Publications: *Table Tennis Illustrated*

Tennis

International Soft Tennis Federation

ISTF

RM 605, Olympic Center 88

Oryun-dong

Song pa-gu

Seoul

KOREA

Telephone: +82 2420 4057

Fax: +82 2420 8089

E-mail: softtennis@sports.or.kr

Web site: www.worldsport.com

Name of Contact Person: Sang Ha Park

Title of Contact Person: President

International Tennis Federation

ITF

Medical Commission, Chair: Dr. Jim Cochrane

Bank Lane

Roehampton

London

SW15 5XZ

UNITED KINGDOM

Telephone: (44.20) 88 78 64 64

Fax: (44 20) 88 78 77 99 or (44.20) 83 92 46 09

E-mail: reception@itftennis.com

Web site: www.itftennis.com

Name of Contact Person: Brian Tobin

Title of Contact Person: President

Membership: 190 affiliated national federations

Founding Date: 1913

Volleyball

International Volleyball Federation

FIVB

The FIVB's mission is to govern and manage all forms of volleyball and beach volleyball worldwide through planning, organizing, marketing, and promotional activities aimed at developing volleyball as a major world sport.

Medical Commission, President: Dr. Peter Adrianus Van Beek

Avenue de la Gare 12

CH-1001 Lausanne Suisse

SWITZERLAND

Telephone: +41 21-340 89 32

Fax: +41 21-320 88 65

E-mail: info@mail.fivb.ch

Web site: www.fivb.ch (or) www.worldsport.com

Name of Contact Person: Dr. Acosta Hernandez Ruben

Title of Contact Person: President

Membership: 218 affiliated national federations; 240 million members

Founding Date: 1947

Publications: *Management and Administration of Sports Organizations* by Dr. Ruben Acosta H; FIVB President; *The Coach Magazine*, *Volleyworld Magazine*

Water Skiing

International Water Ski Federation

IWSF

World Medical Subcommittee, Chair: Dr. Ross Outabridge

CP 5537

BO22

I-40134 Bologna BO

(continued on next page)

(IWSF, continued)

ITALY

Telephone: (39.051) 615 29 56

Fax: (39.051) 615 50 15

E-mail: g.tognala@bo.nettuno.it

Web site: www.iwsf.com (or) worldsport.com

Name of Contact Person: Andrès Botero

Title of Contact Person: President

Calle 48#70.180

Medellin

COLOMBIA

Telephone: +57.426.045.26 (office)/ +57.431.312.22 (home)

Fax: +57.426.045.26

E-mail: IWSF@intic.net

Membership: 80 affiliated national federations

Founding Date: 1946

Wrestling

Fédération Internationale de Sambo

Sambo is a form of wrestling developed in the Soviet Union combining elements of regional Soviet styles.

FIAS

445 Cheyenne Mtn. Blvd, Suite 108

Colorado Springs, CO 80906

UNITED STATES OF AMERICA

Telephone: (807) 133-1160

E-mail: FIAS@sombo.org

Web site: www.worldsport.com

International Federation of Associated Wrestling Styles

FILA

Medical Commission

Av. Juste-Olivier 17

CH-1006 Lausanne

SWITZERLAND

Telephone: (41.21) 312 84 26

Fax: (41.21) 323 60 73

Web site: www.worldsport.com

Name of Contact Person: Milan Ercegan

Title of Contact Person: President

FILA Bureau

Jevremova 40

YU-11000 Belgrade

YUGOSLAVIA

Telephone: +381 11 637 103

Fax: +381 11 181 339

Membership: 136 affiliated national federations

Founding Date: 1912

International Sumo Federation

IFS

Onoya Bldg. 7F

2-20-1 Hyakunincho, Shinjuku-ku

Tokyo 169-0073

JAPAN

Telephone: (81.3) 3360 3911

Fax: (81.3) 3360 4020

Web site: www.AmateurSumo.com

Name of Contact Person: Akira Sasai

Title of Contact Person: President

Membership: 81 affiliated national federations

Founding Date: 1946

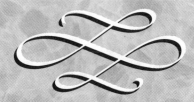

Position
Statements

Introduction

Part III contains the most comprehensive collection of sports medicine position statements available anywhere. These statements have been prepared by sports, medicine, and sports medicine organizations world wide. The position statements are loosely grouped by content into six categories, presented as separate chapters. If readers are aware of position statements that are not included in this collection and would like to see them included, please contact the Sports Medicine Managing Editor at Human Kinetics (see page 36 for contact information).

These position statements, recent updates, and new position statements, are available at **www.esportmed.com**, a sports medicine information site of Human Kinetics.

6
General

Definition of Sports Medicine

American Academy of Family Physicians (AAFP)

www.aafp.org/policy138

Definition

Sports medicine is a body of knowledge in the broad area of health care that addresses the needs of patients in all age groups who exercise as an essential component of health. Sports medicine deals with the medical supervision of recreational and competitive athletes and all others who exercise for prevention and treatment of disease and injury.

1988; 1995 (revised)

AARP Reference Manual

Ethics

FIMS Code of Ethics in Sports Medicine

International Federation of Sports Medicine (FIMS)

Web site: www.fims.org/state.html

1. Medical ethics in general

The same ethical principles that apply to the practice of medicine shall apply to sports medicine. The main duties of a physician include:

- Always make the health of the athlete a priority.
- Never do harm.
- Never impose your authority in a way that impinges on the individual right of the athlete to make his/her own decisions (1).

2. Ethics in Sports Medicine

Physicians who care for athletes of all ages have an ethical obligation to understand the specific physical, mental and emotional demands of physical activity, exercise and sports training.

A different relationship exists between sports medicine practitioners, their employers, official sports organization, professional colleagues and the athletes (2). In sports medicine there is also a link between the pathologic concern and specific recreational and professional activity. An athletic injury has a direct and immediate impact on the participation in this activity that may have psychological and financial implications. The most obvious difference between sports medicine and other aspects of medicine is that the athletes treated are generally healthy.

Ethics in sports medicine should also be distinguished from law as it relates to sport. One refers to morality the other to a set of enforceable social rules (2). Although it is desirable that the law be grounded in moral principles and that matters of moral importance should be given legal backing in many instances, not everything that is illegal is immoral and similarly not every immoral behavior is against the law.

Thus when speaking of ethics in sports medicine, one is not concerned with etiquette or law, but with basic morality.

3. Special Ethical Issues in Sports Medicine

The physician's duty to the athlete must be his/her first concern and contractual and other responsibilities are of secondary importance. A medical decision must be taken honestly and conscientiously.

A basic ethical principle in health care is that of respect for autonomy. An essential component of autonomy is knowledge. Failure to obtain informed consent is to undermine the athlete's autonomy. Similarly, failure to give them necessary information violates the right of the athlete to make autonomous choices. Truthfulness is important in health care ethics. The overriding ethical concern is to provide information to the best of one's ability that is necessary for the patient to decide and act autonomously.

The highest respect will always be maintained for human life and well-being. A mere motive of profit shall never be permitted to be an influence in conducting sports medicine practice or functions (3).

4. The Athlete-Physician Relationship:

The physician shall not allow consideration of religion, nationality, race, party politics or social standing to intervene between his/her duty and the athlete.

The basis of the relationship between the physician and the athlete should be that of absolute confidence and mutual respect. The athlete can expect a physician to exercise professional skill at all times. Advice given and action taken should always be in the athlete's best interest.

The athlete's right to privacy must be protected.

The regulations regarding medical records in health care and medicine shall also be applied in the field of sports medicine. The sports medicine physician should maintain a complete and accurate record of the patient.

In view of the strong public and media interest in the health of athletes, the physician should decide with the athlete what information can be released for public distribution (1).

When serving as a team physician, the sports medicine physician assumes the responsibility to athletes as well as team administrators and coaches. It is essential that each athlete is informed of that responsibility and authorizes disclosure of otherwise confidential medical information, but solely to the specific responsible persons and for the expressed purpose of determining the fitness of the athlete for participation (4).

The sports medicine physician will inform the athlete about the treatment, the use of medication and the possible consequences in an understandable way and proceed to request his or her permission for the treatment.

The team physician will explain to the individual athlete that he or she is free to consult another physician.

5. Training and Competition

Sports medicine physicians should oppose training and practices and competition rules as they may jeopardize the health of the athlete. In general, the physician shall obtain knowledge of the specific and mental demands made of athletes when they participate in sport activities. Relevant aspects in these respect include expertise, effectiveness and efficiency, and safety (5).

If the athletes concerned are children or growing individuals, the physician must take into consideration the special risks that the sport in questions may represent to persons who have not yet reached physical or psychological maturity. When the sports participant is a growing individual, the sports physician must ensure that the training and competition are appropriate for the state of growth and de-

velopment (4). The physician shall contribute to the spreading of information or the special conditions that pertain to young people training and competing. It is vital that this information also reaches the young athletes, parents, guardians, and trainers (1).

6. Education

Sports medicine physicians should participate in continuing education courses to improve and maintain the knowledge and skills that will allow them to provide optimal advice and care to their patient athletes (6). Knowledge should be shared with colleagues in the field.

7. Health Promotion

Sports medicine physicians are obligated to educate people of all ages about the health benefits of physical activity and exercise.

8. Injuries and Athletes

It is the responsibility of the sports medicine physician to determine whether the injured athletes should continue training or participate in competition. The outcome of the competition or the coaches should not influence the decision, but solely the possible risks and consequences to the health of the athlete.

If the physician considers that a certain sport entails major risks he should try to eliminate the risk by exerting pressure on the athletes as well as on the relevant decision makers. Injury prevention should receive the highest priority.

9. Therapeutic Exercise

When supported by scientific research, a detailed exercise prescription should be part of the therapeutic plan for an athlete recovering from injury or disease.

10. Relationship with Other Professionals

The sports medicine physician should work in collaboration with professionals of other disciplines. The sports medicine physician should cooperate with physical therapists, podiatrists, psychologists, sport scientists including biochemists, biomechanists, physiologists, and others. The sports medicine physician has the final responsibility for the health and well-being of the athlete and should therefore coordinate the respective roles of these professionals and those of appropriate medical specialists in the prevention, treatment and rehabilitation of disease and injury. The concept of interdisciplinary team work is fundamental to the practice of sports medicine.

A sports medicine physician should refrain from publicly criticizing fellow professionals who are involved in the treatment of athletes.

A sports medicine physician should behave in relation to his colleagues and coworkers as he would like them to behave towards him.

When a sports medicine physician recognizes that the athlete's problems are beyond his level of expertise, it beholds him to advise the athlete of other persons with the necessary expertise and refer the athlete to such appropriate persons for assistance.

11. Relation to Officials, Clubs, etc.

At a sport venue, it is the responsibility of the sports medicine physician to determine when an injured athlete can participate in or return to an event or game. The physician should not delegate this decision. In all cases, priority must be given to the athlete's health and safety. The outcome of the competition must never influence such decisions.

To enable the sports medicine physician to undertake this ethical obligation the sports medicine physician must insist on professional autonomy and responsibility for all medical decisions concerning the health, safety and legitimate interest of the athlete. No third party should influence these decisions (3).

No information about an athlete may be given to a third party without the consent of the athlete.

12. Doping (see FIMS Position Statement)

The sports medicine physician should oppose and in practice refrain from using methods to improve performance artificially such as those prohibited by the IOC (4).

The physicians have forcefully opposed the use of methods that are not in accordance with medical ethics or scientifically proven experience. Thus, it is contrary to medical ethics to condone doping in any form. Neither may the physician in anyway mask pain in order to enable the athlete's return to practicing the sport if there is any risk of aggravating the injury (1).

13. Research

Research should be conducted following the ethical principles accepted for research in animals and human subjects. Research should never be conducted in a manner which may injure athletes or jeopardize their athletic performance.

References

1. Code of Ethics. Swedish Society of Sports Medicine.
2. Hodge KP. Character building in sport: fact or fiction? *New Zealand Journal of Sports Medicine* 17(2):23-25, 1989.
3. Code of Ethics. Sports Medicine Australia.
4. Principles and Ethical Guidelines of Health Care for Sports Medicine. International Olympic Committee.
5. Code of Ethics. The Netherlands Association of Sports Medicine.
6. Code of Ethics. The American College of Sports Medicine.

September 1997

Physical Activity

Physical Activity and Health

Brazilian Society of Sports Medicine

Introduction

Health and quality of life can be preserved and improved by practicing regular physical activity. Physical inactivity is an undesirable condition and represents a risk for the health. This document, elaborated by exercise and sports medicine physicians, is based on scientific concepts and experience in clinical practice, focusing on apparently healthy individuals. It is not the aim of this document to discuss aspects related to the clinical use of exercise in the management of illnesses, or to aspects about activities of competitive level. The purpose of this text is to guide health professionals in the efficient use of physical activity.

Effect of Regular Physical Activity on Morbidity and Mortality

Epidemiological studies have been demonstrating a close relationship between an active lifestyle, lower death probability and better quality of life. The deleterious effects of sedentary life surpass by far the eventual compli-

---

Main clinical conditions counteracted by regular physical exercise

Coronary Artery Disease

Systemic Arterial Hypertension

Stroke

Periphereal Vascular Disease

Obesity

Type II Diabetes Mellitus

Osteoporosis and Osteoartosis

Cancer: colon, breast, prostate, lung

Anxiety and Depression

---

cations resulting from physical exercise practice, which, therefore, presents a very interesting risk/benefit ratio. Considering the high prevalence, allied to the significant risk of sedentary life to the development of chronic-degenerative diseases, augmenting population's physical activity represents a definitely contribution for public health, with a strong impact in the reduction of treatment costs, including hospitalization, one of the reasons for its considerable social benefits. Researches have been demonstrating that physically fit and/or trained individuals tend to present the majority of the chronic-degenerative illnesses in a minimal incidence, which can be explained by many physiologic and psychological benefits, achieved through regular physical activity.

Pre-Participation Evaluation

The health risks, particularly cardiovascular risks, consequent to moderate-intensity physical exercise are extremely low and can become even more reduced by a criterious pre-participation evaluation that allows for oriented exercise practice. Depending on the evaluated population, the objectives of the physical activity and the availability of facilities and qualified staff, the complexity of the evaluation can vary from the simple application of questionnaires, until sophisticated medical and functional examinations. Symptomatic individuals and/or with important risk factors for cardiovascular, metabolic, pulmonary, and locomotive illnesses, that could be aggravated by physical activity, demand specialized medical evaluation, for objective definition of eventual restrictions and the correct exercise prescription. The PAR-Q (acronym for Physical Activity Readiness Questionnaire) (Figure 2) has been suggested as the minimum standard pre-participation evaluation, because it can identify, when there is a positive answer, the ones who need to be submitted to a previous medical evaluation.

Physical Exercise Prescription

There is a strong dose-dependent relationship between the fitness level and its protective effect, with risk to acquire illness diminishing as the activity level augments. Significant health benefits can be achieved with relatively low intensity activities, common in daily life, as walking, climbing up stairs, riding a bicycle and dancing. Therefore, not only formal physical exercise programs, but also informal activities that develop fitness, are interesting. Both possibilities must be considered, since the combined effect of them facilitates to achieve a certain amount of physical activity.

A regular physical exercise program must include at least three components: aerobic, muscular resistance and flexibility, with emphasis in each one depending on the clinical condition and objectives for each individual. The adequate physical activity prescription must include variables such as: mode, duration, intensity, and weekly frequency. Innumerable combinations of these variables can provide positive results. The combination of some activities must be considered, as the ones in figure 3, in order to provide a caloric weekly expense of at least 2,000 kcal, considered a satisfactory level.

Both the beginning and restarting of activities must be gradual, especially for the elderly individuals. Initially, the duration is increased up to the minimum time accepted. Then, the intensity can be increased. The activity should not induce fatigue in each session of exercise, but it can be perceived as tiring, taking less than one hour to disappear.

The aerobic part of the exercise should be practiced, if possible, every day, with a minimum duration of 30-40 minutes. A practical and very common form for controlling the intensity of aerobic exercise is the measure of heart rate. The information collected during a more detailed functional and medical evaluation, obtaining the direct measure of the maximum oxygen consumption and the identification of anaerobic threshold, contribute for an individualized prescription concerning the exercise intensity.

Exercise for improving muscular function and flexibility is even more important after 40 years of age. They must be repeated at least two to three times per week, including the main muscular groups and joints. Recent data suggest that a set of six to eight exercises carried through during only one series with ten to 12 repetitions or, alternatively, two series with five to six repetitions and a small interval between them are enough for maintenance and improvement of muscular and bone mass and demand little time, what contributes for a better adherence to the resistance training. The flexibility training must involve the main body movements, carried through slowly, until causing slight discomfort, and, then, being kept by 10-20 seconds, and should be performed before and/or after the aerobic part.

Physical Activity Readiness Questionnaire (PAR-Q)—1992

1. A doctor has ever said that you have heart problems and that you should only make physical activity under health professional supervision?

2. Do you feel chest pain when practicing physical activity?

3. During the last month, did you feel chest pain when practicing physical exercise?

4. Do you have balance problems because of dizziness and/or loss of conscience?

5. Do you have any bone or joint problem that could be worsened by physical activity?

6. Are you using any medicine for blood pressure or heart problem?

7. Do you know any other reason why you should not practice physical activity?

Time necessary for a 70kg person to achieve a caloric weekly expent of 2000kcal in some activities (approximated values)

Activity	Weekly time	Daily time (7x week)	Daily time (5x week)
Walking on plan	6h	50min	1h10min
Riding a bike	7h30min	1h05min	1h30min
Run slowly	3h30min	30min	40min
Run fast	2h	20min	25min
Gardening	4h40min	40min	1h
Dancing	9h20min	1h20min	1h50min
Shopping	8h	1hr10min	1h35min
Swimming (crawl slowly)	3h40min	30min	45min
Swimming (crawl fast)	3h	25min	35min
Sweeping a carpet	10h30min	1h30min	2h10min

There must always be conciliation between the maximum benefit with a minimum risk of injuries or complications, in order to establish an interesting risk/benefit relationship.

Conclusions

We recommend that:

1. Health professionals should combat sedentary life, including in their interview specific questions about regular physical activity, competitive or not, making people aware about this subject and encouraging the increment of physical activity, through informal and formal activities;

2. The government, at all levels, should consider physical activity as a basic public health question, spreading related information and implementing programs for oriented practice;

3. The professional and scientific organizations, the media, and the society in general, should contribute to reduce the prevalence of sedentarism and to provide oriented physical exercise practice.

Bibliography

1. American College of Sports Medicine: *ACSM's Guidelines for Exercise Testing and Prescription*, 5th ed., Baltimore, Williams & Wilkins, 1995.

2. Bijnen FCH, Caspersen CJ, Mosterd WL: Physical inactivity as a risk factor for coronary heart disease: a WHO and International Society and Federation of Cardiology position statement. *Bull World Health Organization* 1994; 72: 1-4.

3. Fletcher GF, Balady G, Blair SN, Blumenthal J, Caspersen C, Chaitman B et al: Statement on exercise: benefits and recommendation for physical activity programs for all Americans – A statement for health professionals by the Committee on Exercise and Cardiac Rehabilitation of the Council on Clinical Cardiology, American Heart Association. *Circulation* 1996; 94: 857-62.

4. Paffenbarger Jr RS, Lee I-M: Physical activity and fitness for health and longevity. *Res Q Exerc Sport* 1996; 67 (Suppl 3): 11-28.

5. Pate RR, Pratt M, Blair SN, Haskell WL, Macera CA, Bouchard C et al: Physical activity and public health – A recommendation from the Center for Disease Control and Prevention and the American College of Sports Medicine. *JAMA* 1995; 273: 402-7.

6. Thomas S, Reading J, Shephard RJ: Revision of the Physical Activity Readiness Questionnaire (PAR-Q). *Can J Sports Sci* 1992; 17: 338-45.

7. U.S. Department of Health and Human Services: *Physical Activity and Health – A report of the Surgeon General*, U.S. Government Printing Office, 1996.

8. WHO/FIMS Committee on Physical Activity for Health: Exercise for health. *Bull World Health Organization* 1995; 73: 135-6.

9. Williams PT: Relationship of distance run per week to coronary heart disease risk factors in 8283 male runners – The National Runners' Health Study. *Arch Intern Med* 1997; 157: 191-8.

1996

Originally published in *Revista Brasileira de Medicina do Esporte 1996; 2(4): 79-81.*

Physical Activity for Health

International Federation of Sports Medicine (FIMS) and the World Health Organization (WHO)

Web site: www.fims.org

A Call to Governments of the World

Today there is an enormous waste of human potential that can be attributed to physical inactivity. In addition, men who fail to take sufficient exercise have about twice the risk of coronary heart disease as their more active counterparts. It is also known that many of the infirmities and disabilities of old age appear to be the result of habitual inactivity rather than of aging itself. Sedentary living is, therefore, now recognized to be a major contributor to ill health and unnecessary death.

In the present century mechanization and automation have radically reduced human physical activity. Nowhere has this been more apparent than in highly developed countries, where heavy manual labor has virtually disappeared and labor-saving appliances in homes have drastically reduced physical effort. Increased use of motor cars and more time spent on sedentary leisure activities, such as television viewing, have to a large extent promoted nonactive lifestyles. Such lifestyles first became prevalent in industrialized countries, but are also increasing in the developing countries. This tendency is not restricted to adults, since there are signs that children and adolescents are also becoming less active. Lowering of physical activity is thus becoming a worldwide phenomenon.

Benefits of Physical Activity

The results of extensive research programs lead to the conclusion that physical activity increases longevity and, to a large extent, protects against the development of the major non communicable, chronic diseases such as coronary heart disease, hypertension, stroke, non-insulin-dependent diabetes mellitus, osteoporosis, and coon cancer. Some studies suggest that physical inactivity also increases the risk of prostate cancer, lung cancer, breast cancer, and clinical depression. Furthermore, appropriate levels of physical activity assist in the rehabilitation of patients with cardiovascular and other chronic diseases.

Appropriate activity is necessary at all ages for physiological "fitness", i.e., the capacity for everyday physical effort and movement without undue fatigue or discomfort; for the regulation of body weight and avoidance of overweight and obesity; and for the optimum performance of a wider range of physiological processes, including fat and carbohydrate metabolism and the body's defenses against infection. People function, feel and look better when leading active lives, and their levels of anxiety and depression can be reduced. Among the elderly, limited mobility and loss of independence are widespread; yet there is much evidence to show the value of habitual physical activity in preventing and alleviating these disabilities.

In general, the indications are that great numbers of people are functioning below, often far below, their biological potential for good health because of inadequate physical activity. Compared with the multifarious health gains that can be expected, the hazards of sensible, appropriate physical activity are minimal.

Recommendations

WHO and the International Federation of Sports Medicine note with concern that an estimated half of the world's population is insufficiently active. They, therefore, urge governments to promote and enhance programs of physical activity and fitness, as part of public health and social policy, centered on the following:

• Daily physical activity should be accepted as the cornerstone of a healthy lifestyle. Physical activity should be reintegrated into the routine of everyday living. An obvious first step would be the use of stairs instead of lifts, and walking or cycling for short journeys.

• Children and adolescents should be provided with facilities and the opportunity to take part in daily programs of enjoyable exercise so that physical activity may develop into a lifetime habit.

• Adults should be encouraged to increase habitual activity gradually, aiming to carry out every day at least 30 minutes of physical activity of moderate intensity, e.g., brisk walking and stair climbing. More strenuous activities such as slow jogging, cycling, field and court games (soccer, tennis, etc.) and swimming could provide additional benefits.

• Women must be offered a variety of opportunities and more encouragement to engage in health exercise.

• The elderly, including the oldest citizens whose numbers are increasing worldwide, should be encouraged to lead physically active lives so as to maintain their independence of movement and personal autonomy, to reduce the risks of body injury, and to promote optimal nutrition. Social roles and social relationships will, therefore, also be facilitated.

• People with disabilities or suffering from chronic diseases should be provided with advice on exercise and facilities appropriate to their needs.

• The fact that there are benefits to be gained by starting physical activity at any age should be broadcast more widely.

The responsibility for personal health ultimately lies with the individual and family, but government action is required to create a social and physical environment that is conducive to the adoption and maintenance of physically active lifestyles. The promotion of physical activity must be a part of public policy because the implications are important and far-reaching. Some of the requirements are outlined below:

1. Promoting action across all levels of government—local and central—so that, for example, transport and environmental policies will have to be concerned as much with the needs of walkers and cyclists as of motorists;

and town-and-country planning should encourage physical activity during leisure time and while commuting.

2. Educating and re-educating physicians, other health professionals, and teachers at all levels in order to promote physical activity by advising their patients and pupils and by setting good examples.

3. Providing convenient and affordable facilities by the local authorities and central government, taking into account the requirements of mothers, working women, the elderly, the physically handicapped, and others with special needs.

4. Giving high priority to the prevention and treatment of sports injuries.

5. Establishing tested public education campaigns through the health services and the media, supported by opinion leaders and role models in the community.

6. Linking up with numerous voluntary organizations—social, environmental, sports and recreational—concerned with promoting healthier and more enjoyable lifestyles.

7. Monitoring physical activity and physical fitness at the national level, as well as programs to promote these and avoid sports injuries; baseline levels should be set up now. Owing to existing social inequalities in health and marked variations in physical activity—for example, the better educated and the more affluent are more likely to engage in healthy leisure pursuits—recognizing this difference and making special provisions accordingly.

If these recommendations are followed, the benefit in saving lives and in improving the quality of life of large numbers of people all over the world is likely to be substantial. The time is now ripe for increased action.

This statement may be reproduced and distributed internationally with the sole requirement that it be identified clearly as the Joint Position Statement of the Fédération Internationale de Médecine Sportive (FIMS) and the World Health Organization (WHO).

The Need for Daily Physical Activity

American Academy of Orthopaedic Surgeons (AAOS)

Web site: www.aaos.org/wordhtml/papers position/exercise.htm

Medical research has proven that people can substantially improve their health and quality of life with moderate physical activity. However, 25 percent of American adults report they don't engage in any physical activity in their leisure time and 60 percent don't engage in vigorous activity. This is a problem of national concern because of the aging population and evidence that adults exercise less as they get older. By the year 2030, one in five people will be 65 or older and 12 percent of the elderly will be 85 or older.

Some people may not exercise because they don't like vigorous activity, don't have the time or are worried that it will aggravate a medical condition. However, researchers have found that moderate physical activity at least 30 minutes a day will provide significant health benefits. Even people with chronic conditions such as osteoarthritis and osteoporosis, can improve their health and quality of life with regular, moderate amounts of physical activity.

The American Academy of Orthopaedic Surgeons and the American Geriatrics Society recommend that adults engage in moderate physical activity at least 30 minutes a day on a regular basis.

Regular physical activity slows the loss of muscle mass, strengthens bones and reduces joint and muscle pain. Physical activity also improves mobility, balance and sleep. These factors all reduce the risk of falling and sustaining a serious injury such as a hip fracture.

Physical activity is safe and beneficial for people with arthritis, high blood pressure, osteoporosis and other chronic conditions. In fact, the lack of activity can make the condition worse or, at least, make it difficult to live with.

The American Academy of Orthopaedic Surgeons and American Geriatrics Society recommend that adults engage in a variety of daily activities to ensure continued interest and participation.

While some people may enjoy participating in a regularly-scheduled exercise class, other adults can achieve healthful benefits from daily activities such as brisk walking, bicycle riding, swimming, dancing, housework and gardening.

Adults are encouraged to do different physical activities on different days, and even in short intervals of 15 minutes in the morning and 15 minutes in the afternoon. The healthful benefits of physical activity are cumulative, however, the benefits diminish quickly when physical activity ceases.

Physical Activity and Health in Children and Adolescents

Brazilian Society of Sports Medicine

Introduction

In adults, an active lifestyle is associated to a reduction in the incidence of many chronic diseases, and a reduction in cardiovascular and all-cause mortality. In children and adolescents, a greater physical activity index contributes to improve lipid and metabolic profiles and to reduce obesity prevalence. Also, a physically active child is more likely to become an active adult. In consequence, from public health and preventive medicine perspectives, to promote physical activity in childhood and adolescence is to establish a solid base to reduction of prevalence of physical inactivity in adult age, contributing to a better quality of life. In this context, we emphasize that physical activity is any movement as a result of a skeletal muscle contraction that increases the energy cost above resting values and not necessarily only sports participation.

This document, written by sports and exercise medicine specialists, is based on scientific concepts and clinical experience, having as objectives: 1) to establish the benefits of physical activity in children and youth; 2) to characterize the parameters of assessment and exercise prescription for health in this age; 3) to encourage the recommendation and the practice of physical activity in children and adolescents, even with chronic diseases, as absolute contraindications are rare.

Epidemiological Aspects

The aging process is accompanied by a tendency to reduce the average daily energy expenditure in consequence of a diminished physical activity. This happens basically for behavioral and social factors, like the increase of school and/or professional demands. A few factors contribute to a less active lifestyle. Availability of technology, lack of security, and the progressive reduction of free spaces in urban centers (where the major part of the Brazilian children live) reduce the opportunities of leisure and a physically active life, thus facilitating sedentary activities, like: watching television, playing videogames and operating computers.

There is a strong association among physical inactivity, obesity and dyslipidemias, and obese children are more likely to grow as obese adults. In consequence, to promote an active lifestyle in children and adolescents may reduce the incidence of obesity and cardiovascular diseases in adult age. Physical activity may produce other long-term benefits, like those related to the skeletal muscle system. Intense physical activity, mainly involving impact, induces an increase in bone mineral density in adolescence and may prevent the risk of osteoporosis in more advanced ages, principally in post-menopausal women.

Exercise Physiology

The general principles that apply to the body responses and adaptations to exercise are the same for children, adolescents and adults. Nevertheless, there are some particularities of exercise physiology in children that are consequent to the increase of body mass (growth) and the maturation that accelerates during puberty (development).

There is an absolute increase in maximal oxygen uptake (VO_2max) with age, with a more rapid increase in boys than in girls. This increase in VO_2max is closely related to the increase in muscle mass, such that if one considers VO_2max corrected by indicators of muscle mass, there is no increase with age in male children and adolescents (VO_2max/body mass remains constant), while there is a progressive decrease in female children and adolescents (VO_2max/body mass decreases).

Anaerobic power augments with age in a greater proportion than the increases in muscle mass, evidencing an effect of maturation on anaerobic metabolism. Anaerobic power does not differ in pre-puberty boys and girls, but increases more rapidly in boys after puberty. Thus, the raise in anaerobic power is a consequence of the increase in muscle mass, and the effect of hormonal maturation on the functional characteristics of the skeletal muscle. Also, lactate production is more developed in adults than in children, a reason why children recover more promptly after high-intensity and short duration exercises, being earlier ready for another bout of exercise. Other characteristic that develops with sexual maturation is the buffering capacity of the muscle acidosis that is more efficient with age, allowing for more intense lactic exercises.

There are some characteristics in thermoregulation in children that must be emphasized. The transfer of heat with the environment is greater in children than in adults, as they have a greater body surface corrected for body mass. Thus, children lose heat in cold environments and gain heat in high temperatures more rapidly than adults, being more prone to thermal complications. Also, children tend to have less thirst than adults, dehydrating and decreasing blood volume more easily, with impairment in physical performance and thermoregulation mechanisms.

Pre-Participation Examination

From a public health perspective, children and adolescents may participate in low and moderate-intensity activities, recreational and leisure activities, with no need of a formal pre-participation examination. It is important that some basic health conditions—as an adequate nutrition—are present to implement physical activity.

When the objective is competitive exercise participation or high-intensity activities, the child must undergo a medical and functional assessment, including a clinical evaluation, body composition assessment, aerobic and anaerobic power tests, among others. The main objective of pre-participation evaluation is to assure a favorable risk/benefit relationship, and one must consider the child objectives, and the facilities and personnel available. The risk of cardiovascular complications in children is extremely low, except for congenital cardiovascular diseases and acute illnesses. The presence of some clinical conditions indicates the need for special recommendations and they must be identified and quantified, like asthma, obesity and type I diabetes mellitus.

The bones of children are under development and growth processes until the end of the second decade. The growth plates are vulnerable to lesions consequent to acute trauma and overuse. Anatomic characteristics that may predispose to lesions must be identified.

Prescription

The main objective of physical activity prescription in children and adolescents is to create the habit and interest for physical activity, and not to train aiming performance. Thus, it must be emphasized the inclusion of physical activity in the day-to-day life and to promote school physical education that encourages life-long physical activity, in a pleasant way, integrating the children and not discriminating the less fit.

Competitive sports participation may offer educational and social benefits because it provides experiences of group activities, permitting the child to face situations of winning and losing. However, the objective for performance, mainly when there is excessive pressure by parents and coaches, may produce undesirable consequences, as aversion to physical activity. For this reason, the recreational component of physical activity must be more important than the competitive component when prescribing physical activity to children. Also important is to offer alternatives to sports participation, to consider the individual interests and the development of different motor abilities, contributing to the development of talents.

A formal program of physical activity should consider at least three components: aerobic, muscular strength and flexibility varying the emphasis in each one according to the clinical condition and the objectives of the child. When the objective is the aerobic conditioning, prescription must consider the following variables: mode, duration, intensity and frequency following the general principles of training. The strength training should be performed with moderate loads and a greater number of repetitions, emphasizing the motor learning, as this type of activity contributes to an increase in muscle strength and bone mass. The risk of orthopedic lesions in children performing strength exercises is lower than in children performing contact sports, provided that submaximal leads are used with an adequate professional supervision. In flexibility training, it should involve the main joint movements, and each movement should be performed slowly until the point of mild discomfort and then maintained for 10 to 20 seconds.

Recommendations

The implementation of physical activity in children and adolescents must be considered as a priority in our society. Thus, we recommend that:

1. Healthcare professionals must combat physical inactivity in children and adolescents, encouraging regular practice of physical activity in the daily life and/or formally with sports participation, even in the presence of diseases, as absolute contraindications to exercise are rare;

2. The professionals involved with children and adolescents that practice physical activity must emphasize the recreational aspects over the competitive aspects and should avoid participation in extremes of temperature;

3. School physical education must be considered essential and an integral part of the global process of education of children and adolescents;

4. The governments at their different levels, the professional and scientific institutions, and the media must consider physical activity in children and adolescents as a public health question, helping to disseminate this information and to implement programs to oriented practice of physical activity.

Recommended References

1. American Academy of Pediatrics Committees on Sports Medicine and School Health. Physical fitness and the schools. *Pediatrics* 1987;80:449-50.

2. American College of Sports Medicine. Opinion statement on physical fitness in children and youth. *Med Sci Sports Exerc* 1988;20:422-3.

3. Caspersen CJ, Nixon PA, Durant RH. Physical activity epidemiology applied to children and adolescents. In: Holloszy JO, ed. *Exerc Sport Sci Rev* 1998;26:341-403.

4. Chan K-M, Micheli LJ, eds. *Sports and Children*. Hong Kong: Williams & Wilkins, 1998.

5. Confederación Panamericana de Medicina del Deporte. Physical activity and health in the children of the Americas / Atividad física y salud en los niños de las Americas. *Boletin COPAMEDE* 1997;1:3.

6. Fédération Internationale de Médecine Sportive. FIMS Consensus Statement on Organized Sports for Children. In: Chan K-M, Micheli LJ, eds. *Sports and Children*. Hong Kong: Williams & Wilkins, 1998.

7. Pate RR. Physical activity in children and adolescents. In: Leon AS, ed. *Physical Activity and Cardiovascular Health - a National Consensus*. Champaign: Human Kinetics, 1997.

8. Sallis JF, Patrick K. Physical activity guidelines for adolescents: Consensus statement. *Ped Exerc Sci* 1994;6:302-14.

9. U.S. Department of Health and Human Services. Physical activity and health: a report of the Surgeon General. Atlanta, GA: U.S. Department of Health and Human Services, Centers for Disease Control and Prevention, National Center for Chronic Disease Prevention and Health Promotion, 1996.

10. U.S. National Institutes of Health. Physical activity and cardiovascular health. NIH Consensus Development Panel on Physical Activity and Cardiovascular Health. *JAMA* 1996;276:241-6.

1998

Originally published in *Revista Brasileira de Medicina do Esporte* 1998; 4(4):107-9.1

Physical Activity and Health in the Children of the Americas

The Pan American Confederation of Sports Medicine (COPAMEDE) in collaboration with The International Federation of Sports Medicine (FIMS)

Web site: www.copamede.org/eng position.html or www.fims.org

Although there is a great deal of information about the beneficial effects of physical activity on the health of adults, less is known about the effects of an active lifestyle during childhood and adolescence on one's health as an adult. There is limited evidence on the short-term benefits of increased physical activity during the early years, especially in children who are at high risk for developing chronic illness in later years. Adults who have a sedentary lifestyle are at a higher risk for several chronic diseases. If activity patterns learned in childhood and adolescence can carry over into adulthood, the risk for disease should be reduced. Thus, it is important to find ways to motivate young people to maintain an active lifestyle throughout life.

Physical activity plays a key role in psychological and social development, as well as in linear growth, body size, motor development, and fitness of young children. Therefore, physical activity is very important at this age, especially because more activity may be demanded of children in developing countries.

There is a large disparity in socioeconomic levels, as well as ethnic and cultural differences, within and between countries in the Americas. These differences are associated with variations in the pattern and quantity of food consumption, opportunities for physical activity, and patterns of body growth and development. Overweight Latin American children have lifestyle-related disorders similar to those of overweight children from the United States and Canada. As well, there is little or no difference in physical fitness when Latin American children from middle and upper socioeconomic levels are compared to children of the same socioeconomic class from industrialized countries.

There is now convincing evidence that general well-being and health can be greatly enhanced by achievable improvements in physical activity, nutrition, and lifestyle. Although there is not sufficient information on the activity of children in Latin America, it does not seem that it is the location (rural or urban) of the children that is as important as their access to and opportunity for sports and physical activity. Thus, there is a need to improve physical education because schools have a major role in enhancing the quantity and quality of physical activity in children by guaranteeing that proper medical and teacher supervision is provided. COPAMEDE feels strongly that all national and local organizations interested in the health, fitness, and productivity of its citizens shall increase their efforts to educate them and to provide increased opportunities for proper nutrition and physical activity.

Physical activity cannot be considered in isolation from factors such as nutrition. Although it is an oversimplification of the complex relationship between nutrition and physical activity in children, it would appear that:

1. Children with adequate levels of nutrition need to maintain nutritional intakes while either maintaining or increasing physical activity:

2. Children with excessive intake of calories need to reduce caloric intake while in-

creasing physical activity to minimize the risk of developing chronic lifestyle diseases; and

3. Children with inadequate intake of calories, protein, and micronutrients need to improve nutrition and maintain physical activity. In some cases, children who are undernourished will be able to increase physical activity if they are able to increase their dietary intake of nutrients.

COPAMEDE believes that children have the right to be active and healthy. COPAMEDE recommends that governments, schools, and private institutions look at all levels of nutritional intake to decide on proper action for each. A more bountiful supply of all food groups is needed for the undernourished. By the same token, for those who are overnourished and underactive, the excesses found in their lifestyles and diets should be avoided. Regular and varied physical activity should be part of daily life for all children.

There is a lack of information on many aspects of physical activity and health in the children of the Americas. For example, surveys of habitual physical activity of Latin American children are not available. COPAMEDE requests more research on the many interrelated areas of physical activity, nutrition, and health.

Selected References

1. Executive Committee of the International Conference on Nutrition and Physical Fitness. Declaration of Olympia on nutrition and fitness. *Bulletin of the Panamerican Health Organization.* 27: 90-94, 1993.

2. Haas, J, S Murdoch, J Rivera, and R Martorell. Early nutrition and later physical work capacity. *Nutrition Reviews.* 54: S41-S48, 1996.

3. Kemper, HCG, and H Coudert (eds) Physical health and fitness of Bolivian boys. *International Journal of Sports Medicine.* 15 (Suppl. 2): S71-S114, 1994.

4. Malina, R. Cardiovascular health status of Latin American children and youth. In: *Issues in Pediatric Exercise Science.* C Blimkie and O Bar-Or, Editors. Champaign, Human Kinetics, 1994. p. 191-216.

5. Matsudo, VKR. Measuring nutrition status, physical activity, and fitness with special emphasis on populations at nutritional risk. *Nutrition Reviews.* 54: S79-S96, 1996.

6. de Onis, M, C Monteiro, J Akré, and G Clugston. The worldwide magnitude of protein-energy malnutrition: an overview from the WHO Global Database on Child Growth. *Bulletin of the World Health Organization.* 71: 1-14, 1993.

7. Parízková, J. *Nutrition, Physical Activity, and Health in Early Life.* Boca Raton, CRC Press, 1996. p. 295.

8. Spurr, G. Physical activity and energy expenditure in undernutrition. *Progress in Food and Nutrition Science.* 14: 139-192, 1990.

9. Sallis, JF. (ed.) Physical activity guidelines for adolescents. *Pediatric Exercise Science* 6(4), 1994.

10. U.S. Department of Health and Human Services. *Physical Activity and Health: a Report of the Surgeon General.* Atlanta, GA: Dept. of Health and Human Services, CDC, National Center for Chronic Disease Prevention and Health Promotion, 1996.

A Physically Active Lifestyle—Public Health's Best Buy?

International Federation of Sports Medicine (FIMS)

Web site: www.fims.org

Times have changed. Many people spend most of their working time in the office, sitting behind computer terminals, PCs or laptops. Death is no longer from a monocausal infectious disease, but by multicausal chronic diseases. Lifestyle factors such as smoking, excessive alcohol intake, poor nutrition (for example, too high an intake of dietary fat or an excessive intake of polysaturated fatty acids, or both), and physical inactivity play an important part in the etiology of chronic diseases such as coronary heart disease (CHD), hypercholesterolemia, hypertension, stroke, non-insulin-dependent diabetes mellitus (NIDDM), and certain forms of cancer.

The first three factors are considered "classic" independent risk factors for multicausal chronic disease. The role of physical inactivity as an independent lifestyle risk factor has been the subject of debate and controversy. This debate, however, seems to have come to an end with the publication of consensus statements (1–3) and policy documents (4–6) on the health benefits of a physically active lifestyle.

Not only will the individual person's health benefit from a reduced risk of the chronic diseases mentioned above, but the public health status of a nation will benefit tremendously from a physically active lifestyle. The public health burden of a sedentary lifestyle can be quantified by calculating the population attributable risk (PAR) of such a lifestyle. PAR is an estimate of the proportion of the public health burden caused by a particular risk factor, for example, a sedentary lifestyle. By calculating PAR we may estimate the proportion of deaths from chronic diseases (CHD, NIDDM, cancer, etc.) that would not occur if everyone in a population was sufficiently physically active (7).

To calculate PAR, we need to know the relative risk (as a measure of the strength of the relation between a risk factor and the public health burden) and the prevalence of the risk factor. The "true" relative risk is constant because it is biologically determined and will therefore not change, even though estimates of relative risk may change because of improvements in scientific measurement (7). Consequently, changes in PAR are highly dependent on changes in prevalence and not on changes in relative risk.

Based on available information on both relative mortality risks and prevalence of a sedentary lifestyle, Powell and Blair (7) estimated the PAR of sedentary living for mortality from CHD, colon cancer, and diabetes mellitus to be 35, 32, and 35%, respectively, meaning that 35% of the CHD deaths, 32% of the colon cancer deaths, and 35% of the diabetes mellitus deaths could be theoretically prevented if everyone was vigorously active.

Recently in the Netherlands (8,9) similar PAR calculations were made for chronic disease mortality, not only for a sedentary lifestyle but also for other lifestyle (related) risk factors. These calculations were based on recent population data. For CHD the following PARs were calculated for men and women, respectively: smoking, 42 and 44%; saturated fatty acid intake (exceeding 10% of total energy intake), 13 and 12%; obesity (body mass index > 30), 13 and 15%; and sedentary lifestyle, 40 and 40%.

From these PARs it seems that for CHD mortality the public health burden caused by a sedentary lifestyle is at least of the same magnitude as that caused by smoking, and about three times as great as the public health burden caused by obesity and the excess intake of saturated fatty acids, respectively. From a public health perspective, it may be more appropriate to encourage a physically active lifestyle, second only to restriction of smoking habits, rather than to put emphasis on a further improvement of the dietary habits or on a reduction of body weight.

Stimulating a physically active lifestyle has other related benefits: a physically active lifestyle (i.e., regular exercise) helps to maintain body weight, leads to favorable dietary habits, and leads to a decline in the number of smokers (10). Knowing this, it seems that stimulating a physically active lifestyle is the public health's best buy.

If stimulating a physically active lifestyle is the public health's best buy, the next question is, How do we do that? To answer this question, one has to be aware of the determinants of physical activity behavior. Many models are used to explain health related physical activity behavior. In general these models include three sets of determinants: (1) knowledge and attitude, (2) social influence, and (3) barriers and self-efficacy (11).

Knowledge about, and attitudes toward, a physically active lifestyle seem to be sufficiently present in the general population (10). It therefore seems that stimulating a physically active lifestyle should predominantly be a matter of favorable changing social influence, influencing a person's self-efficacy in a positive way, and breaking down the barriers that keep people from being physically active. Dealing with the variety of physical activity determinants requires different preventative strategies and approaches, varying from mass media educational campaigns to political activism to changing our society's system.

Health care personnel should play an important role in getting more people more active, and in this respect a promising approach—the PACE (Physician-based Assessment and Counseling for Exercise approach)—is thus based on the Stages of Change model (12). This model describes the changes that need to take place for a more physically active lifestyle. The PACE approach aims at overcoming barriers to counsel patients about physical activity behavior for them to become physically more active. In pilot projects, PACE programs have proven to be both feasible (13) and effective (14). From a public health standpoint, further implementations and evaluation of PACE-like projects deserve wide attention within the common (para-) medical practice.

Finally, an argument brought up regularly against promoting physical activity is the risk of injury and the direct and indirect cost to society. But in a recent macroeconomic analysis on information derived from a representative sample of the Dutch population, the health benefits of a physically active lifestyle, in terms of a reduced use of the health care system and a reduction in sick leave from work because of better health, outweigh the negative effects, in terms of cost of medical treatment and sick leave compensation caused by sports injuries sustained (15).

In this study, the positive macroeconomic balance in favor of a physically active lifestyle increases with increasing age. To conclude, no time to waste, everybody should become more active now. It is everyone's concern.

References

1. Anonymous. Exercise for health. WHO/FIMS Committee on Physical Activity for Health. *Bull. World Health Organ.* 1995; 733: 135-6.

2. Pate, RR, Pratt M, Blair SN, Haskell WL, Macera CA, Bouchard C, et al. Physical activity and public health: *A recommendation from the Centers for Disease Control and Prevention and the American College of Sports Medicine. JAMA.* 1995; 273: 402-7.

3. *NIH Consensus Development Panel on Physical Activity and Cardiovascular Health. Physical activity and cardiovascular health. JAMA.* 1996; 276: 241-6.

4. Killoran AJ, Fentem P, Caspersen CJ. *Moving on. International perspectives on promoting physical activity.* London: Health Education Authority, 1994.

5. Anonymous. *Recommendation No. R (95) 17 of the Committee of Ministers to the Member States on the Significance of Sport for Society*. Council of Europe. Strasbourg: CDDS (95) 58, 1995; 8-10.

6. *U.S. Physical activity and health; A report of the surgeon general*. Atlanta, GA: U.S. Dept. of Health and Human Services, National Centers for Disease Control and Prevention, USA, 1996.

7. Powell KE, Blair SN. *The public health burden of sedentary living habits: Theoretical but realistic estimates. Med Sci Sports Exerc* 1994; 26: 851-6.

8. Ruwaard D, Kramers PGN, eds. *Volksgezondheid Toekomst Verkenning*. Den Haag: SDU, 1993.

9. Ruwaard D, Kramers PGN, eds. *Volksgezondheid Toekomst Verkenning 1997. De som der delen*. Utrecht: Elsevier/DE Tijdstroom, 1997.

10. Vuori I, Fentem P. *Health, position paper. In: Vuori I, Fentem P, Svoboda B, Patriksson G, Andreff W, Weber W, eds. The significance of sport for society*. Strasbourg: Council of Europe Press, 1995; 11-90.

11. Van Mechelen W. *Can running injuries be effectively prevented?* Sports Med 1995; 19: 161-5.

12. DiProchaska JO, Markus BH. *The transtheoretical model: Applications to exercise. In: Dishman, RK, ed. Advances in exercise adherence*. Champaign, IL: Human Kinetics, 1994; 161-80.

13. Long BJ, Calfas KJ, Wooten W, Sallis JF, Patrick K, Goldstein M, et al. *A multisite field test of the acceptability of physical activity counseling in primary care. Am J Prev Med* 1996; 12: 73-81.

14. Calfas KJ, Long BJ, Sallis JF, Wooten W, Pratt M, Patrick K. *A controlled trial of physician counseling to promote the adaptation of physical activity. Prev Med* 1996;25: 225-33.

15. Stam PJA, Heldebrandt VH, Backx FJG, Velthuijsen JW. *Sportif bewegen en gezondheidsaspecten: een verkennde studie naar kosten en baten*. Amsterdam: SEO, 1996.

Willem Van Mechelen

Institute for Research in Extramural Medicine and Department of Social Medicine

Faculty of Medicine

Vrije Universiteit

Van der Boechorststraat 7

NL-1081 BT Amsterdam, The Netherlands

1997

Originally published in: *British Journal of Sports Medicine*, 1997; 31:264-265.

CHAPTER

7

Injury Prevention &
Rehabilitation

Prevention

Rehabilitation

Prevention

ATV

All-Terrain Vehicles

American Academy of Orthopaedic Surgeons (AAOS)

Web site: www.aaos.org/wordhtml/papers position/atvs.htm

All-terrain vehicles (ATVs) are three- or four-wheeled motorized vehicles designed primarily for off-the-road use. They have handlebars like a motorcycle, and the rider straddles the body of the vehicle. With large, soft tires, ATVs have a relatively high center of gravity. Some can reach speeds of 50 mph.

Very few states require a license to operate an ATV, most of which are used for recreation. There are no mandatory national safety standards for their construction and only a few states have issued regulations for their use. ATVs are often operated by children, some as young as age five.

ATVs have been involved in an alarming number of injuries and deaths, particularly among young people. Numerous groups have questioned the inherent danger of the design of these vehicles, and in December 1987, the U.S. Consumer Products Safety Commission issued a consent decree with ATV manufacturers. Some of its provisions are: three-wheeled ATVs may no longer be manufactured and new three-wheeled ATVs may not be sold in the United States, and retailers may not sell either three- or four-wheeled ATVs with an engine size greater than 90 cubic centimeters for use by children under age 16.

In light of statistics that show an inordinate number of injuries and deaths resulting from the use of ATVs, the American Academy of Orthopaedic Surgeons considers ATVs to be a significant public health risk.

During the past five years, more than 200 deaths a year related to ATV use have been re-corded. Almost 40 percent of the dead were children 16 years of age or younger; 17 percent were under the age of 12.

From 1984 to 1985, the number of ATV-related injuries treated in hospital emergency departments in the U.S. increased from 63,900 to 85,900. After the Consumer Products Safety Commission consent decree of December 1987, that number dropped to 51,700 injuries treated in 1990 and 51,200 injuries treated in 1991. Almost 40 percent of the injuries were to children under the age of 16.

The American Academy of Orthopaedic Surgeons supports the Consumer Products Safety Commission consent decree issued December 1987 that ends the sale and production of new three-wheeled ATVs in the United States.

The three-wheeled ATV is inherently unstable. When the operator executes a sharp turn at even moderate rates of speed, the high center of gravity of the vehicle, the short wheel base, and the short turning radius combine in many cases to cause the vehicle to turn over. The rider may be thrown from the vehicle or crushed beneath it as it rolls.

Many other risk factors, such as the use of alcohol and the lack of safety equipment, can contribute to accidents on ATVs. However, the basic design of the three-wheeled models make them hazardous to anyone who rides them.

The American Academy of Orthopedic Surgeons supports the Consumer Products Safety Commission consent decree issued December 1987 that ends the sale and production of new three-wheeled ATVs in the United States.

Four-wheel ATVs have some of the same design features as the three-wheel models, including a high center of gravity, short wheelbase, short turning radius and high-powered engine. They are difficult machines to operate, even if somewhat less likely to roll over than the three-wheeled versions. Moreover, as off-the-road vehicles, they are generally used on rough or uneven ground. Uneven surfaces can cause them to turn over, largely due to the high center of gravity. When used on hills, they are capable of flipping over from front to back, as the rear wheels can lift the front wheels off the ground when excessive power is applied. Studies have shown that almost 60 percent of accidents involving four-wheel ATVs result from tipping and overturning. Drivers can be thrown from these ATVs or can be crushed beneath them, just as with three-wheel models. In fact, since the Consumer Product Safety Commission restrictions on three-wheeled ATVs have taken effect, nearly 60 percent of ATV-related deaths have involved four-wheeled ATVs.

Operators should be licensed on the basis of demonstrated competence in handling the vehicle and knowledge of the safety hazards that are presented by driving an ATV. With few laws governing the use of these vehicles, at present, almost anyone of any age or level of skill or training can legally operate an ATV. Although ATVs with a 90 cc or greater engine size may not be sold to or for the use of children under the age of 16, once an ATV has been purchased and taken home it is difficult to prevent small children from driving the ATV. No person should operate such a machine without some demonstration of training, knowledge and maturity.

The minimum age of 16 for operating an ATV on or off the road should be enforced. Children under the age of 12 generally possess neither the body size and strength, nor the motor skills and coordination necessary for the safe handling of an ATV. Children under age 16 generally have not yet developed the perceptual abilities or the judgment required for the safe use of highly powered vehicles. *Operators should be required to wear safety equipment.* While sturdy clothing and leather gloves can help, in a modest way, to prevent or mitigate cuts and abrasions associated with falls from the vehicle, the key piece of safety equipment is a safety helmet that meets standards set for helmets used by motorcycle riders. As with motorcycle riders, the helmet provides the best protection available against death or serious, disabling injury. In 80 percent of the deaths from accidents involving ATVs, the driver was not wearing a helmet.

ATVs should be used only during daylight hours. Most ATVs are marketed and used as off-the-road, recreational vehicles. In the varied terrain in which they are most commonly used, good visibility is required. Riding after dark is especially dangerous because lights attached to a vehicle cannot provide enough properly directed illumination when the vehicle is bouncing or turning.

Only one person at a time should ride an ATV. Adding a passenger to the ATV increases the propensity of the vehicle to tip or turn over, because the passenger, to a significant extent, increases the high center of gravity. In almost a third of ATV accidents (31 percent), more than one person was riding the vehicle.

October 1987; December 1992 (revised)

American Academy of Orthopaedic Surgeons

Document Number: 1101

This material may not be modified without the express written permission of the American Academy of Orthopaedic Surgeons.

For additional information, contact the Public and Media Relations Department, Joanne L. Swanson at (847)384-4142 or email: swanson@aaos.org; or Paula Poda at (847)384-4139 or email: poda@aaos.org.

Motorized Recreational Vehicles

American Academy of
Family Physicians (AAFP)

Web site: www.aafp.org/policy/136.html

The Academy recommends that family physicians become well educated with the potential dangers associated with the use of motorized recreational vehicles (including minibikes, all terrain vehicles, snowmobiles and personal watercraft) and advise patients about their safe use.

1973; 1996
   AAFP Reference Manual

Boxing

Sport of Boxing

American Academy of Family Physicians (AAFP)

Web site: www.aafp.org/policy/8.html

The American Academy of Family Physicians recommends to its members that physicians make greater effort to discourage their patients from participating in the sport of boxing and also recommends communicating to the media their opposition to the sport of boxing.

1984; 1996

AAFP Reference Manual

Participation in Boxing by Children, Adolescents, and Young Adults (RE9703)

American Academy of Pediatrics (AAP), Committee on Sports Medicine and Fitness

Web site: www.aap.org/policy/re9703.html/

ABSTRACT. Because boxing may result in serious brain and eye injuries, the American Academy of Pediatrics opposes this sport. This policy statement summarizes the reasons.

1997

American Academy of Pediatrics

Breakaway Bases

Use of Breakaway Bases in Preventing Recreational Baseball and Softball Injuries

American Academy of Orthopaedic Surgeons (AAOS)

Web site: www.aaos.org/wordhtml/papers position/bases.htm

Softball and baseball are our nation's leading recreational sports, with more than 40 million Americans playing organized softball and another 3 million participating in Little League, high school and college baseball. It is not surprising, therefore, that softball and baseball account for a large number of sports injuries, with softball players being the most frequently hurt. Since many of these injuries are serious enough to require emergency room treatment, the costs for medical care is estimated at more than $2 billion annually. This estimate does not include the hidden costs of lost work time, lower work productivity, restriction of future athletic activity, medical-legal services, permanent impairment and escalating insurance premiums for the injured player, his or her employer, the field owner and the softball or baseball league.

Injuries occur while sliding into bases, these mishaps and their resulting costs could be significantly lowered by installing breakaway bases on all playing fields. A study conducted at the University of Michigan found that using breakaway bases in recreational softball games reduced sliding injuries by 98 percent and associated medical care costs by 99 percent. The federal government has recommended the installation of breakaway bases on playing fields at all military installations and federal prisons.

A traditional stationary base bolted to a metal post and sunk into the ground becomes a rigid obstacle for an athlete to encounter while sliding. In contrast, a breakaway base is snapped onto grommets attached to an anchored rubber mat which holds it in place during normal play. Although it can be dislodged by a sliding runner, the breakaway base is stable and will not detach during normal base running.

The American Academy of Orthopaedic Surgeons believes the deployment of breakaway bases at all levels of baseball and softball could dramatically reduce injuries to athletes and therefore reduce health care costs. The Academy recommends that breakaway bases be installed on all playing fields and further recommends that physicians involved with sports activities around the country actively promote the use of breakaway bases in their local community.

May 1997

American Academy of Orthopaedic Surgeons

Document Number: 1140

For additional information, contact the Public and Media Relations Department, Joanne L. Swanson at (847) 384-4035 or email: swanson@aaos.org; or Paula Poda at (847) 384-4034 or email: poda@aaos.org.

The Role of Breakaway Bases in Preventing Recreational Baseball and Softball Injuries

American Orthopaedic Foot and Ankle Society (AOFAS)

The American Orthopaedic Foot and Ankle Society (AOFAS) believes that the deployment of breakaway bases at all levels of baseball and softball could have a dramatic affect on the health and fitness of athletes and the reduction of health care costs nationally. Therefore, the Society recommends that breakaway bases be installed on all amateur playing fields.

The American Orthopaedic Foot and Ankle Society further recommends that physicians involved with sports activities around the country actively promote the use of breakaway bases in their local communities.

More than 40 million Americans participate in recreational softball leagues. Another three million play Little League, high school and college baseball. Softball and baseball are our nation's leading sports and also the leading cause of all recreational sports injuries.

Most of these injuries occur when players slide into bases. Recreational softball players sustain more than 1.7 million base-sliding injuries a year, 360,000 of them serious enough to require hospital emergency room treatment. Medical treatment for these injuries costs the public $2.1 billion annually. This does not include the costs due to lost work time, lowered work productivity, restriction of future athletic activities, permanent impairment, and escalating insurance premiums for the injured player, his or her employer, the field owner, and the softball or baseball league.

These costs could be virtually eliminated simply by installing breakaway bases on all playing fields. A study conducted at the University of Michigan found that using breakaway bases in recreational softball games reduced sliding injuries by 98 percent and associated health care costs by 99 percent. Another study demonstrated similar results among college and professional athletes that used breakaway bases.*

Breakaway bases work very simply. Seated on grommets attached to anchored rubber mats holding them in place during normal play, they pop off when a player slides into them. They do not detach during routine base running. In contrast, the traditional stationary base, bolted in a metal post sunk into the ground, is a rigid, fixed base that takes five times as much force to dislodge as a breakaway base.

Breakaway bases have been shown to be highly effective in reducing injury, have a negligible effect on how the game is played and do not rely on the judgement or skill of players, coaches or umpires to achieve their effectiveness. Given the economic costs and personal inconvenience and suffering caused by stationary bases, it is hard to justify their continued use at any level of amateur play. For that reason, the federal government has recommended the installation of breakaway bases on playing fields at all military installations and federal prisons. A resolution being introduced to Congress calls for breakaway bases to be installed on all federal playing fields. The American Orthopaedic Foot and Ankle Society supports these measures and recommends that these efforts be expanded to all amateur playing fields across the country.

Recreational softball and baseball are the nations most popular sports. Given the high direct and indirect cost in health care dollars, lost work time, and pain and physical impairment resulting from these injuries, a cost-effective solution to prevent them would be of significant benefit to society as a whole.

Collision Sports

Collision Sports

American Academy of Family Physicians (AAFP)

www.aafp.org/policy/138

The American Academy of Family Physicians recommends that family physicians become well educated with the risks of all collision sports (boxing, football, hockey, lacrosse, etc.) and fully advise patients regarding the risks of these competitive activities.

1990; 1996

AAFP Reference Manual

Eye Protection

Eye Injuries and Eye Protection in Sports

International Federation of Sports Medicine (FIMS)

Web site: www.fims.org/state.html

The International Federation of Sports Medicine (FIMS) calls attention to the fact that, while injuries in sports can be relatively frequent, they are almost completely preventable. Loss of sight, even in one eye, involves changes in lifestyle for the individual and serious financial and social consequences both for the individual and for society as a whole. It is imperative that sport eye injury risk be reduced to as low a level as possible by enforcement of existing safety rules or by rules changes, where applicable. All athletes should be prescribed eye protectors where appropriate to the sport. Sports can be classified on the basis of low risk, high risk, and extremely high risk for eye injury. Most sports that pose risk for unprotected eyes can be made quite safe with the use of appropriate protective devices. Eye examination and counseling should play an important part in the screening physical examination for every athlete prior to sports participation. The athlete deserves a careful explanation of the risk of eye injury, both with and without various types of eye protectors in the proposed sport. Athletes who are functionally one-eyed must have their status diagnosed and appropriate eye protection prescribed. Glass lenses, ordinary plastic lenses, and open (lensless) eyeguards do not provide adequate protection for those involved in active sports. In many situations, their use can increase the risk for and the severity of eye injury. As contact lenses do not protect the athlete from serious eye injury, they should only be worn in combination with recommended sport eye protectors.

Eye Injury Risk in Sports

Eye injury risk is almost totally related to the particular type of sport. Low risk sports do not involve a thrown or hit ball, a bat or a stick, or close aggressive play with body contact. Examples include track and field, swimming, gymnastics, and rowing. Sports with high risk of eye injury (when protective devices are not being worn) involve a high speed ball (or puck), the use of a bat or stick, close aggressive play with intentional or unintentional body contact and collision, or a combination of these factors. Examples include hockey (ice, field, and street), the racket sports (racquetball, squash, tennis, badminton), lacrosse (men's and women's), handball, baseball, basketball, football (U.S., Canadian, Australian), soccer, and volleyball. The incidence of serious eye injury in these spots is a source of great concern, but adequate eye protective devices are available. Sports involving extremely high risk for eye injury are the combative sports such as boxing and full-contact karate for which effective eye protective devices are not available. The functionally one-eyed athlete should be strongly advised against participation in such sports.

Other Risk Factors

It is suspected but not yet proven that risk for eye injury may also be related to physical development, skill level, and existing visual impairment. It is believed that a beginner is more prone to injuries than are intermediate or advanced players because beginners have not yet learned or refined the necessary skills to master the sport. However, in such sports as hockey, squash, and racquetball, highly skilled athletes play a faster game with more aggressiveness and, thus, may be subject to higher eye injury risk than other participants. Any eye condition that could be made worse if the eye were to be struck places that athlete at increased risk of serious eye injury. Athletes with retinal degenerations, thin schlera, prior eye surgery (including cataract surgery, retinal detachment surgery, and radial keratotomy), prior serious eye injury, or eye disease should seek consultation with an ophthalmologist before participating in a sport.

The Functionally One-Eyed Athlete

Sports participants with one good eye are at particular risk since a serious injury to the good eye could leave the person with a severe visual handicap or permanently blind. Any person with good vision in only one eye should consult with an ophthalmologist on whether or not to participate in a particular sport. If a decision is made to participate, then the person should wear maximum protection for the particular sport for all practice sessions and for competition. A person is functionally one-eyed when loss of the better eye would result in a significant change in lifestyle due to poorer vision in the remaining eye. There is no question that a person with 6/60 (20/200) or poorer best-corrected vision in one eye is functionally one-eyed since loss of the good eye would result in legal or total blindness, with its attendant burden both to the individual and society. One the other hand, ophthalmologists believe that most persons with one eye function quite well with 6/12 (20/40) or better vision in that eye. Every athlete who tests less than 6/12 (20/40) with glasses, if worn, on the screening examination should be evaluated by an optometrist or an ophthalmologist to determine if the subnormal vision is simply due to a change in refraction. If the best-corrected vision in either eye is less than 6/12 (20/40) after refraction, ophthalmological evaluation to obtain a definitive diagnosis of the visual deficit is indicated. If the athlete is functionally one-eyed, the potential serious, long-term consequences of injury to the better eye should be discussed in detail.

Eye Protectors

Most eye (and face) injuries could be prevented or, at least, the effects of such injuries minimized by using protective eyewear. Normal "streetwear" eyeglass frames with 2 mm polycarbonate lenses give adequate, cosmetically acceptable protection for routine use by active people. Such protective glasses are recommended for daily wear by the visually impaired or functionally one-eyed athlete. They are also satisfactory for athletes in competition who wear eyeglasses and participate in low risk sports. Molded polycarbonate frames and lenses (plano/non-prescription protective eyewear) are suggested for contact lens wearers and athletes who ordinarily do not wear glasses but participate in moderate to high-risk, non-contact sports (e.g., racket sports, baseball, basketball). In high risk contact or collision sports, they can be used in combination with a face mask or helmet with face protection for additional protection. Such protective glasses are recommended to the functionally one-eyed athlete who does not require prescription protective eyewear in the good eye to be used in combination with a facemask and helmet for higher risk contact sports. Face masks or helmets with face protection are required for use in the high-risk contact or collision sports (e.g., ice hockey, U.S. football). The facemask may consist of metal wire, coated wire, or a transparent polycarbonate shield. When protective eyewear has been employed in racket sports and face protection devices employed in hockey, eye injuries have been eliminated.

Routine Examination

General practitioners providing medical screening for athletes should have facilities for vision testing and basic eye examination at their disposal and be aware of both the basic principles of eye protection ins sports and the available protective eyewear. It is recommended that athletes have their vision tested and eyes examined on a regular basis. Vision or eye problems are best corrected by an eye care specialist when detected early. An examination also offers an opportunity to discuss any sports vision needs and the most appropriate type of protective eyewear.

Fluids

Exercise and Fluid Replacement

American College of Sports Medicine (ACSM)
Web site: www.acsm.org

Summary

American College of Sports Medicine. Position Stand on Exercise and Fluid Replacement. *Med. Sci. Sports Exerc.*, Vol. 28, No. 1, pp. i-vii, 1996. It is the position of the American College of Sports Medicine that adequate fluid replacement helps maintain hydration and, therefore, promotes the health, safety, and optimal physical performance of individuals participating in regular physical activity. This position statement is based on a comprehensive review and interpretation of scientific literature concerning the influence of fluid replacement on exercise performance and the risk of thermal injury associated with dehydration and hyperthermia. Based on available evidence, the American College of Sports Medicine makes the following general recommendations on the amount and composition of fluid that should be ingested in preparation for, during, and after exercise or athletic competition: 1) It is recommended that individuals consume a nutritionally balanced diet and drink adequate fluids during the 24-h period before an event, especially during the period that includes the meal prior to exercise, to promote proper hydration before exercise or competition. 2) It is recommended that individuals drink about 500 ml (about 17 ounces) of fluid about 2 h before exercise to promote adequate hydration and allow time for excretion of excess ingested water. 3) During exercise, athletes should start drinking early and at regular intervals in an attempt to consume fluids at a rate sufficient to replace all the water lost through sweating (i.e., body weight loss), or consume the maximal amount that can be tolerated. 4) It is recommended that ingested fluids be cooler than ambient temperature [between 15° and 22°C (59° and 72°F)] and flavored to enhance palatability and promote fluid replacement. Fluids should be readily available and served in containers that allow adequate volumes to be ingested with ease and with minimal interruption of exercise. 5) Addition of proper amounts of carbohydrates and/or electrolytes to a fluid replacement solution is recommended for exercise events of duration greater than 1 h since it does not significantly impair water delivery to the body and may enhance performance. During exercise lasting less than 1 h, there is little evidence of physiological or physical performance differences between consuming a carbohydrate-electrolyte drink and plain water. 6) During intense exercise lasting longer than 1 h, it is recommended that carbohydrates be ingested at a rate of 30-60 g · h-1 to maintain oxidation of carbohydrates and delay fatigue. This rate of carbohydrate intake can be achieved without compromising fluid delivery by drinking 600-1200 ml · h-1 of solutions containing 4%-8% carbohydrates (g · 100 ml-1). The carbohydrates can be sugars (glucose or sucrose) or starch (e.g., maltodextrin). 7) Inclusion of sodium (0.5-0.7 g · l-1 of water) in the rehydration solution ingested during exercise lasting longer than 1 h is recommended since it may be advantageous in enhancing palatability, promoting fluid retention, and possibly preventing hyponatremia in certain individuals who drink excessive quantities of fluid. There is little physiological basis for the presence of sodium in an oral rehydration solution for enhancing intestinal water absorption as long as sodium is sufficiently available from the previous meal.

January 1996

Med. Sci. Sports Exerc. Vol.28, No. 1, pp i-vii, 1996.

American College of Sports Medicine

Helmet Use

Helmet Use by Motorcycle Drivers and Passengers, and Bicyclists

American Academy of Orthopaedic Surgeons (AAOS)

Web site: www.aaos.org/wordhtml/papers
position/mhelmet.htm

The American Academy of Orthopaedic Surgeons endorses laws mandating the use of helmets by motorcycle drivers and passengers, and bicyclists.

Orthopaedic surgeons, the medical specialists most often called upon to treat injuries to motorcyclists, believe a significant reduction in fatalities and head injuries could be effected through the implementation of laws mandating the use of helmets by all motorcycle and bicycle drivers and passengers. The American Academy of Orthopaedic Surgeons strongly endorses such mandatory helmet laws.

Numerous studies in various parts of the United States have shown that helmet use reduces the severity and cost associated with injuries to motorcycle riders. Federal efforts beginning with the Highway Safety Act of 1966 achieved the passage of state laws mandating helmet use and by 1975, 47 states had enacted such laws. With the Highway Safety Act of 1977, however, Section 208 of which relaxed the pressure on states to have helmet laws, the federal government created the opportunity to measure the effectiveness of helmet use when 27 states repealed their helmet laws in the following three years.

In 1991, the U.S. Congress attached a provision to its federal highway legislation dictating that states lacking mandatory comprehensive motorcycle helmet laws after September 30, 1993 will have 1.5 percent of their federal highway construction funds for the following fiscal year reallocated to safety programs. If a state still does not have the mandatory laws in place by September 30, 1994, the safety program re-

allocation will rise to 3 percent. In the mid-1980s, Congress used a similar provision to force all states to raise their legal drinking age to 21. Congressional opponents of the bill have attempted to introduce other legislation that would repeal this provision.

Objective analysis of data from the mid-1970s (when helmet laws were widespread) and the late 70s (when more than half the states had repealed such laws) shows clearly that head injuries and fatalities of motorcycle riders are reduced when motorcyclists wear helmets. Moreover, the costs associated with treating motorcycle riders head injuries have been demonstrated to be significantly reduced—up to 80 percent in one university study—when helmet laws are in effect.

The American Academy of Orthopaedic Surgeons believes that issues of personal freedom should be seen in the context of the fact that the public at large incurs a major part of the cost for injuries to motorcycle riders.

The repeal of helmet laws in many states was based on issues involving some motorcyclists' claims that mandatory use laws infringed on their right to personal freedom. While it can be argued that the states' laws mandating that motorcyclists be licensed to operate the vehicle are a similar infringement, the more important issue is the cost borne by society when a motorcyclist is injured in an accident. Numerous studies have shown that in cases involving motorcyclists who were not wearing helmets, head injuries were more severe, requiring longer, more expensive hospitalization and rehabilitation. Moreover, it has been shown that the public at large bears a major portion of these increased costs, both in the cases where the injured patients' insurance does not cover all the costs associated with care and through the increasing cost of medical insurance premiums. Society must evaluate the claim of infringement on freedom versus the funding of these costs.

The American Academy of Orthopaedic Surgeons believes that the current diversity of state helmet laws provides too little protection for motorcycle riders and for society at large.

Currently, 25 states have comprehensive motorcycle helmet laws in place requiring helmet use by all riders. Another 25 require helmet use for certain riders, usually these under age 18. Three states—Illinois, Iowa, and Colorado—have no helmet requirements at all. With federal statistics showing that a motorcycle driver or passenger is twice as likely to receive a head injury in an accident if he or she is not wearing a helmet, such inconsistencies in state laws seem an egregious lack of responsibility by the legislatures in many states.

The American Academy of Orthopaedic Surgeons believes that mandatory helmet laws should be expanded to cover bicyclists as well as motorcycle riders.

In the past several years, thousands of Americans of all ages have taken up bicycling for fun, health and fitness benefits, and as a mode of transportation. With this increase in popularity, however, has come an increase in bicycle-related injury and death. In 1997, 813 bicyclists were killed, 75 percent of those are in collisions between bicycles and motor vehicles. In addition, more than 57,860 bicycle-related injuries were treated in 1997.

Too few bicycle enthusiasts protect themselves from injury with safety helmets. Three-fourths of bicycle-related deaths and one-third of the injuries involve injury to the head or face. Although studies show that bicycle helmets can reduce head injuries by up to 95 percent, the U.S. Centers for Disease Control and Prevention reports that fewer than 10 percent of all cyclists wear protective helmets, and fewer than 2 percent of those under the age of 15 wear them.

Because one-third of bicycle-related deaths and two-thirds of the injuries involve children under the age of 15, most bicycle safety programs in the United States have been targeted at children. Fifteen states and several more counties currently require the use of bicycle helmets, generally for children under age 16. There are two national safety standards for bicycle helmets sold in this country. Only helmets labeled as meeting the safety requirements of the Snell Memorial Foundation of the American National Standards Institute (ANSI) should be purchased and worn. Bicycle safety programs must also focus on wearing the proper clothing, proper maintenance of the bicycle, and understanding and following the rules of the road.

1981; 1996 (revised)

AAFP Reference Manual

Document Number: 1110

For additional information, contact Public and Media Relations Department, Joanne L. Swanson at (847) 384-4142 or email: swanson@aaos.org; or Paula Poda at (847) 384-4139 or email: poda@aaos.org

Bicycle Helmets

International Federation of Sports Medicine (FIMS)

Web site: www.fims.org/state.html

Bicycles are owned by 1 in 10 people and are involved in more accidents per kilometer than any other vehicle excluding motorcycles (1). In a study by Begg et al., 57 of 848 cyclists reported 62 (6.7%) accidents with 40 (4.7%) injuries (2). In an earlier paper by Kilburz et al., accidents, defined in a broader sense, were reported by 46% of 492 cyclists with 9% requiring hospitalization and 23% having lost days from work (3). In total, the bicycle injury rate is 163 per population of 100,000. Forty-two of these are head injuries, the most serious bicycle related injury (4,1).

Head injuries in children are most frequently caused by bicycles and, according to various authors, result in 70 to 90% of bicycle related deaths (6,7,8) and 50% of significant injuries (9). Only 20% of bicycle injuries involve the head, but these account for 70% of bicycle related hospitalizations (5,7,13). The frequency of bicycle accidents is greatest in the 13 to 16 year old age group and 40% of bicycle deaths occur between the ages of 3 and 14 (14,15). Ninety percent of the fatalities involve a motor vehicle; 50% take place at an intersection (11).

Helmet use plays a significant role in reducing the severity of trauma to the head, particularly when those approved by SNELL (Snell Memorial Foundation), CSA (Canadian Standards Association), or ASI (American National Standards Institute) are worm (5). A study by Benz et al. showed that in a 1.5 meter fall, forces acting on the head were reduced fivefold from 547-1078 g to 122209 g with the use of a helmet (10). Another report states that, at 15 kilometers per hour, the energy absorbed by the head is lessened by 90% if a helmet is worn (5). Helmet use has been shown to reduce the Injury Severity Score (ISS) from 18 to 3.8; serious head injury from 47 to 5.2%; mortality from 60 to 0.9%; the occurrence of head injury by 85 to 95% (1,13,14); brain injury by 88% (13); skull fractures from 11 to 1%; soft tissue facial injuries from 18 to 5% (5,15).

While literature is inconsistent, reports by various authorities clearly reflect the positive impact of helmet use on prevention. These describe decreases in injury rates ranging from 39 to 90% (1,11,16,17). As well, reductions of 86% in loss of consciousness (17), 40% in fatalities, 20% in total injuries (18), and a protection factor of 3.25 (11% versus 4% head injuries) (10) are reported.

These estimates support observations that a bicycle helmet was not worn by any child who sustained a head injury (5,9) or died (5) as a result of a head injury. Cooke et al. report that, in Western Australia, helmets reduced deaths by eight-fold (20). It appears that a cyclist traveling on a hard surface at 25 kilometers per hour will be protected from head injury by a standard helmet (21). The overall effect of bicycle helmets has been compared to that of a car seat belt (22,23). Consequently, various authorities recommend regular use of helmets by cyclists of all ages (5,24,25).

Compliance with bicycle helmet use can be improved through education and legislation. Increases ranging from 8 to 13% (26) and 5 to 62% (27) have been attributed to campaigns in education and the media. Education has been most successful in elementary schools, resulting in a 70% compliance rate (28). Other factors affecting helmet use include subsidization of helmet costs (29,31,32) and cultural influences (33). The history of previous injury did not affect compliance (30). Several references in recent literature describing the various aspects of public campaigns and education report that 20 to 73% of the populations studied eventually used helmets (26,27,28,29,31,32,33, 34,35,36,37). Two such campaigns resulted in limited, 8 to 43% (26), or no effect on compliance (29,33). Legislation has been the strongest influence, credited with increases ranging from 47% to 90% (28,31,38).

Summary and Conclusions

Bicycle helmets reduce the incidence of head, face, and brain injuries. Both educational campaigns and legislation have improved child, adolescent, and adult compliance, but legislation is more effective. It is important that bicycle helmet education and legislation be promoted by all health care providers.

October 1996

This statement may be reproduced and distributed with the sole requirement that it be identified clearly as a Position Statement of the International Federation of Sports Medicine.

Motorcycle and Bicycle Helmet Laws

American Academy of Family Physicians (AAFP)

Web site: www.aafp.org/policy/136.html

The American Academy of Family Physicians endorses the concept of legislative measures to require the use of helmets when riding or driving a motorcycle or bicycle, and the AAFP urges constituent chapters to support the enactment of or preservation of state motorcycle and bicycle helmet laws.

1981; 1996
AAFP Reference Manual

Mandatory Use of Bicycle Helmets

Canadian Association of Sports Medicine (CASM)

Background

Bicycles have been widely used for fitness, recreation and as a means of transportation for over a century. While the benefits of cycling from the health and environmental perspective is well recognized, each year in Canada there are between 100 and 130 bicycle deaths, and an estimated 50,000 injuries requiring medical attention. As a result, there has been increasing attention paid to cycling injuries and bicycle safety issues. While it is recognized that this is a multi-faceted problem, the Canadian Academy of Sport Medicine has formulated this position paper to examine the role of bicycle helmets in injury prevention, and provide information for the medical practitioner and public supporting the mandatory use of bicycle helmets.

Recommendations

The Canadian Academy of Sport Medicine position regarding bicycle helmet use includes:

1. That all Provincial and Territorial governments be encouraged to enact legislation mandating that bicyclists wear helmets

2. That physicians providing medical coverage, require the use of bicycle helmets at all activities involving the use of bicycles

3. The Canadian Academy of Sport Medicine recommends only ANSI, CSA or SNELL approved helmets

4. The Canadian Academy of Sport Medicine supports programs to promote bicycle helmet usage and affordability

Epidemiology

The danger of the injury posed by bicycling is related to the relative instability of bicycles and bicyclists, exposure to motor vehicles, and a hard road surface, and inexperience of both bicyclists and motorists. As a result of the mechanics of bicycle design, bicycle riders are actually in greater danger of significant head injury than motor cyclists, a group that has been targeted in the past for head injury prevention through the use of helmet legislation. Head injuries account for 70% of the cases of hospitalization from cycling injuries, although they account for only 20% of the total injuries. Wearing an approved bicycle helmet reduces the risk of head injury by 85% and brain injury by 88%. Head injuries are the major cause of death in 70 to 80% of all bicycle related deaths, and cycling is the single most common cause of head injuries in children. Bicycles must be regarded as a transportation vehicle, with all the risks of sharing the road as multi-vehicle crashes, (car to bicycle) represent 90% of the fatal bicycle crashes.

The bicycle death rate rises rapidly from about 5 years of age, and is highest in the 13 to 16 year old group. Forty percent of the deaths from cycling occur in the 5 to 14 year old group. Deaths are not the only serious outcome of unprotected bicycling head injuries. Those who survive with brain injuries may suffer from epilepsy, permanent intellectual and memory impairment, and personality changes.

In a review from Calgary, none of the patients sustaining cerebral trauma were wearing helmets. In a similar study from Florida, none of the patients who died from a head injury were wearing a helmet. An estimated 50 deaths and 6,000 injuries a year could be prevented in Canada if helmets were worn by all cyclists.

Helmet wearers also experience significantly fewer facial soft tissue injuries (5% versus 18%), and have a lower incidence of serious injuries to the midface, nose, eye and orbit.

Helmet Standards

Accepted standards for helmets include ANSI (American National Standards Institute), SNELL (Snell Memorial Foundation), and CSA (Canadian Standards Association). At speeds of 15 kilometres per hour (a common cycling speed), helmets meeting these safety standards have a capability to reduce the energy absorbed by the skull by over 90%. Despite the ample evidence to support the use of helmets, relatively few bicyclists utilize them. Figures vary from as low as 2% of elementary and secondary school children to 30% of the adult population.

Changing Behaviour

Educational campaigns to promote helmet usage have resulted in only modest increases in usage. Physician counseling resulted in no significant increase in helmet purchase when compared to a control group. Even multi-discipline, intensive promotion at a community level resulted in modest increases in helmet ownership, but no observed change in helmet use. An additional study from Virginia demonstrated that the increased use in helmet usage following an intensive multi-discipline promotional campaign was transient, and neighbourhood helmet use rates fell to nearly zero (baseline values) shortly after the program.

By comparison, the beneficial effects of bicycle helmet legislation, in addition to an education program, has been well demonstrated. In the Maryland experience, helmet use rates increased from 5% to 47% post helmet law. In Victoria, Australia, legislation resulted in substantial increases in helmet use rates, rising to between the 70% and 90% level. Preliminary data has also shown that the number of bicyclists with head injuries has also dropped in the period since legislation came into effect.

There are many reasons why cyclists do not use helmets, including inadequate knowledge about the need and effectiveness of helmets, price, comfort and convenience. In children in particular, peer pressure is cited as the most common reason why helmets are not worn. Children obviously need particular direction, but adults remain important role models. In addition to all of the safety reasons outlined, this is an important reason why policy must be directed at all bicycle users.

References

1. Traffic Injury Research Foundation, Ottawa. Halpern, J.S. Bicycle Helmets for Children. *J. Emerg Nurs*. 1990; 16:36-40.

2. McDermott, F.T., Klug, G.L. Head Injury Predominance: Pedal-cyclists vs Motor-cyclists. *Med. J. Aust*. 1985; 143(6): 232-34.

3. Thompson, R.S., Rivers, F.P., et al. A. Case-Control Study of the Effectiveness of Bicycle Safety Helmets. *New Eng J Med*. 1980; 320:1361-67.

4. Ivan, L.P., Choo, S.H., Ventureyra, E.C. Head Injuries in Childhood: A Two Year Survey. *Can Med Assoc Journal* 1983; 128:281-84.

5. Facts, 1991 Edition. Arlington, VA: *Insurance Institute for Highway Safety*; 1991.

6. Accident Facts, National Safety Council, Chicago 1982: 45-91.

7. Guichon, D.M.P., Myles, T.S. Bicycle Injuries: One Year Sample in Calgary. *J. Trauma*. 1975: 15:504-06.

8. Weiss, B.D. Preventing Bicycle-Related Head Injuries. *N.W. State Med. J* 1987; 87(6):310-20.

9. Wasserman, R.C., Buccini, R.V. Helmet Protection from Head Injuries Among Recreational Bicyclists. *The Am J Sports Med*. vol 18, No. 1990: 96-7.

10. Thompson, D.C., Thompson, Rivara, F.P., Wolf, M.E. A Case-Control Study of the Effectiveness of Bicycle Safety Helmets in Preventing Facial Injury. *Am J Public Health*, 1990; 80:1471-1471.

11. Mills, N.J., Protective Capability of Bicycle Helmets, *Br J Sports Med*. 1990; 24:55-60.

12. Cushman, R.A., Down, J., MacMillan, N., Waclawik, H. Bicycle Helmet Use in Ottawa. *Can Fam Physician*. 1990; 36:697-700.

13. Weiss, D.B., Bicycle Helmet Use by Children. *Pediatrics*. 1986; 77:677-679.

14. DiGuiseppi, C.G., Rivara, F.P., Koepsell, T.D. et al: Bicycle Helmet Use by Children: Evaluation of a Community-Wide Helmet Campaign. *JAMA* 1989; 262:2256-61.

15. Cushman, R., Down, J., MacMillan, N., Waclawik, H. Helmet Promotion in the Emergency Room Following a Bicycle Injury: A Randomized Trial. *Pediatrics* 1991; 88:43-47.

16. Towner, P., Marve, M.K. A School-Based Intervention to Increase the Use of Bicycle Helmets. *Fam Med* 1992; 24:156-8.

17. Winn, G.L., Jones, D.F., Bonk, C.J. Taking it to the Street, Helmet Use and Bicycle Safety as Components of Inner-City Youth Development. *Clinical Pediatrics*. Nov. 1992. 672-677.

18. Vulcan, A.P., Cameron, M.H., Watson, W.L. Mandatory Bicycle Helmet Use: Experience in Victoria, Australia. *World J. Surg*. 1992 16:389-397.

19. Cote, T.R., Sacks, J.J., Lambert-Huber, D.A., Dannenberg, A.L. Kresnow, M., Lipsitz, C.M., Schmidt, E.R. Bicycle Helmet Use Among Maryland Children: Effect of Legislation and Education Pediatrics 1992; 89:1216-1220.

In-line Skates

Protective Equipment Policy for In-Line Skating and Skate Boards

American Academy of Family Physicians (AAFP)

www.aafp.org/policy/136

The American Academy of Family Physicians supports the use of protective equipment while using in-line skates and skateboards. Protective equipment *to include, but not be limited to, safety helmets, elbow and knee pads, and wrist braces.*

1995

AAFP Reference Manual

In-Line Skating

International Federation of Sports Medicine (FIMS)

Web site: www.fims.org

The number of people participating in in-line skating in Canada and the United States exceeds 24 million. [12] In 1995 over 100,000 skaters sustained injuries requiring emergency room care. [12] While fractures of the distal radius are the most common ranging in frequency from 25% to 75%, [3,7,9,10,12] a 2%-12.8% incidence of head injuries [1,6,7,10] as well as the occurrence of severe lower extremity injuries [3,8] has been reported. A study of 61 children who fell while in-line skating reported that 1 in 8 sustained a fracture during the first attempt at the sport. [9]

It is becoming increasingly evident that an appreciable proportion of in-line skating injuries are in fact severe. In a comparison of data obtained from the Canadian Hospital Injury Reporting and Prevention Program Database concerning sport related injuries in children, a significantly greater number of fractures (55% versus 21%) and upper extremity injuries occurred in in-line skating than in other sports. Compared to the database overall, in-line skaters sustained more serious injuries and required more extensive care. [5] A London, Canada survey showed that major injuries occurred in almost one-half of the patients presenting to the emergency department with in-line skating injuries. Seventy one percent of these involved the upper extremity and 79% were fractures requiring an average of 2.7 follow-up visits and 3.9 radiographs. These injuries resulted in significant functional impairment as measured by the Functional Independence Mean as well as significant amounts of time lost from work and participation in sports. [11]

The broad accessibility of in-line skating with the subsequent rapid growth in participation makes prevention of injuries a particularly difficult challenge for health care professionals. Risk factors include easily achievable high speeds, difficult stopping techniques, and the hazards presented by the public pathways or roads that in-line skaters share with pedestrians, cyclists and motor vehicles.

Most studies recommend the use of protective equipment and report that it is underused.

[1,3,6,8-10,12,13] One study reports 4 cases of open forearm fractures associated with the use of wrist splints. [2] Protective equipment alone is not a guaranteed injury measure prevention. The importance of instruction for beginner skaters is pointed out. [4,6] Loss of control is identified as a major factor contributing to injury. [4,5]

The following recommendations are suggested based on the Canadian Academy of Sports Medicine (CASM[14]), The American Academy of Orthopedic Surgeons (AAOS[15]), and other available information:

1. Wear complete protective gear.
2. Learn the basics.
3. Anticipate hazards.
4. Avoid, if possible, public roads and obey road rules if you must use public ways.
5. Skate in safe areas and under good conditions.
6. Do not skate while being towed.
7. Make sure to use highly visible clothing and use fluorescent clothing and illumination in the dark.

References

1. Adams SL, Wyte CD, Paradise MS, delCastillo J. A prospective study of in-line skating: observational series and survey of active in-line skaters...injuries, protective equipment, and training. *Acad. Emerg Med* 1996; 3:303-311.

2. Cheng SL, Rajaratnam K, Raskin KB, Hu RW, Axlerod TS. "Splint-top" fracture of the forearm: a description of an in-line skating injury associated with the use of protective wrist splints. *J. Trauma* 1995; 39: 1194-1197.

3. Eingartner C, Jockheck M, Krackhardt T, Weise K. Injuries due to in-line skating. *Sporverletzung Sporschaden* 1997; 11:48-51.

4. Ellis JA, Keirulf JC, Klassen TP. Injuries associated with in-line skating from the Canadian hospitals injury reporting and prevention program database. *Can J Public Health* 1998; 86: 133-136.

5. Frankowvich R, Petrella R, Stewart M, Osman T. In-line skating injury patterns and protective equipment use. Presented at Sport Med '96, January 1996, Toronto.

6. Jaffe MS, Dijkers MP, Zametis M. A population-based survey of in-line skaters. *Arch Phys Med Rehabil* 1997; 78: 1352-1357.

7. Majetschak M, Kock HJ, Neudeck F, Schmit-Neuerburg KP. Causation and injury pattern in in-line skating. *Unfallchirurg* 1997; 23: 171-178.

8. Malanga GA, Smith HM. Lower extremity injuries in in-line skaters. *J Sports Med Phys Fitness* 1996; 36: 304-311.

9. Mitts KG, Hennrikus WL. In-line skating fractures in children. *J Pediatr Orthop* 1996; 15: 640-643.

10. Powell EC, Tanz RR. In-line skate and rollerskate injuries in childhood. *Pediat Emerg Care* 1996; 12:259-262.

11. Rampersaud R, King G. In-line skating injury survey. Presented at the 25th Clinical Seminar in Orthopaedic Surgery, London Ontario, May 1997

12. Scheiber RA, Branche-Dorsey CM, Ryan Gw, Rutherford GW, Stevens JA, O'Neil J. Risk factors for injuries from in-line skating and the effectiveness of safety gear. *New Eng J Med* 1996; 335: 1630-1635.

13. Williams-Avery RM, MacKinnon DP. Injuries and the use of protective equipment among college in-line skaters. *Accid Anal Prev* 1998; 28: 779-784.

14. Position Statement, 1997. Canadian Academy of Sport Medicine, 1600 James Naismith Drive, Suite 502, Gloucester Ontario, KIB 5N4 CANADA.

15. Position statement, 1995. American Academy of Orthopaedic Surgeons. 300 North River Road Rosemont, IL 60018-4262, USA.

Injuries from In-Line Skating

American Academy of Orthopaedic Surgeons (AAOS)

Web site: www.aaos.org/wordhtml/papers
position/inline.htm

The American Academy of Orthopaedic Surgeons believes that the public should be informed of the dangers and injuries that can occur in the recreational sport called in-line skating and strongly urges proper precautions to prevent and minimize those injuries.

More than 26 million Americans have taken up the new sport of in-line skating, which combines roller skating with ice skating by aligning rollers in the shape of a single blade. In-line skaters may easily reach speeds of more than 25 mph. Whether skating fast or standing still, many in-line skaters have sustained injuries that are preventable.

The number of injuries due to in-line skating is rapidly increasing. Hospitals, clinics, ambulatory surgery centers and doctors offices reported 269,194 in-line skating injuries in 1997. More than 35% of these injuries were a fracture or dislocation, 25% were injuries of the wrist, and nearly 5% were injuries of the head. Although head injuries are relatively less common, they can be life threatening, very expensive, and cause long-term disability. The estimated yearly cost of medical treatment due to in-line skating injuries is $4.8 billion. This does not include bruises and scrapes that were never seen or treated.

To reduce the risk of serious injury, the American Academy of Orthopaedic Surgeons strongly urges in-line skaters to follow these safety measures:

- learn the basic skills of the sport **particularly how to stop properly**, before venturing into vehicular or pedestrian traffic

- wear a helmet, wrist protectors, and knee and elbow pads
- always put on protective gear before putting on your skates
- perform warm-up exercises before and after skating
- obey traffic signals, stay at the right side of the road and don't weave in and out of lanes
- avoid skating in crowded walkways

Skate boots must fit properly to avoid irritation. The following tips should be considered.

- Don't buy boots that put too much pressure on any area of your foot; the pressure can cause blisters.
- Choose the boot size at the end of the day or after training, when feet will be at their largest.
- When selecting the size of the boot, wear the same type of sock that will be worn when skating.
- Kick both feet into the back of the boots before buckling and skating.
- Be certain the heel doesn't move up and down in the boot during skating.

February 1995; December 1998 (revised)

American Academy of Orthopaedic Surgeons

Document No. 1127

In-line Skating Injuries in Children and Adolescents (RE9739)

American Academy of Pediatrics (AAP), Committee on Injury and Poison Prevention and Committee on Sports Medicine and Fitness

Web site: www.aap.org/policy/re9739.html

ABSTRACT. In-line skating has become one of the fastest-growing recreational sports in the United States. Recent studies emphasize the value of protective gear in reducing the incidence of injuries. Recommendations are provided for parents and pediatricians, with special emphasis on the novice or inexperienced skater.

© April 1998

American Academy of Pediatrics

April 1998, pp 720-722

In-Line Skating

Canadian Academy of Sport Medicine (CASM)

The Canadian Academy of Sport Medicine (CASM) has concerns about injuries and safety in in-line skating. The CASM's recommendations for safe in-line skating are based on the current limited scientific literature, experience from groups involved in in-line skating and knowledge of safety issues in similar sporting activities.

Recommendations

1. Wear complete protective gear

The CASM recommends the use of a regulation helmet, (ANSI, CSA, or SNELL), wrist guards, knee pads and elbow pads. Equipment should fit properly and be secured in place before each excursion). Protective equipment is most effective when ALL the gear is worn together.

2. Learn the basics.

The CASM recommends that an individual must learn proper in-line skating techniques. When beginning to take up the sport, take the time to learn how to stop and maintain balance while skating. Practice in a flat area free from obstacles and vehicles. Avoid hills until you feel comfortable controlling your speed and have learned to stop effectively.

3. Anticipate hazards.

Be alert for pedestrians, vehicles, and cyclists. Look for obstacles on the ground like uneven pavement and tree branches. Proceed with caution if a potential hazard is identified especially going downhill and approaching blind corners.

4. Obey the rules of the road.

Traffic signals should be adhered to and signs posted in parks should be followed. This is especially important in crowded areas.

5. Skate in safe areas under good conditions.

Skate in parks, playgrounds, and roller rinks. Avoid wet conditions and always skate during daylight hours.

6. Do not skate while being towed.

It is dangerous to be pulled by cars, bicycles or pets. Excessive speeds are generated which can not be easily controlled. The risk of injury and the severity of the injury increases when vehicles are involved.

For More Information

For further information on in-line skating issues or to obtain a copy of supporting documentation, please contact:
Telephone: 613-748-5851
Fax: 613-748-5792
Unit 14 - 1010 Polytek Street Gloucester, Ont. K1B 5N4

Specific Information about the Position Statement on In-Line Skatine: Dr. Jamie Kissick General Information about CASM: Ms. Jacqueline Burke Webmaster (for Web Page suggestions): ishrier@med.mcgill.ca

Mouth Protection

A Properly Fitted Mouthguard

Academy for Sports Dentistry

"A mouthguard is a resilient device or appliance placed inside the mouth (or inside and outside) to reduce mouth injuries particularly to the teeth and surrounding structures." (ASTM) For the optimal safety and wellbeing of athletes competing in the 21st Century, the Academy for Sports Dentistry has adopted the position that the single word "mouthguard" must be replaced by the term "a properly fitted mouthguard."

The criteria for the fabrication or adaptation of "a properly fitted mouthguard" must include the following considerations:

1. Pertinent Medical History
2. Dental Status
   a. Dental Caries
   b. Periodontal Status
   c. Developmental Occlusion
   d. Orthodontic or Prosthodontic Appliances
   e. Congenital/Pathological Conditions
   f. Jaw Relationship
3. Demographic Factors

With these considerations, knowledgeable persons in the field of sports dentistry should advise the athlete and/or parents of the special design for the "properly fitted mouthguard" and the individual. A fitting of a mouthguard is best accomplished under the supervision or direction of a dentist. The end product should have the properties that include:

1. Adequate thickness in all areas to provide for the reduction of impact forces.
2. A fit that is retentive and not dislodged on impact.
3. Speech considerations equal to the demands of the playing status of the athlete.
4. A material that meets the FDA approval (1).
5. Preferably a wearing length of time equal to one season of play.

References

1. NCAA Football Rules and Interpretations

December 1998

Approved by the Academy of Sports Dentistry Board of Directors

Mouthguard Mandates

Academy for Sports Dentistry

The Academy for Sports Dentistry recommends the use of a properly fitted mouthguard; encourages the use of a custom-fabricated mouthguard made over a dental cast and delivered under the supervision of a dentist; and supports a mandate for use of a properly-fitted mouthguard in all collision and contact sports.

When considering the enactment of mandatory mouthguard regulations, one should consider the following items:

Education
Timing
Manpower
Cost
Liability

January 1999

See ASD Newsletter Vol 14, #3, Pg. 7-8, Jan 1999

Sledding

Sledding Safety

> **American Academy of Orthopaedic Surgeons (AAOS)**
>
> Web site: www.aaos.org/wordhtml/papers position/sledding.htm

Every year, thousands of youths and adults are injured sledding down hills in city parks, streets and resort areas. In 1995, hospital emergency rooms treated 54,727 injuries related to sleds, toboggans, and inflated or plastic tubes and disks used in sledding, according to the National Electronic Injury Surveillance System of the U.S. Consumer Product Safety Commission. The medical, legal, insurance costs were $365 million. Half of all emergency visits were for injuries to arms and legs; 17 percent, spine; 15 percent, head; and 11 percent facial injuries.

Two-thirds of the injuries were sustained by youths age 14 and younger. Younger children have proportionally larger heads and higher centers of gravity than do older children and adolescents. When the injuries to youths and young adults age 15-24 are included, the 0-24 age group accounts for 85 percent of the total injuries and more than 80 percent of the total cost. From 1991 through 1995, there were 250,361 injuries related to sledding treated in hospital emergency rooms. The economic impact was $1.79 billion.

The American Academy of Orthopaedic Surgeons recommends the following safety guidelines to improve sledding safety:

Essential

- Sled only in designated areas free of fixed objects such as trees, posts and fences.

- Children in these areas must be supervised by parents or adults.

- All participants must sit in a forward-facing position, steering with their feet or a rope tied to the steering handles of the sled. No one should sled head-first down a slope.

- Do not sled on slopes that end in a street, drop off, parking lot, river or pond.

Preferred

- Children under 12 years old should sled wearing a helmet.

- Wear layers of clothing for protection from injuries.

- Do not sit/slide on plastic sheets or other materials that can be pierced by objects on the ground.

- Use a sled with runners and a steering mechanism, which is safer than toboggans or snow disks.

- Sled in well-lighted areas when choosing evening activities.

For additional information, contact the Public and Media Relations Department, Joanne L. Swanson at (847) 384-4142 or email: swanson@aaos.org; or Paula Poda at (847) 384-4139 or email: poda@aaos.org.

Soccer

Injuries in Youth Soccer:
A Subject Review (RE9934)

American Academy of Pediatrics
(AAP), Committee on Sports Medicine

Web site: www.aap.org/policy/re9934.html

ABSTRACT. The current literature on injuries in youth soccer, known as football worldwide, has been reviewed to assess the frequency, type, and causes of injuries in this sport. The information in this review serves as a basis for encouraging safe participation in soccer for children and adolescents.

© March 2000

American Academy of Pediatrics

Volume 105, Number 3, pp 659-661

Swimming

Infant Swimming Programs

> ### American Academy of Pediatrics (AAP), Committee on Sports Medicine
> Web site: www.aap.org/policy/re9940.html

ABSTRACT. Infant and toddler aquatic programs provide an opportunity to introduce young children to the joy and risks of being in or around water. Generally, children are not developmentally ready for swimming lessons until after their fourth birthday. Aquatic programs for infants and toddlers have not been shown to decrease the risk of drowning, and parents should not feel secure that their child is safe in water or safe from drowning after participating in such programs. Young children should receive constant, close supervision by an adult while in and around water.

April 2000

American Academy of Pediatrics

Volume 105, Number 4, pp 868-870

Residential Pool Safety

> ### American Academy of Family Physicians (AAFP)
> Web site: www.aafp.org/policy/136.html

The American Academy of Family Physicians supports residential pool safety measures including the following:

1. Permanent perimeter protection of pool by an approved safeguard to limit or delay access of children to the pool. Approved safeguards may include but are not limited to: fencing with self-closing and self-latching gates, stand alone walls; building walls; screen enclosures, natural topography or an approved pool safety cover. Where a building wall serves as a barrier, all doors and windows with direct access to the pool shall have approved locks, alarms or other devices to limit or delay access to the pool.

2. Training of household adults, older children and other adult supervisors in CPR.

3. Telephone access pool side with visible emergency numbers.

4. Constant adult supervision of young children at all times. Reliance on a child's water safety classes or floatation device provides a false sense of security and is not a substitute for adult supervision.

1989; 1995 (revised)

AAFP Reference Manual

Trampoline

Trampolines and Trampoline Safety

American Academy of Orthopaedic Surgeons (AAOS)

Web site: www.aaos.org/wordhtml/papers
position/trampoli.htm

The number and severity of injuries resulting from the use of trampolines is significant and increasing. Hospital emergency rooms treated 52,103 trampoline injuries sustained by children under age 15 in 1995. The estimated cost of medical, legal, insurance and disability costs and other expenses in 1995 was $272.6 million. Even very young children ages 5 to 9 are at risk; 19,454 injuries related to trampolines were treated in emergency rooms at a cost of $99.8 million. The most common injuries are sprains and fractures, often severe, which usually result from a fall through the trampoline or an uncontrolled maneuver. Although severe or life-threatening injuries are not common, they do occur and can result in paralysis or, rarely, death. Use of the trampoline by more than one child further increases the risk of injury through collisions among jumpers or the catapulting of jumpers off the trampoline.

In an effort to reduce the number and severity of injuries resulting from the use of trampolines, the American Academy of Orthopaedic Surgeons recommends routine observation of the following guidelines:

- Use of trampolines for physical education, competitive gymnastics, diving training and other similar activities requires careful adult supervision and proper safety measures.

- Trampolines should not be used for unsupervised recreational activity.

- Competent adult supervision and instruction is needed for children at all times.

- Only one participant should use a trampoline at any time.

- Spotters should be present when participants are jumping.

- Somersaults or high risk maneuvers should be avoided without proper supervision and instruction; these maneuvers should be done only with proper use of protective equipment, such as a harness.

- The trampoline jumping surface should be placed at ground level.

- The supporting bars, strings and surrounding landing surfaces should have adequate protective padding.

For additional information, contact the Public and Media Relations Department, Joanne L. Swanson at (847) 384-4035 or email: swanson@aaos.org; or Paula Poda at (847) 384-4034 or email: poda@aaos.org.

Trampolines at Home, School, and Recreational Centers (RE9844)

American Academy of Pediatrics (AAP), Committee on Injury and Poison Prevention and Committee on Sports Medicine and Fitness

Web site: www.aap.org/policy/re9844.html

ABSTRACT. The latest available data indicate that an estimated 83 400 trampoline-related injuries occurred in 1996 in the United States. This represents an annual rate 140% higher than was reported in 1990. Most injuries were sustained on home trampolines. In addition, 30% of trampoline-related injuries treated in an emergency department were fractures often resulting in hospitalization and surgery. These data support the American Academy of Pediatrics' reaffirmation of its recommendation that trampolines should never be used in the home environment, in routine physical education classes, or in outdoor playgrounds. Design and behavioral recommendations are made for the limited use of trampolines in supervised training programs.

May 1999

American Academy of Pediatrics

Pediatrics, Vol. 103, No. 5, p. 1053-1056

Underwater Diving

Breath-hold Underwater Diving

YMCA of the USA Medical Advisory Committee

The practice of extended breath-hold underwater diving has become a popular competitive event, but has significant dangers associated with it, including brain damage and death. Individuals who perform this activity competitively train themselves to resist the urge to breathe to see how far they can swim underwater while holding their breath. This activity is not a safe practice in YMCA aquatic programs. To increase awareness and safety within YMCA aquatic facilities and programs, the Medical Advisory Committee of the YMCA of the USA recommends the following safety precautions and recommendations:

1. YMCAs should prohibit extended underwater breath-hold diving. For training purposes in programs such as swim teams and skin/scuba diving, under the direct supervision of a coach or instructor, moderate underwater breath-hold swimming that is normal and reasonable is permissable.

2. Under no circumstances should a YMCA allow the practice of "static apnea" (motionless underwater or face-down on the surface and holding one's breath). This activity is performed to see how long one can hold his or her breath. Due to the extreme physiological danger of latent anoxia (blackout), this activity should be prohibited.

3. Hyperventilation (more than four rapid inhalations and exhalations) prior to underwater swimming can be dangerous and should be discouraged.

4. At no time should even moderate underwater breath-hold swimming, snorkeling or skin diving occur without the direct, uninterrupted supervision of a coach, instructor or swimming partner. Extended underwater breath-hold diving is not recommended at any time.

November 1999

Disclaimer: These recommendations were developed by the YMCA of the USA Medical Advisory Committee for the exclusive use by YMCAs in United States. As they were developed with the specific needs of the YMCAs in mind, they may not be applicable to other organizations. These recommendations are consistent with the mission and values of the YMCA.

Youth Baseball

Youth Baseball

American Academy of Orthopaedic Surgeons (AAOS)

Web site: www.aaos.org/wordhtml/papers position/throw.htm

The American Academy of Orthopaedic Surgeons believes that parents should be informed about the risks and injuries which occur in youth baseball as a result of excessive throwing, and strongly urges compliance with the recommendations for throwing restriction in youth baseball to minimize such injuries.

More than 4.6 million children in the United States play youth baseball under the supervision of adult coaches, administrators and parents. More than 30 years ago, physicians recognized the risk to the upper extremity, particularly the shoulder and elbow, in the growing child. These significant risks include pain which limits activity, loss of motion and strength, damage to the growth centers of the shoulder and elbow, and other X-ray changes that may be permanent.

A number of studies have documented 20 percent of children eight to 12 years of age and 45 percent of those 13 to 14 years of age will have arm pain during a single youth baseball season. Documentation of these injuries resulted in the institution of rules by youth baseball in the United States which control the number of innings pitched by an individual player. These rules allow the player to pitch from four to 10 innings per week as a maximum. In spite of these rules, there are growing concerns that parents and coaches avoid these restrictions by allowing children to play on multiple teams or in multiple leagues.

The American Academy of Orthopaedic Surgeons recommends the following safety guidelines to decrease the risk of injury to the upper extremity in the growing athlete who participates in youth baseball:

- Follow the guidelines about the number of innings pitched as specified by the individual's baseball association (a maximum of four to 10 innings a week) not by the number of teams played on.

- While there is no concrete guideline for the number of pitches allowed, a reasonable approach is to count the number of pitches thrown and use 80 to 100 pitches as a maximum in a game, and 30 to 40 pitches in a practice.

- Any persistent pain, loss of motion (especially extension) or documented X-ray abnormalities should disqualify a child from playing until these findings abate or are clarified by a physician.

- Coaches and players in youth baseball should be taught proper throwing technique.

- Coaches should educate players to the importance of and techniques for stretching and strengthening the upper extremity.

For additional information, contact the Public and Media Relations Department, Joanne L. Swanson at (847) 384-4035 or email: swanson@aaos.org; or Paula Poda at (847) 384-4034 or email: poda@aaos.org.

Rehabilitation

Family Physicians

Family Physician's Role

> **American Academy of Family Physicians (AAFP)**
>
> www.aafp.org

Broad knowledge and experience uniquely qualify the family physician to practice sports medicine. Preparticipation assessment, team physician function, and the diagnosis and treatment of exercise-related injuries are best incorporated into comprehensive medical management of the total person. Family physicians recognize that a program of regular exercise contributes to good health and a patient's sense of well-being.

1988; 1994 (revised)
  AAFP Reference Manual

Family Physician as Team Physician

> **American Academy of Family Physicians (AAFP)**
>
> www.aafp.org

Family practice training and experience, with broad medical, psychosocial and management skills in the delivery and coordination of medical services, make the family physician uniquely qualified to care for the athlete and the team.

1988; 1995 (revised)
  AAFP Reference Manual

Heel Surgery

Endoscopic and Open Heel Surgery

American Orthopaedic Foot and Ankle Society (AOFAS)

Web site: www.aofas.org/endoscopic.htm

1. Nonsurgical treatment is recommended for a minimum of 6 months and preferably 12 months.

2. More than 90% of patients respond to nonsurgical treatment within 6 to 10 months.

3. When surgery is considered in the remaining patients, then a medical evaluation should be considered prior to surgery.

4. Patients should be advised of complications and risks if an endoscopic or open procedure is not indicated.

5. If nerve compression is coexistent with fascial or bone pain, then an endoscopic or open procedure should not be attempted.

6. The AOFAS does not recommend surgical procedures before nonoperative methods have been utilized.

7. The AOFAS does support responsible, carefully planned surgical intervention when nonsurgical treatment fails and work-up is complete.

8. The AOFAS supports cost constraints in the treatment of heel pain when the outcome is not altered.

9. The AOFAS recommends heel padding, medications and stretching prior to prescribing custom orthoses, and extended physical therapy.

10. This position statement is intended as a guide to the orthopaedist and is not intended to dictate a treatment plan.

Knee Braces

The Use of Knee Braces

American Academy of Orthopaedic Surgeons (AAOS)

Web site: www.aaos.org/wordhtml/papers position/kneebr.htm

Orthopaedists are the medical specialists most often called upon to diagnose and treat injuries to the knee joint. Through the American Academy of Orthopaedic Surgeons, orthopaedists have undertaken the continuing review of the effectiveness of knee braces in the prevention and treatment of knee injuries. The Academy's goal has been to provide physicians and others in the medical community with an informed assessment of the state of the art of knee bracing and to provide guidance to physicians and others in the use of knee braces.

The Academy's 1984 *Knee Braces Seminar* Report classified existing knee braces into three groups:

- **prophylactic knee braces** which are designed to prevent or reduce the severity of knee injuries

- **rehabilitative knee braces** which are designed to allow protected motion of injured knees or knees that have been treated operatively

- **functional knee braces** which are designed to provide stability for the unstable knee.

The 1984 seminar has been followed by continuing examination of the developments in knee bracing and of the published literature in the field. Based on this examination by individual physicians, faculty at continuing medical education programs and by relevant Academy committees, the Academy has adopted the following statement.

AAOS believes that the routine use of prophylactic knee braces currently available has not been proven effective in reducing the number or severity of knee injuries. In some circumstances, such braces may even have the potential to be a contributing factor to injury.

Because knee injuries are common in many sports, particularly contact sports such as football, there is a widespread concern about their impact on players and teams. Non-contact stresses in many other sports also can produce significant knee injuries. Tears of the ligaments and menisci and damage to the articular cartilage of the knee may result in lost playing time and may lead to permanent disability. Most players, coaches, athletic trainers and physicians would welcome a device such as a brace that would reduce the incidence and/or the severity of injuries to the knee. Current prophylactic knee braces are intended to, and may mistakenly be believed, to meet those goals.

Scientific studies undertaken to demonstrate the effectiveness of prophylactic knee braces in reducing the frequency and severity of knee injuries have failed to show consistent findings regarding the braces that are currently available. Moreover, few studies in this field have included objective data collected over a significant period of time. Injuries to the medial collateral ligament have been the most studied, and no consistent reduction in these injuries attributable to the use of a particular brace has been demonstrated. No reduction in injuries to the anterior evidence that the use of a prophylactic knee brace on a "normal" knee in an athletic situation cruciate ligament or the menisci have been demonstrated. In some studies there has been actually increased the severity of certain injuries.

AAOS believes that to require players to use knee braces "just in case they might help," is not sup-

ported by the studies that have examined the effectiveness of such braces.

The intent of this statement is not to argue that prophylactic knee braces do not work and never will. Instead it is to state that medical science has not demonstrated that, as currently constructed and used, they are effective today. There is no credible, long-term, scientifically conducted study that supports using knee braces on otherwise healthy players. The Academy is concerned that significant amounts of money are being expended in schools in the United States for equipment that is, at best, only hoped to be effective in reducing the frequency or severity of knee injuries.

In regard to other categories of braces, AAOS believes that rehabilitative knee braces and functional knee braces can be effective in many treatment programs, and that this efficacy has been demonstrated by long-term scientifically conducted studies.

Types of braces other than prophylactic knee braces have different structural designs and have been developed to help treat specific problems stemming from injury or disease. *Rehabilitative knee braces* have been designed to provide a compromise between protection and motion. That is, they allow the knee to move, but within specific limits, which has been shown to be beneficial to the injured knee. Rehabilitative knee braces generally are more effective in protecting against excessive flexion and extension than in protecting against anterior and posterior motion.

Functional knee braces aid in the control of unstable knees. Studies have shown that some of the currently available braces are very effective in controlling abnormal motions under low load conditions but not under high loading conditions that occur during many athletic activities. Most studies designed to test whether functional knee braces protect against the knee "giving way" have demonstrated some beneficial effect of the brace. However, the patient and the physician must guard against a false sense of security evoked by the use of such a brace; bio-mechanical studies show that functional knee braces do not restore normal knee stability under high forces related to certain activities. However, when it is properly fitted, used in conjunction with a knee rehabilitation program, and the patient modifies his or her activities appropriately, a functional knee brace can provide an important adjunct in the treatment of knee instability.

October 1997

American Academy of Orthopaedic Surgeons

Document Number: 1124

This material may not be modified without the express written permission of the American Academy of Orthopaedic Surgeons.

For additional information, contact the Public and Media Relations Department, Joanne L. Swanson at (847) 384-4142 or email: swanson@aaos.org; or Paula Poda at (847) 384-4139 or email: poda@aaos.org

Massage Therapy

Massage Therapy in YMCAs

YMCA of the USA Medical Advisory Committee

Massage therapy spans a wide variety of therapeutic approaches which work to improve an individual's health and well-being through the manipulation of muscles and other soft tissues of the body. Massage therapy is designed to enhance blood flow to soft tissues and facilitate the removal of metabolic wastes from muscle tissue. For many, massage has the added benefits of reducing mental stress and reducing anxiety levels.

Therapeutic massage methods used today have both Eastern and Western origins. Early records of massage date back 3,000 years to early Chinese folk medicine and ancient medicine of India. Shiatsu acupressure and reflexology techniques evolved from these Eastern sources, as have other contemporary massage methods. Modem Western massage is credited primarily to a 19th century Swedish approach of hands-on techniques with active movements which became known as Swedish massage, one of the most commonly used methods today.

The growing emphasis on wellness in the United States has led to a growth in the massage therapy profession. Some health insurance plans have begun to provide coverage for massage therapy for patients. While massage services have been offered in YMCAs for many years, recently there has been an increase in the availability of traditional health salon spa services, those relaxing amenities which includes massage therapy. Following are guidelines for YMCAs offering massage therapy services:

1. YMCAs offering massage programs and services should employ a professionally trained and certified massage therapist to provide such amenities. YMCAs should check their state and local health department codes to insure compliance with requirements concerning the licensure of massage therapists (licensing is required in most states).

2. YMCAs offering massage services should make every effort to provide massage programs that meet the personal interests and needs of members.

3. YMCAs offering massage should have a registration system available at a membership control area for massage appointments and payment.

4. The massage area should have a minimum of 120 square feet of floor space and should be suitably equipped with massage tables, towels and massage supplies, proper lighting, and a sink.

5. Massage tables should have the following features:

   - Adjustable height (24-34 inches)
   - Width of at least 30 inches
   - Adjustable face cradle
   - Double padding under double-stitched vinyl
   - Cervical pillows and lumbar rolls

6. To insure adequate illumination, the massage room should have a lighting system that can adjust levels from 0 foot-candles to 30 to 50 foot-candles at the surface of the floor. Ideally this system should use indirect lighting sources.

7. Appropriate temperature, humidity, and air circulation levels should be maintained in the massage area. The following levels are recommended:

   - Temperature: 72 to 78 degrees Fahrenheit

- Humidity: 60 percent or less
- Air circulation: 6 to 8 exchanges per hour

A qualified massage therapist should either be nationally certified or be able to document professional training in massage therapy at an accredited institution. The American Massage Therapy Association (AMTA) is an organization of massage therapists who have demonstrated a level of skill and expertise through testing and/or education. All AMTA members agree to abide by the organization's Code of Ethics. For more information, contact the AMTA at (847) 864-0123.

October 1998

Disclaimer: These recommendations were developed by the YMCA of the USA Medical Advisory Committee for the exclusive use by YMCAs in United States. As they were developed with the specific needs of the YMCAs in mind, they may not be applicable to other organizations. These recommendations are consistent with the mission and values of the YMCA.

CHAPTER

8

Medicine

Body Composition

Bioelectrical Impedance Analysis by YMCAs

YMCA of the USA Medical Advisory Committee

Bioelectrical impedance analysis (BIA) is a widely used method for estimating body composition. The technology is relatively simple, quick, and noninvasive. BIA is currently used in diverse settings, including private clinicians' offices, health clubs, and hospitals, and across a spectrum of ages, body weights, and disease states. Despite a general public perception that BIA measures "body fat", the technology actually determines the electrical impedance of body tissues, which provides an estimate of total body water. Using the estimated values of total body water derived from BIA, one can then estimate fat-free mass and body fat.

Bioelectrical impedance analysis measure the opposition of body tissues to the flow of a small (less than I mA) alternating current. Many equations are available to estimate total body water and fat-free mass as of function of impedance, weight, height, gender, and age. In actual use, however, BIA calculations of an individual's body fat may vary by as much as 10 per cent of body weight because of differences in machines and methodologies used. Equations and their variables differ, as does the choice of a reference method.[1]

The attractiveness and marketability of BIA is its speed (about 3 minutes per subject), its ease of operation, and its self-explanatory computer printouts. Participant compliance with suggestions to improve health is boosted by the "printout mystique," the belief that computers are infallible. The provider's image may also benefit by association with this very visible high-tech equipment.

However, the output of a computer is no more accurate than its input. In the case of BIA, as the assumptions and formulas used in the computer program have not been proven to be valid, many of the parameters printed out may have a poor relationship to what was measured. The validity and reliability of BIA continues to be studied.

The National Institutes of Health (NIH) held a Technology Assessment Conference on December 12-14, 1994, titled "Bioelectrical Impedance Analysis in Body Composition Measurement", with 33 national experts in the field presenting current data on this topic. The statement from this conference has the following conclusions:

- Bioelectrical impedance analysis provides a reliable estimate of total body water under most conditions. Subsequent estimation of fat-free mass and the percentage of body fat vary in validity depending on the population or individual studied and on the applicability of the prediction equation used to estimate these parameters of body composition.

- Bioelectrical impedance analysis can be a useful technique for body composition analysis in healthy individuals and in those with a number of chronic conditions such as mild-to-moderate obesity, diabetes mellitus, and other medical conditions in which major disturbances of water distribution are not prominent.

- The ability of bioelectrical impedance analysis to accurately predict adiposity in severely obese individuals is limited. In addition, bioelectrical impedance analysis is not useful in measuring short-term changes in body composition (i.e., in response to diet or exercise) among individuals.

- Bioelectrical impedance analysis values are affected by numerous variables including body position, hydration status (amount of water in the body), consumption of food and beverages, ambient air and skin temperature, recent physical activity, and conductance of the examining table. Reliable bioelectrical impedance analysis requires standardization and control of these variables.

• A systematic evaluation of some safety considerations is warranted, especially as related to implanted defibrillators.

• A specific, well-defined procedure for performing routine bioelectrical impedance analysis measurements is not practiced. Therefore, the NIH panel recommended that a committee of appropriate scientific experts and instrument manufacturers be formed with the goal of setting instrument standards and procedural methods.

• Further research is recommended by the NIH in bioelectrical impedance analysis, the basic science of impedance measurements, determinations of intra- and extracellular water, and correlations with clinical outcome in specific patient populations.

The YMCA of the USA Medical Advisory Committee agrees with these conclusions, and acknowledges that bioelectrical impedance analysis can be reasonably reliable with proper equipment, procedures, and interpretation of results. BIA appears to fall within the same range of accuracy as other methods of estimating body composition, such as skinfolds, infrared technology, and body mass index. YMCAs are encouraged to consider the relative cost of BIA compared to these other methods, and may wish to wait for standardization of the BIA industry prior to purchasing and using this equipment.

The YMCA of the USA Medical Advisory Committee awaits the results of further research on this issue and the publishing of industry standards before giving a final recommendation on its use in YMCAS.

November 1988; October 1995 (revised)

Disclaimer: These recommendations were developed by the YMCA of the USA Medical Advisory Committee for the exclusive use by YMCAs in United States. As they were developed with the specific needs of the YMCAs in mind, they may not be applicable to other organizations. These recommendations are consistent with the mission and values of the YMCA.

Chronic Obstructive Pulmonary Disease (COPD)

Ventilatory muscle training in patients with chronic obstructive pulmonary disease (COPD)

International Federation of Sports Medicine (FIMS)

Web site: www.fims.org

Respiratory reserve does not affect the ability of healthy individuals to exercise unless there are loads of very high intensity. [1,2] However, respiratory reserve does become a factor that limits physical activity if there is a deterioration in lung function with age or disease. [3] In patients with COPD, decreased pulmonary function and respiratory reserve lead to a sedentary lifestyle, inactivity and eventual deconditioning of the musculoskeletal and cardiovascular systems. [2,4]

Dyspnea experienced by almost all patients with COPD, is the main cause of inactivity. Pulmonary function is impeded by increased respiratory load, [5,6] ineffective ventilatory muscle function, [5,6,7,8] geometrical changes in the lungs associated with hyperinflation and incomplete emptying with each respiratory cycle, and increased in pressure to overcome intrinsic positive pressure and expiratory pressure. [6] The prolonged use of corticosteroids in COPD patients induces a catabolic process and an eventual deterioration in ventilatory muscle function, strength and endurance. [9,17,18]

Respiratory muscle training improves respiratory muscle strength and endurance in healthy individuals [10] and ventilatory capacity in quadriplegic patients, [11] those with neuromuscular disease [12], and in cardiac patients treated prophylactically prior to open heart surgery. [13]

Decreased respiratory reserve in patients with COPD places them at a high risk for serious complications, frequent exacerbations of lung disease that may be compounded by bacterial or viral infractions or inflammation, [14] allergic reactions, [15] excessive secretions, [14] cor pulmonale [14] and surgery and/or trauma. [16]

The benefits of respiratory muscle training are well-documented. Belman and Mittman [19] were the first to demonstrate that ventilatory muscle training enhances ventilatory muscle strength, endurance and exercise capacity in patients with COPD.

Their observations were subsequently confirmed by many other investigators. [19, 20] Goldstein et al. [21] and Reis et al [22] clearly demonstrated a reduction in symptoms of dyspnea and fatigue after a respiratory exercise program. Other studies have demonstrated that respiratory muscle training is a successful adjunct to protocols used to wean patients form mechanical ventilation. [23,24, 25]

The various ventilatory training methods have been used:

1. resistive breathing training. [11]
2. isocapneic hyperventilation. [10, 20]
3. threshold pressure training. [27]

In addition to preventing exacerbations in patients with COPD, ventilatory muscle training has been show to be advantageous as prophylactic pre-operative treatment. [13] There have been good results shown with respiratory rehabilitation programs of mild to moderate intensity. [26]

Based on this information it is recommended that:

1. ventilatory muscle training be routinely incorporated into respiratory rehabilitation programs.
2. ventilatory muscle training be a primary component in the management of all stages of COPD.

References

1. Bye PT, Esau SA, Wally KR, Macleton PT, Pardy RL: Ventilatory Muscles During Exercise in Air and Oxygen in Normal Men; *J Appl Physiol*; 56:464-471, 1984.

2. Jones N, Campbell MEJ, Edwards HT, Robertson DG: *Clinical Exercise Testing*; pp. 21-40, WB Saunders, Philadelphia, 1975.

3. Jones N, Campbell MEJ, Edwards HT, Robertson DG: *Clinical Exercise Testing*; pp. 125-129, WB Saunders, Philadelphia, 1975.

4. Wasserman K, Whipp BJ: Exercise Physiology in Health and Disease; *Amer Rev Resp Dis*; 112: 219-249, 1975.

5. Pengeli LD, Rebuck AS, Campbell MEJ: *Loaded Breathing*; pp. 14-90, Churchill Livingston, 1974.

6. Rochester DF, Brain NM: Determinants of Maximal Respiratory Pressure in Chronic Obstructive Pulmonary Disease; *Am Rev Resp Dis*; 132:42-47, 1976.

7. Arora MS, Rochester DF: COPD and Human Diaphragm Muscle Dimensions; *Chest*; 91:719-724, 1987.

8. Belmore F, Grassino A: Force Reserve of the Diaphragm in Patients with COPD; *J Appl Physiol*; 15:8-15, 1983.

9. Weiner P, Azgad X, Weinner M, Ganen R: Inspiratory Muscle Training Combined with General Exercise in Patients with COPD; *Chest*; 102: 1351-1356, 1992.

10. Leith DE, Bradley ME: Ventilatory Muscle Strength and Endurance Training; *J Appl Physiol*; 41: 508-516, 1976.

11. Gross D, Ladd H, Riely E, Macklem P, Grassino A: The Effect of Training on Strength and Endurance on the Diaphragm in Quadriplegics; *Amer Journ Med*; 66: 27-35, 1980.

12. Gross D, Meiner Z: The Effect of Ventilatory Muscle Training on Respiratory Function and Capacity in Ambulatory and Bed Ridden Patients with Neuromuscle Diseases; *Monaldi Archives Chest Disease*; 48: 322-326, 1993.

13. Gross D, Applebaum A: Respiratory Muscle Training in Health and Disease; eds Grassimo A, Rampulla C, Ambrossimo N, Fracchia C; *Current Topics in Rehabilitation: Chronic Pulmonary Hyperinflation*; Springer Verlag, New York, pp. 160-169, 1991.

14. Burrows B: Airways Obstructive Disease: Pathogenetic Mechanisms and Natural Histories of the Disorders; *Med Clin North Amer*; 74: 547-559, 1990.

15. Verdal S: Outdoor Air Pollution and Obstructive Airway Disease; *Europ Respir Rev*; 5: 323-326, 1995.

16. Latumer RG, Dickman M, Day WC, Cann MC, Schmidt DC: Ventilatory Pattern and Pulmonary Complication After Upper Abdominal Surgery Determined by Pre-operation and Post-operation Computerized Spirometry and Blood Gas Analysis; *Amer Journal Surg*; 122: 622-623, 1972.

17. Weiner P, Asgad Y, Weiner N: The effect of Corticosteroid on Respiratory Muscle Performance in Humans; *Chest*; 104:1788-91, 1993.

18. Nisa M, Walshow M, Eans JS, Pearson MG, Cavely PMA: Assessment of Reversibility of Airway Obstruction in Patients with Chronic Obstructive Airway Disease; *Thorax*; 45:190-194, 1990.

19. Belman M, Wittman O: Ventilatory Muscle Training Improves Exercise Capacity in Chronic Obstructive Pulmonary Disease Patients; *Amer Rev Resp Dis*; 121: 273-280, 1980.

20. Pardy RL, Rivington RN, Depas PJ, Macklem PT: The Effect of Aspiratory Muscle Training on Exercise Gas Performance and Chronic Airflow Limitation; *Amer Rev Resp Dis*; 123: 426-433, 1981.

21. Godestein RS, Gort EH, Stubbing D, Avendano MA, Guyatt GH: Randomized Controlled Trial of Respiratory Rehabilitation; *Lancet*; 344:1394-1397, 1994.

22. Reis AL, kaplan RM, Limberg TM, Prewit LM: Effects of Rehabilitation on Physiological and Psychological Outcomes in Patients with Chronic Obstructive Pulmonary Disease. *Ann Int Med*; 122: 823-832, 1995.

23. Aldrich TK, Karpel JP, Uhlass RM, Sparupani MA, Eramo D, Ferranti R: Weaning from mechanical ventilation: Adjunctive use of inspiratory muscle resistive training. *Crit Care Med*; 17: 143-174, 1989.

24. Gross D, Shenkman Z, Krieger D: The effect of resistive breathing training in a weaning protocol for very difficult patients. *Europ Respir J*, 7:1908, 1994.

25. Belman MJ: Respiratory failure treated by ventilatory muscle training (VMT): A report of two cases. *Eur J Resp Dis*; 62:391-395, 1981.

26. Lonsdorfer J, Lambert E, Mettauer B, Hoppler H, Schnedecker B, Clotte J, Geny B, Haberey P: Exercise, hyperventilation and fatigue in heart transplant. *Eur Respir Rev*; 5:18-23, 1995.

27. Flynn MG, Baxter CE, Nosworthy JC, Prett JJ, Rochford PD, Peirce RJ: Threshold Pressure Training, Breathing Pattern and Exercise Performance in Chronic Airflow Obstruction; *Chest*; 95: 535-540, 1989.

The Scientific Commission acknowledges the contribution of Dr. Ditza Gross, Sorosky Medical Center, Tel Aviv, Israel.

Coronary Artery Disease

Exercise for Patients with Coronary Artery Disease

American College of Sports Medicine

Web site: www.ascm.org

Summary

Exercise training improves functional capacity and reduces clinical symptoms in patients with coronary artery disease. However, such patients are at increased risk for cardiovascular complications during exercise; therefore, appropriate safeguards should be employed to minimize these risks. Based on the documented benefits and risks of exercise for patients with coronary artery disease, it is the position of the American College of Sports Medicine that most patients with coronary artery disease should engage in individually designed exercise programs to achieve optimal physical and emotional health.

1994

"Exercise for Patients With Coronary Artery Disease." *Med. Sci. Sports Exerc.*, Vol. 26, No. 3, pp. i-v, 1994.

Diabetes Mellitus

Diabetes Mellitus and Exercise

International Federation of Sports Medicine (FIMS)

Web site: www.fims.org

Introduction

Diabetes mellitus is a common metabolic disease characterized by insulin insufficiency resulting in impaired ability to transport glucose across the cell membrane for its subsequent oxidation. Also, muscle and liver glycogen resynthesis, triglyceride synthesis in adipose cells, inhibition of their breakdown (antilipolytic effect), as well as protein synthesis and storage (anabolic effects) are being impaired. Insulin insufficiency thus leads to metabolic disturbances leading to such common symptoms as fatigue, weakness, weight loss, hunger, overeating, polyuria, and signs of glycosuria, and ketosis.

Though being clinically silent for many years, diabetes mellitus often leads to serious pathological complications of various organ systems (eyes, kidneys, peripheral nerves, coronary and peripheral arteries) which may substantially impair quality of life and reduce life expectancy.

There are two distinct forms of diabetes, termed insulin dependent diabetes mellitus (IDDM) and non-insulin dependent diabetes mellitus (NIDDM).

IDDM is an autoimmune disease in which the body attacks and ultimately destroys insulin producing pancreatic beta cells. In addition to a genetic component, evidence supports a viral infection triggering an autoimmune process either due to similarities with beta cell protein or sensitization to destructed beta cells.

The key pathogenetic factor of NIDDM is relative insufficiency of insulin due to insulin resistance and/or defective insulin secretion. Insulin resistance is often associated with hypertension, lipid disturbances, and obesity. Apart from genetic dispositions, diet and obesity, animal experiments as well as epidemiological data suggest that a lack of physical activity may also contribute to a relative deficiency of insulin.

Diabetes may be precipitated by, or a similar syndrome brought about by endocrine disorders (e.g., hypercorticosteroidism, acromegaly, hyperthyroidism, pheochromocytoma), drugs (e.g., glucocorticoids, thyroid hormones, contraceptives, thiazides), and pancreatic or liver disease.

Rationale for Exercise in Prevention and Therapy

Due to an insulin-like effect on muscle contraction (an increase of membrane permeability to glucose) exercise has a potential to increase insulin sensitivity, lower blood glucose and increase its utilization. Improved glucose tolerance positively influences the glycemic profile that can be detected by lower concentration of glycosylated hemoglobin. A better glycemic profile may postpone and reduce the risk of late complication. Since this effect is rather short-lived, regular frequent exercise sessions are needed to maintain such a benefit.

Also reducing body fat due to the increased energy expended and its effect on the basal metabolic rate may, indirectly, but significantly decrease insulin resistance.

In addition to obesity, exercise has the potential to favorable alter other risk factors of cardiovascular disease, namely elevated blood lipids and hypertension. In this way an already increased risk of coronary heart disease (3 times higher than general population) may be reduced.

Last but not least, exercise may reduce psychological stress, positively influence a feeling of well being, and improve the quality of life.

Exercise Guidelines

Clearance by a knowledgeable physician is recommended prior to the initiation of an exercise program. In addition to a general assessment, screening should include an exercise stress test to detect latent cardiovascular disease. Requisites include an absence of ketoacidosis and glycemia under 300 mg. When late complications are evident such as hypertension or renal impairment, the risks and benefits should carefully be considered.

During the initial stages of an exercise program, close medical supervision which includes blood glucose monitoring is strongly recommended in order to adjust diet and medication (insulin or PAD doses) to the exercise altered metabolic situation.

Modes of Exercise

Aerobic activities carried out at moderate intensity such as brisk walking, cycling, jogging or running, or cross country skiing are preferred modes of exercise. Since the majority of diabetics are obese, non-weight bearing exercise like cycling and swimming may pose less stress on the locomotor system and contribute to better compliance. General daily activities or a habitual nature are encouraged in addition to the exercise sessions.

In the past, resistance exercise has not been recommended because of the potential for a dangerous increase in blood pressure, especially in those with vascular complications. Recent findings indicate that appropriate forms of resistance exercise are safe and may potentiate the positive effects of aerobic exercise. A circuit training approach aimed at all major muscle groups is recommended. The resistances should allow 10 to 12 comfortable repetitions.

Intensity of Exercise

The exercise intensity should be between 50 and 70% of VO_2max. Higher intensities excessively activate the sympathoadrenal system with subsequent increase of glycemia. With caution, hear rate can be used as an indicator of intensity. In patients with autonomic neuropathy, heart rate may not accurately reflect exercise intensity. As an alternative, perceived exertion of METs (metabolic equivalents) should be used for the exercise prescription.

Duration of Exercise

Exercise sessions between 20 and 60 minutes are recommended. Less than 20 minutes yields little cardiovascular benefit, longer exercise tends to increase the risk of hypoglycemia.

Frequency of Exercise

Daily exercise is suggested because such an approach enables easier insulin adjustment and diet planning. A more realistic and practical goal may be 4 to 6 sessions a week.

Practical Remarks

- Patients should be educated about the effects and potential risks of exercise, namely hypoglycemia.
- The participants should wear identification indicating their diabetic condition and should exercise with a knowledgeable partner in case of hypoglycemia including loss of consciousness.
- When possible exercise should be performed at the same convenient time with similar intensity and duration.
- Because of the pro insulin effect of exercise, insulin dependent diabetics should reduce insulin doses by 20% or adequately increase food intake upon initiating an exercise program.
- To avoid hypoglycemia a small carbohydrate snack should be eaten 30 minutes prior to exercise. During more prolonged activity a 10 g carbohydrate snack (fruit, fruit juice, or soft drink) should be ingested for each 30 minutes of exercise.
- Pay careful attention to the feet of the exercising diabetic patient. Loss of sensation due

to neuropathy and/or impaired peripheral circulation increases the risk of injuries. Good footwear and careful foot hygiene are essential to avoid injuries like calluses, corns and blisters that may lead to serious complications.

- Warm up and cool down periods should be an integral part of an exercise program.

Suggested Reading

1. Chisholm, D.J. Diabetes mellitus, in Bloomfield, J., Fricker, P.A., and Fitch, K.B. (eds) *Textbook of Science and Medicine in Sports*, Blackwell Science Ltd., Oxford, pp. 560, 1992.

2. Schneider, S.H., Ruderman, N.B. Exercise and NIDDM. *Diabetes Care*, 13, 785-789, 1990.

3. Wallberg-Henriksson, H. Exercise and diabetes mellitus. *Exer. Sport Rev.*, 20, 339-368, 1992.

October 1996

This statement may be reproduced and distributed with the sole requirement that it be identified clearly as a Position Statement of the International Federation of Sports Medicine.

Foot Injuries

Women's Shoes and Foot Problems

American Orthopaedic Foot and Ankle Society (AOFAS)

The American Orthopaedic Foot and Ankle Society (AOFAS) believes that foot problems resulting from poorly fitting shoes have reached epidemic proportions and pose a major health risk for women in America.

A 1991 AOFAS Council on Women's Footwear survey of 356 women found that almost 90 percent wore shoes too small for feet and that about 80 percent had foot problems. Most women wear shoes a width to two width sizes too small. As a result, many suffer from bunions, hammertoes, bunionettes, coms, and other disabling foot problems.

The lack of availability of a variety of width sizes partially explains this problem. Men's shoes on the whole are available in a greater variety of widths and conform more closely to the outer dimensions of their feet. The failure of shoe purchasers to obtain proper shoe fit also contributes to the problem. The Council on Women's Footwear study found that three quarters of the women surveyed had not had their feet measured in the last five years and many of those who had their feet measured were measured incorrectly.

Neither shoe manufacturers nor shoe purchasers can be blamed for what is a complex societal and attitudinal problem. The national obsession with beauty has created a demand for shoes that make the foot seem smaller, daintier and narrower. Narrow, pointy-toed shoes and high heeled shoes that make the foot look smaller by placing it in a more vertical position are the height of fashion. Furthermore, few women receive instruction in proper shoe fit. The results are devastating. Women have about 90 percent of surgeries for conunon foot problems such as bunions, bunionettes, hammertoes, and neuromas. These surgeries cost the American public at least $3.5 billion for surgery and 15 million lost work days annually.

The only real solution to this problem is the intelligent construction, selling and purchasing of sensible, comfortable, roomy shoes.

Because the problem is so complex, it only can be solved through the cooperation of three important groups: 1) the shoe manufacturer; 2) the shoe sales person; and 3) the shoe purchaser. The American Orthopaedic Foot and Ankle Society (AOFAS), the National Shoe Retailers Association (NSRA), and the Pedorthic Footwear Association (PFA) took the first step by initiating a public awareness campaign on the importance of proper shoe fit. This collaboration resulted in the production of a "Ten Points of Shoe Fit" brochure and countertop display, which have been widely distributed to physicians' offices and shoe stores around the U.S.

Heat and Cold Illnesses

Heat and Cold Illnesses During Distance Running

American College of Sports Medicine (ACSM)
Web site: www.acsm.org

Summary

Many recreational and elite runners participate in distance races each year. When these events are conducted in hot or cold conditions, the risk of environmental illness increases. However, exertions hypertherrnia, hypothermia, dehydration, and other related problems may be minimized with pre-event education and preparation. This position stand provides recommendations for the medical director and other race officials in the following areas: scheduling; organizing personnel, facilities, supplies, equipment, and communication; providing competitor education; measuring environmental stress; providing fluids; and avoiding potential legal liabilities. This document also describes the predisposing conditions, recognition, and treatment of the four most common environmental illnesses: heat exhaustion, heatstroke, hypothermia, and frostbite. The objectives of this position stand are: 1) To educate distance running event officials and participants about the most common forms of environmental illness including predisposing conditions, warning signs, susceptibility, and incidence reduction. 2) To advise race officials of their legal responsibilities and potential liability with regard to event safety and injury prevention. 3) To recommend that race officials consult local weather archives and plan events at times likely to be of low environmental stress to minimize detrimental effects on participants. 4) To encourage race officials to warn participants about environmental stress on race day and its implications for heat and cold illness. 5) To inform race officials of preventive actions that may reduce debilitation and environmental illness. 6) To describe the personnel, equipment, and supplies necessary to reduce and treat cases of collapse and environmental illness.

December 1996

HIV and Athletes

Human Immunodeficiency Virus and Other Blood-borne Viral Pathogens in the Athletic Setting (RE9821)

American Academy of Pediatrics, Committee on Sports Medicine and Fitness

Web site: www.aap.org/policy/re9821.html

Abstract. Because athletes and the staff of athletic programs can be exposed to blood during athletic activity, they have a very small risk of becoming infected with human immunodeficiency virus, hepatitis B virus, or hepatitis C virus. This statement, which updates a previous position statement of the American Academy of Pediatrics, discusses sports participation for athletes infected with these pathogens and the precautions needed to reduce the risk of infection to others in the athletic setting. Each of the recommendations in this statement is dependent upon and intended to be considered with reference to the other recommendations in this statement and not in isolation.

December 1999

© American Academy of Pediatrics

Volume 104, Number 6, pp1400-1403

AIDS and Sports

International Federation of Sports Medicine (FIMS)

Web site: www.fims.org

Introduction

A consensus statement by the International Federation of Sports Medicine (FIMS) and the World Health Organization (WHO) on "AIDS and Sports" was presented and circulated in 1989. Recently acquired information has stimulated revisions to this document. The following is based primarily on the joint position of the American Medical Society for Sports Medicine (AMSSM) and the American Orthopaedic Society for Sports Medicine (AOSSM) entitled, "Human Immunodeficiency Virus (HIV) and Other Blood Borne Pathogens in Sports" (1995). The FIMS Position Statement presents a summary of presently available information directed at physicians and other health-care providers involved in the field of sports medicine and is intended to serve as a guide toward:

1. understanding HIV as it relates to sports,

2. implementing practical preventive measures that further minimize the low risk of transmission of this pathogen,

3. developing effective educational initiatives among athletes and others involved in

sport regarding this infection, its transmission and prevention, and

4. providing guidance for the care of HIV-infected athletes.

Definition

Typically with AIDS, there is a decline in immunologic function that, over an extended period of time, may be associated with clinically obvious symptomatology (5,6). Because of the progressively worsening nature of this process, the HIV-1 spectrum disease should be considered as chronic with three clearly definable stages. Of these, AIDS represents the final, fatal stage. Initial infection is often unrecognized and it usually takes from 4-12 weeks for the person to become HIV-1 seropositive (2,10). The first phase of HIV-1 spectrum disease can last as long as 10-15 years and is asymptomatic (15). Fifty percent of HIV-infected patients develop AIDS within 8 years of infection and during this time, are capable of transmitting the virus to others (19). Once individuals begin to experience symptoms such as night sweats, unintentional substantial weight loss, thrush, herpes zoster, swollen lymph nodes, chronic diarrhea, fever of unexplained origin, and recurrent upper respiratory tract infections, they have progressed to the second stage of HIV disease (often referred to as early symptomatic pre-AIDS). Only when immunocompetence is severely impaired or unusual, and opportunistic infections such as pneumocystis cirinii pneumonia, cryptoccocal meningitis, toxoplasmosis or herpes simplex encephalitis are present, is the individual diagnosed with AIDS (11).

Epidemiology

According to the WHO, an estimated 2 million people worldwide have developed AIDS and an estimated 10-12 million people have been infected with HIV, the virus that causes AIDS. It has also been projected by WHO that 30-40 million people will be infected with HIV-1 by the year 2000 (14).

Transmission of HIV

The HIV is transmitted through sexual contact, parenteral exposure to blood and blood components, contamination of open wounds or mucous membranes by infected blood, and perinatally from an infected mother to fetus or infant.

While the virus may be present in a variety of body fluids, only blood poses any degree of risk of transmission in athletic settings. The virus cannot be transmitted by giving blood, or by mosquitoes or other insects (9). Tears, sweat, urine, sputum, vomitus, saliva, and respiratory droplets have not been implicated in the transmission of infection.

Transmission of HIV Through Sports

At present, there are no well-documented epidemiological studies assessing the transmission of HIV or other blood-born pathogens during sport activity. However, despite the negative data, the theoretical chance for HIV transmission in sport situations where significant blood exposures to open wounds may occur is not zero.

Participation in the bloodiest sports, such as boxing, wrestling, and tae kwon do presents the greatest risk. Playing basketball, field hockey, ice hockey, judo, soccer, and team handball is of moderate risk and involvement in sports which require little physical contact such as baseball, gymnastics, and tennis presents the lowest risk (8).

It should be recognized that contact and collision sports have a higher risk of significant blood exposure than do other sports. Athletes competing in such sports need to be aware of the small theoretical risk of blood-borne pathogen transmission. The infected athlete who continues to participate in this form of competition has special responsibilities.

The greatest risk to the athlete for contracting any blood-borne pathogen infection originated not in the sporting arena, but through sexual activity and parenteral drug use.

Education

In the absence of a cure for HIV or a vaccine to prevent it, education and prevention techniques remain the primary means of controlling its spread (1). Sports medicine practitioners should play an important role in educational activities directed at athletes, their families, athletic trainers, other health care-providers, coaches, officials and others involved in sports. Abstinence or monogamous sex between uninfected partners is the only certain strategy for protection against sexual transmission. In other sexual relationships, the use of condoms with water based lubricants is recommended. The effectiveness of spermicides containing nonoxynol-9 is still being reviewed; these may serve as adjuncts to condoms. Also, the athlete is susceptible to transmission via shared contaminated needles and syringes associated with drug use. This includes the use of ergogenic aids such as anabolic steroids as well as drugs that are illegally abused, such as heroin. Tattoo applications at parlours that do not use disposable needles or adequately sterilize needles between clients also present a needle transmission risk (19). When traveling, athletes should be aware that they may be exposed to a population with a higher prevalence of these viruses. As well, they could be offered possibly risky medical treatment, such as unscreened blood transfusion or injections with a contaminated needle. These (16), as well as practices of sharing personal items such as razors, toothbrushes and nail clippers may place individuals as an increased risk. Athletes should be made aware of these potential dangers.

Education regarding the risk of transmission during sports competition is important. The risk of such transmission, though highly improbable, can be further minimized by such common sense hygienic measure as the prompt application of first aid to bleeding injuries. Athletes should be made aware that it is in their best interest to report significant injuries to the appropriate official, coach or caregiver in a timely manner. Caregivers should be trained in and adhere to universal precautions.

Physicians involved in sports medicine can play important roles in general education aimed at reducing the fear and misconceptions concerning blood-born pathogen transmission among athletes, their families, and all persons associated with sports. Athletic organizations, as well as individual athletes, can make meaningful contributions to the community's overall educational effort. Many sports organizations have already developed policies that provide information about precautionary procedures to decrease blood-borne transmission in sports (1).

The HIV-Infected Athlete

Physicians involved in sports medicine must be knowledgeable about the issues concerning the management of HIV-infected athletes. Given the continuing epidemic of HIV infection worldwide, it will be diagnosed more frequently in athletes. Although HIV is an extremely serious health problem, it must be recognized that it is a chronic disease. Its natural history frequently allows the infected person many years of excellent health and productive life.

Meanwhile, no studies have assessed the effect of strenuous exercise on an HIV-positive athlete. Very strenuous exercise has been shown to suppress the immune system of even those healthy, elite athletes who are not HIV-positive.

The decision to recommend continued athletic competition should be made on an individual basis and should involve the athlete, the athlete's personal physician, and the sports medicine practitioner. Variables to be considered in reaching this decision include:

1. the athlete's current state of health and the status of the HIV infection
2. the nature and intensity of training,
3. the potential contribution of stress from athletic competition, and
4. the potential risk of HIV transmission.

Based on current medical and epidemiological information, the presence of HIV infection alone is not sufficient grounds to prohibit sports competition.

Exercise and the HIV-Infected Sedentaries

Although no reliable data are yet available regarding exercise training for individuals infected with HIV who are symptomatic, several studies (7,12,17,18) seem to indicate that moderate levels of supervised physical activity are safe throughout the course of the disease. Therefore, caution is still warranted in this area (13).

Long term effects of acute, exhaustive exercise in people who have chronic illnesses are not clear. Thus, HIV-infected patients whose immune systems are suppressed, as indicated by low CD4+/CD8+ lymphocyte ratios, should probably not exercise to exhaustion (14). A moderate exercise training program may improve mental health and forestall a decline in immunity in individuals infected with HIV. In fact, exercise appears to offer an adjunctive therapeutic technique that may play an important role in the management of the HIV disease (13).

Everyone infected with HIV should have a complete physical examination prior to beginning any type of physical activity program. Exercise training programs should be discussed with a physician and exercise specialist. It is further recommended that individuals infected with HIV should begin an exercise program while still healthy. By following these simple recommendations, moderate exercise training can be a safe and beneficial activity for many individuals with HIV infections (13).

Mandatory HIV Testing

Mandatory testing or widespread blood-borne pathogen screening is not justified for medical reasons as a condition for athletic participation or competition (3). Any consideration of a blood-borne pathogen testing program in the athletic setting must address the practical, medical, scientific, and ethical problems that such a program poses.

First, the issue of whom should be tested may be unclear. In addition, it would be necessary to determine the frequency of testing. A negative test does not guarantee of invulnerability. Although most people test positively 4 months after being exposed to HIV, in others, the virus can take a year to become evident. For this reason, testing should be done several months following the potentially risky activity. A negative result 12 or more months after the possible exposure indicates that the person is not infected (8). Other factors in mandatory testing include overwhelming costs, as well as legal and ethical considerations for populations that may comprise minors. These issues further suggest that there is no rational basis for supporting blood-borne pathogen tests in sports.

Voluntary HIV testing

Voluntary testing should be suggested to athletes as well as nonathletes who may have been exposed to transmission. This would include those who have had:

1. multiple sexual partners,
2. injections of non-prescription drugs such as drugs of abuse or ergogenic aids,
3. sexual contacts with at-risk persons,
4. sexually transmitted disease including HBV, or
5. blood transfusions before 1985.

When obtaining informed consent and reviewing the positive and negative results, federal, or local guidelines must be followed. (Guidelines may vary.)

Personal knowledge of blood-borne serum status, combined with pre- and post-test counseling, can be a helpful adjunct to preventive education.

Knowledge of one's infection is helpful for a variety of reasons. These include availability of therapy for asymptomatic patients in the case of HIV, modification of behavior that can prevent transmission of blood-borne pathogens to others, and appropriate counseling regarding exercise and sports participation. Early knowledge of a positive test will enable timely medical intervention that may prolong life (1). The International Federation of Sports Medicine urges that applicable public health measures for handling an epidemic should be implemented with the HIV-infected persons.

Other Blood-Borne Pathogens

Hepatitis B (HBV) and Hepatitis C (HCV) are spread through the same routes as HIV. The chronic hepatitis B carrier presents the greatest concern for transmission. Hepatitis delta virus (HDV) requires the presence of HBV for expression of the disease. The HDV results in a more virulent course of the disease than HBV alone. Risk factors for the two diseases are similar. HBV is far more concentrated in blood, thus it is more readily transmitted than HIV.

In the general health-care setting, the risk of HBV transmission from parenteral exposure is much greater than that of HIV. It may be presumed that the sports-related transmission risk for HBV is greater than the risk for HIV.

Accurate laboratory blood tests are available for HBV and HCV screening. There is no evidence that intense, highly competitive training is a problem for the asymptomatic HBV carrier (acute or chronic).

Vaccination for HBV is now available and should be considered particularly by health care workers. No recommendation has been specifically made regarding immunizations against HBV for athletes. However, several groups now endorse universal immunization against HBV of both newborn and young adults.

The recommendations for HIV are also appropriate to reduce the risk of other blood-borne pathogens, including HBV and HCV (16).

Legal Considerations

Confidentiality dictates that medical information is the property of the patient. Exceptions include medical conditions that are reportable by regulation and statute. Therefore, the responsibility of the physician is very clear. The physician is not liable for failure to warn the uninfected opponent. That legal responsibility lies with the HIV-infected athlete. However, the uninfected athlete must be aware that he or she assumes some of the risk (albeit small) of contacting HIV or other blood-borne pathogen disease in sports activities because it cannot be assumed that his or her competitors are HIV (or other blood-borne pathogen) free. This does not differ from other injuries that are inherent in sports.

The responsibility for the sexual transmission of HIV lies with the HIV infected person. As yet, there has been no legal activity regarding transmission of HIV in sports competition. The physician is advised to be aware of local and federal statues, and regulations concerning confidentiality.

Specific Management and Preventive Measures for Sport Events

Any risk of blood-borne pathogen transmission in sports is exceedingly small. However, all those involved with sports will help further reduce the risk of transmission by following guidelines that are both practical and simple to implement. A major component to these is common sense and adherence to basic principles of hygiene.

Because the risk of blood-borne pathogen transmission in sports is confined to contact with blood, body fluids and other fluids containing blood, preventive measures should be focused on the recognition and immediate treatment of bleeding.

The following recommendations are designed to minimize the risk of blood-borne pathogen transmission in the context of athletic events and provide treatment guidelines for caregivers:

1. Proper care for existing wounds is essential. Abrasions, cuts, or oozing wounds that may serve as a source of bleeding or as a portal of entry for blood-borne pathogens should be covered with an occlusive dressing that will

withstand the demands of competition. Likewise, care providers with healing wounds or dermatitis should have these areas adequately covered to prevent transmission to or from a patient.

2. Necessary equipment and/or supplies, important for compliance with universal precautions, should be available to caregivers. These supplies include latex or vinyl gloves, disinfectant, bleach (freshly prepared in a 1:10 dilution with tap water), antiseptic, designated receptacles for soiled equipment or uniforms (with separate waterproof bags or receptacles appropriately marked for uniforms and equipment contaminated with blood), bandages or dressings, and a container for appropriate disposal of needles, syringes, or scalpels.

3. During the sports event, early recognition of bleeding is the responsibility of officials, athletes, and medical personnel. Participants with active bleeding should be removed from the event as soon as is practical. Bleeding must be controlled and the wound cleansed with soap and water or an antiseptic. The wound must be covered with an occlusive dressing that will withhold the demands of the activity. When bleeding is controlled and any wound properly covered, the player may return to competition. Any participant whose uniform is saturated with blood, regardless of source, must have that uniform changed before returning to competition.

4. Athletes must be advised that it is their responsibility to report all wounds and injuries including those recognized before the sporting activity in a timely manner. In contact sports, it is the athlete's responsibility to wear appropriate equipment, including a mouth protector, at all times.

5. The care provider managing an acute blood exposure must follow universal precautions. Appropriate gloves should be worn when direct contact with blood, body fluids, and other fluids containing blood is anticipated. Gloves should be changed after treating each individual participation and, as soon as practical after glove removal, hands should be washed with soap and water or antiseptic.

6. Minor cuts or abrasions commonly occur during sport. These do not require interruption of play or removal of the participant from competition. Minor cuts and abrasions that are not bleeding should be cleansed and covered at the next scheduled break in play. Likewise, a small amount of blood staining a uniform does not necessitate removal of the participant or a uniform change.

7. Lack of protective equipment should not delay emergency care for life-threatening injuries. Although HIV is not transmitted by saliva, medical personnel may prefer using airway devices. These devices should be made available whenever possible.

8. Any equipment or area (e.g., wrestling mat) soiled with blood should be wiped immediately with paper towels or disposable cloths. The contaminated areas should be disinfected with a solution prepared daily of one part household bleach to ten parts water. The cleaned area should be dry before re-use. Gloves should be worn by persons cleaning equipment or collecting soiled linen.

9. Post-event considerations should include re-evaluation of any wounds sustained during the sporting event. Further cleaning and dressing of the wound may be necessary. Also, blood-soiled uniforms or towels should be collected for eventual washing in hot water and detergent.

10. Procedures performed in the training room are also governed by adherence to universal precautions. Gloves should be worn by care providers. Any blood body fluids or other fluids containing blood should be cleaned in a manner as described previously. Equipment handlers, laundry personnel and janitorial staff should be advised to wear gloves whenever contact with bloody equipment, clothing or other items are anticipated. Appropriate containers for the disposal of needles, syringes, or scalpels should be available.

Many athletic contests and practices, especially at the community or scholastic level, occur without medical personnel in attendance. The above guidelines apply not only to physicians, athletic trainers, and physical therapists involved in the coverage of sports, but also to coaches and officials who may be present as the primary caregivers. All personnel involved with sport should be trained in basic first aid and infection control, including the preventive measures outlined.

June 1997

Joint position statement of the American Medical Society for Sports Medicine (AMSSM) and The American Orthopaedic Society for Sports Medicine (AOSSM), "Human Immunodeficiency Virus (HIV) and Other Blood-Borne Pathogens in Sports" (1995).

HIV in Sport

Canadian Academy of Sport Medicine (CASM)

Introduction

The Canadian Academy of Sport Medicine (CASM) recognizes the importance of clarifying issues related to Human Immunodeficiency Virus (HIV) in sport. CASM feels that it is important to educate the sport community on the implications of HIV infection and transmission. CASM feels that it is also important to include discussion on Hepatitis B and C as these are viruses that have a similar mechanism of transmission to HIV.

Definitions of HIV, HBV and HCV

Human Immunodeficiency Virus (HIV) is the cause of Acquired Immunodeficiency Syndrome (AIDS). HIV infects and seriously damages the body's immune system. Without the protection of the immune system people with AIDS suffer from fatal infections and cancers. People can be infected with HIV for many years before becoming symptomatic.

Hepatitis B (HBV) and Hepatitis C (HCV) are also virus infections. The Hepatitis viruses infect the liver causing serious illness. The complications of hepatitis may be fatal. HIV, HBV and HCV are all transmitted in similar ways.

Prevalence

It is estimated that there are 600,000 AIDS cases world wide and that by 1993 there will be 5 to 10 million HIV infected people. It is esti-

mated that there are currently more than 50,000 Canadians living with HIV infection.

Transmission

Transmission of HIV occurs in the following ways:

1. Sexual activity; mainly by penetrating sexual intercourse with exchange of semen and/or vaginal and cervical secretions. This is the major way that HIV is transmitted.

2. Parenteral inoculations; occurs when virus infected body fluids enter another person's blood system in the following ways:

   a. Blood transfusion; only with blood that has not been screened. (In Canada all blood has been screened for HIV since November 1985).

   b. Percutaneous injuries; punctures wounds by contaminated needles and other sharp objects.

   c. Blood into an open wound; the risk from this route is very small, less than any other type of transmission.

3. Perinatal; from infected mother to fetus/infant.

Most of the knowledge of non-sexual HIV transmission has been studied in the health-care setting. In the study of 2042 percutaneous injuries involving HIV infected blood, 6 health-care workers were infected. Of these six cases, five were related to injuries with sharp objects or needles. One was related to blood exposed in an open wound. All cases involved a large quantity of HIV infected blood.

Body fluids implicated in the transmission of HIV include the following: blood, semen, breast milk, vaginal and cervical secretions. Body fluids not implicated in the transmission of HIV include the following: tears, saliva, sweat, urine, sputum, respiratory droplets. HIV is not transmitted through handshaking, skin contact, swimming pool water, communal bath water, toilet seats, food or drinking water (World Health Organization, 1989). No known cases of HIV transmission have occurred from contact with contaminated surfaces such as wrestling mats, taping tables, toilet seats, sinks or other surfaces. Although HIV, HBV and HCV are all transmitted similarly, they are not identical. HBV and HCV are more easily transmitted than HIV.

Risk of HIV Transmission In Sport

The risk of transmission of HIV in the sport setting is exceedingly low. This statement is based on the evidence in the health-care setting and the type of exposure that occurs in sport. To date there has been only one unconfirmed case reported of an athlete who acquired HIV in sport by contact of bloody wound to bloody wound.

Participants in sport, are subject to the same risks of HIV infection as any other individual in the general population. The greatest risk of transmission continues to be through sexual activity.

Athletes travelling should be aware that they may be exposed to a population with a higher prevalence of these viruses. They could be offered medical treatment for example, unscreened blood transfusion or injections with a contaminated needle, that may put them at increased risk for acquiring these viruses.

Prevention

The following recommendations are intended to reduce the risk of transmission of HIV. Although these recommendations are directly applicable to HIV, they are also appropriate to reduce the risk of other viruses and infectious diseases including HBV and HCV.

General Prevention

Safe sex and abstinence from sex play the major role in decreasing HIV transmission.

1. Vaccination for HBV is now available and should be considered by athletes, coaches, officials and health-care workers. Vaccinations for the other viruses should be considered if they become available.

2. Instruments designed for piercing the skin, such as needles and syringes used for injections, ear-piercing, tattooing, acupuncture and suturing should be sterile, used one time and not shared.

3. Personal items that may pierce the skin or mucous membranes should not be shared. This includes items like razors, toothbrushes, and nail clippers.

4. Blood and blood products must be screened for HIV before transfusing. Blood and blood products must also be screened for HBV and HCV.

5. Sport participants travelling should confirm the medical precautions required for each destination.

Sport Specific Prevention

1. Primary prevention for bloody injuries includes the use of appropriate protective equipment. Protective equipment should be designed and maintained to prevent bloody injuries. Equipment designed to prevent open wounds such as mouth pieces to prevent penetration of another participants skin should be considered for all contact sports.

2. Dealing with a bloody wound;

a. If bleeding occurs where other participants may be exposed to blood, the individual's participation must be interrupted until the bleeding has been stopped. The wound must both be cleansed with antiseptic and securely covered.

b. All clothing soiled with blood must be replaced prior to the athlete resuming training or competition. Clothing soiled with blood and other body fluids must be washed in hot, soapy water.

c. All equipment and surfaces contaminated with blood and other body fluids should be cleaned with a solution of one part household bleach to nine parts water. This solution should be prepared fresh daily.

While cleaning blood or other body fluid spills, the following must be done:

- wear waterproof gloves
- wipe up fluids with paper towel or disposable cloths
- disinfect the area as described in 2c
- place all soiled waste in a plastic bag for disposal
- remove gloves and wash hands with soap and water

3. Other wounds including abrasions and all skin lesions and rashes on athletes, coaches and officials must be reviewed by medical personnel. All wounds, skin lesions, rashes must be confirmed as noninfectious and be securely covered prior to the athlete starting or continuing participation.

Prevention For Medical Staff And First Aid Administrators

These recommendations are directed at physicians, therapists and other medical personnel involved in sport. Coaches and officials should also follow these recommendations where applicable.

1. Wear waterproof gloves for direct contact with another individuals blood or body fluids. Change gloves after treating each individual.

2. Wash hands with soap and water after removing gloves.

3. When a blood or body fluid spill occurs as a result of medical treatment on an injury, wash the blood or body fluids from the skin or wound as soon as possible with antiseptic or soapy water.

4. Sharps and syringes should be considered as potentially infectious and handled with extraordinary care in order to prevent accidental injuries. After they are used, syringes, needles and other sharp items should be placed in a puncture-resistant container for disposal in the approved manner for medical waste. Needles and blades should not be purposefully bent, broken, removed or otherwise manipulated by hand.

5. Care providers with weeping skin lesions, open wounds or dermatitis must routinely wear waterproof gloves when treating people.

6. Treatment for life threatening injury including control of bleeding and mouth-to-mouth resuscitation can proceed without gloves or mouth pieces, although they should be used if available.

Incident Follow-Up

If an event occurs where an athlete is at risk of virus infection a physician should be contacted as soon as possible to assess the situation and institute appropriate action.

Testing

Accurate laboratory blood tests are available for HIV, HBV and HCV. Mandatory testing of athletes is unwarranted. Individuals may consider voluntary testing. This testing should include informed consent, pre and post test counseling and be confidential.

HIV+ Individuals In Sport

1. An HIV+ individual should not be excluded from participating in sport exclusively on the basis of his/her HIV infection.

2. An HIV+ individual should seek medical care primarily to assess his/her own health and benefit from possible treatment to discuss and further participation in sport.

Education

Sport organizations, clubs and groups must be made aware of the above recommendations and ensure that all participants, officials and ancillary personnel are aware of them. In addition, this may provide the opportunity for reviewing general hygienic practices related to sport. (WHO, 1989).

For More Information

For further information on this issue contact the Canadian Academy of Sport Medicine Task Force on Infectious Disease in Sport. For further information on HIV and AIDS contact the following:

- Your doctor
- Your Public Health Unit or Community Health Centre
- Your local Community AIDS Organization
- The National AIDS Secretariat

  17th Floor Jeanne Mance Building Tunney's Pasture Ottawa, Ontario K1A 0K9

  Tel. (613) 957-7580
- AIDS Education and Awareness Program Canadian Public Health Association 400 - 1565 Carling Avenue Ottawa, Ontario K1Z 8R1
  Tel. (613) 725-3769
  Fax. (613) 725-9826

February 1994

Hypertension

Physical Activity, Physical Fitness, and Hypertension

American College of Sports Medicine

Web site: www.acsm.org

Summary

American College of Sports Medicine Position Stand: "Physical Activity, Physical Fitness, and Hypertension." *Med. Sci. Sports Exerc.* Vol. 25. No. 10. pp. i-x. 1993. Hypertension is present in epidemic proportions in adults of industrialized societies and is associated with a markedly increased risk of developing numerous cardiovascular pathologies. There is a continuing debate as to the efficacy of aggressive pharmacological therapy in individuals with mild to moderate elevations in blood pressure. This has led to a search for nonpharmacological therapies, such as exercise training, for these individuals. The available evidence indicates that endurance exercise training by individuals at high risk for developing hypertension will reduce the rise in blood pressure that occurs with time. Thus, it is the position of the American College of Sports Medicine that endurance exercise training is recommended as a nonpharmacological strategy to reduce the incidence of hypertension in susceptible individuals. A large number of studies indicate that endurance exercise training will elicit a 10 mm Hg average reduction in both systolic and diastolic blood pressures in individuals with mild essential hypertension (blood pressures 140-180/90-105 mm Hg). Endurance exercise training also has the capacity to improve other risk factors for cardiovascular disease in hypertensive individuals. Endurance exercise training appears to elicit even greater reductions in blood pressure in patients with secondary hypertension due to renal dysfunction. The mode (large muscle activities), frequency (3-5 d/wk),

duration (20-60 min and intensity (50-85% of maximal oxygen uptake) of the exercise recommended to achieve this effect are generally the same as those prescribed for developing and maintaining cardiovascular fitness in healthy adults. Exercise training at somewhat lower intensities (40-70% $V\dot{O}_2$max appears to lower blood pressure as much, or more, than exercise at higher intensities, which may be important in specific hypertensive populations. Physically active and fit individuals with hypertension have markedly lower rates of mortality than sedentary, unfit hypertensive individuals. Thus, it seems reasonable to recommend exercise as the initial treatment strategy for individuals with mild to moderate essential hypertension. A follow-up period should assess the efficacy of the patient's exercise program, and adjunct therapies should be implemented according to the individual patient's blood pressure and CAD risk factor goals. Individuals with more marked-elevations in blood pressure (< 150/105 mm Hg) should add endurance exercise training to their treatment regimen only after initiating pharmacologic therapy. Resistive, or strength, exercise training is not recommended to lower blood pressure in individuals with hypertension when done as their only form of exercise training. It is recommended when included as one component of a well-rounded fitness program, such as circuit training done in conjunction with endurance exercise training. Exercise testing is not advocated to determine normotensive individuals with an exaggerated exercise blood pressure response who might be at high risk of developing hypertension in the future. However, if exercise test results are available, they can be used to provide some indication of risk stratification and the need for appropriate lifestyle behavior counselling that might ameliorate this risk.

© 1993

American College of Sports Medicine

MSSE, 25:10, 1993, pp. i-x

Athletic Participation by Children and Adolescents Who Have Systemic Hypertension (RE9715)

American Academy of Pediatrics (AAP), Committee on Sports Medicine and Fitness

Web site: www.aap.org/policy/re9715.html

ABSTRACT. Children and adolescents who have systemic hypertension may be at risk for complications when exercise causes their blood pressures to rise even higher. The purpose of this statement is to make recommendations concerning the athletic participation of individuals with hypertension using the 26th Bethesda conference on heart disease and athletic participation and of the second task force on blood pressure control in children as a basis.

April 1997

American Academy of Pediatrics

Volume 99, Number 4, pp 637-638

Nutrition

Promoting Healthy Nutrition for Youth in YMCA Programs

YMCA of the USA Medical Advisory Committee

Proper nutrition is essential for the healthy growth and development of young people. YMCA facilities, programs, and activities which provide food and/or snacks for youth should do so in a safe, clean, and pleasant environment, and in a responsible manner. While most eating habits begin at home and families are primarily responsible for teaching children to make healthy food choices, YMCAs can support this effort whenever food is served as part of a program or activity.

The U.S. Department of Agriculture and the Department of Health and Human Services have published the following dietary guidelines for all Americans:

- Eat a variety of foods
- Maintain desirable weight
- Avoid a diet too high in saturated fats and cholesterol (after age 2)
- Consume a diet high in fruits, vegetables, and grains
- Avoid too much sugar
- Avoid too much salt

The Medical Advisory Committee endorses these general guidelines, and urges YMCAs to use them when planning food and/or snacks to youth as well as adults in YMCA programs. In addition, they offer the following specific recommendations:

1. When providing food and/or snacks for YMCA events and programs, avoid high fat, high sugar products. Complex carbohydrates are excellent choices as snacks.

2. Encourage good eating habits through the availability of healthy choice items in vending machines, such as: unsweetened fruit juices, water, fresh fruit, pretzels, raw vegetables, low-fat granola bars, raisins, nut mixes, frozen yogurt bars.

3. Youth programs such as child care, camping, and sports are encouraged to include a nutrition curriculum that promotes proper nutrition and stresses healthy food choices.

4. Fund raising activities that sell foods are encouraged to sell food products that are consistent with the USDA dietary recommendations.

November 1997

Disclaimer: These recommendations were developed by the YMCA of the USA Medical Advisory Committee for the exclusive use by YMCAs in United States. As they were developed with the specific needs of the YMCAs in mind, they may not be applicable to other organizations. These recommendations are consistent with the mission and values of the YMCA.

Osteoporosis

Scientific Commentary: Osteoporosis and Exercise

International Federation of Sports Medicine (FIMS)

Web site: www.fims.org

FIMS acknowledges and congratulates the American College of Sports Medicine (ACSM) for their extensive publication on Osteoporosis and Exercise. This commentary summarizes this document for a worldwide audience and also includes new information on the subject.

Osteoporosis is a disease characterized by low bone mass and the microarchitectural deterioration of bone tissue leading to an increase in bone fragility and the consequent risk of fracture. Prevention of osteoporotic fracture should therefore be focused on the preservation or enhancement of the material and structural properties of bone, the prevention of falls, and the increase of overall lean tissue mass. While forces applied to bone during daily activity in part develop and maintain its load bearing capacity, additional exercise and functional loading exert a positive influence on bone mass. However, the extent of this benefit, and the types of programs that will induce the most effective osteogenic stimulus remain uncertain. Results vary according to age, hormonal status, nutrition and exercise prescription.

It has long been recognized that deterioration of bone mass occurs more rapidly with unloading than with increased loading. This is a particular problem in older individuals who may find it impossible to continue with activities that provide an adequate load-bearing stimulus to maintain bone mass. On the other hand, it appears that strength and overall fitness can be improved at any age through a carefully planned exercise program. At the present time there is no conclusive evidence that exercise alone or in combination with added calcium intake prevents a rapid decrease in bone mass in the immediate post-menopausal years. However, the additional benefits of regular exercise to general health and well-being are numerous and all healthy women should be encouraged to participate in physical activities regardless of their osteogenic component.

Based on this information the following recommendations are made:

1. Weight-bearing physical activity is essential for normal development and maintenance of a healthy skeleton. Activities that focus on increasing muscle strength may also be beneficial, particularly for non weight-bearing bones.

2. Recent evidence demonstrating that growing bone is more responsive to mechanical loading and physical activity than mature bone suggests that regular exercise during early life may be an important factor in the prevention of osteoporosis in later life.

3. Excessive endurance training may induce hormonal changes, menstrual disturbances and even adversely affect bone structure.

4. Exercise cannot be recommended as a substitute for hormone replacement therapy during menopause.

5. Activities that improve strength, flexibility and coordination may indirectly but effectively decrease the incidence of osteoporotic fractures by reducing the likelihood of falling. These should be included in an optimal exercise program for older women.

References

1. *Medicine and Science in Sports and Exercise.* Vol. 27. No. 4 pages i-vii. 1995.

2. D.A. Bailey: The Saskatchewan Pediatric Bone Mineral Accrual Study: Bone Mineral Acquisition During Growing Years, presented at the symposium "Problems and Solutions in Longitudinal Research" Aug. 31 to Sept. 2, 1996 Noordwijkerhout, Netherlands. In press: *Int J. Sp. Med.*

Sun Dangers

Statement on Sun Dangers for the Lifeguard

International Life Saving Federation Medical Commission

Background

The nature of the profession of lifesaving requires significant time outdoors. This leads to exposure to the elements which includes sunlight. Extensive exposure to the ultraviolet rays in sunlight leads to premature aging, skin damage, skin cancer, and eye damage. This risk is significantly increased in fair skinned individuals, or those who have suffered severe sunburn in early childhood.

Skin cancer is the most common of all cancers and can be deadly. The three main types are squamous cell carcinoma, basal cell carcinoma, and the most aggressive type, melanoma. The prevalence of skin cancer increases with sun exposure, burning or tanning.

Ninety-five percent of skin cancer can be cured if detected early. Therefore, individuals such as lifeguards who have significant sun exposure should have regular screening for skin cancer, at least once per year.

New moles, changing moles, or scaly, crusty, raised skin lesions should be evaluated by a qualified physician. Enlargement, notching, itching, bleeding or color change in a pre-existing mole is a warning sign.

Avoidance of sun exposure especially during peak times of the day is helpful in reducing skin damage and cancer risk. This can be accomplished by appropriate shelter at guard stations, tightly woven long sleeve clothing, wide brimmed hats, and frequent and thorough use of water resistant sun screen. Sunscreen should be a minimum SPF 30 or greater. It should be applied 15 to 30 minutes prior to sun exposure and should be used even on cloudy days as UV light penetrates clouds and causes skin burn-

ing. Sun screen should be applied with extra care to the lips, ears, nose, shoulders and head. It should be reapplied every 2–3 hours or more often if swimming, or sweating profusely.

Lifeguards and other personnel who experience significant skin cancer may not in some instances be able to continue employment in outdoor activities. This situation may have a substantial financial impact on the individual and the organization.

The UV rays in sunlight can also seriously damage the eyes. Sun damage can contribute to cataracts, macular degeneration, corneal damage, and pterygiums. Eye protection should consist of good quality sunglasses in addition to shade and hats. Sunglasses should offer 99 - 100% protection from UVA and UVB light as well as screening out 75 - 95% of the visible light. They should be breakage resistant with brown, gray, green, or amber lenses. Wraparound style and polarization are advised to help reduce glare and eye fatigue, but must not obstruct peripheral vision.

Statement

1. Lifeguarding is a high-risk occupation for the development of skin cancer due to extensive sun exposure. All professional and volunteer lifeguard organizations should have mandatory sun protection policies. These policies should include:

   a. Appropriate education on the dangers of sun exposure.

   b. Mandatory requirements for the use of wide brim hats, tightly woven 50 (or more) rated clothing, minimum SPF 30 sunscreen.

c. The mandatory provision of minimum SPF 30 sunscreen and adequate natural or artificial shade for all personnel on duty.

d. Yearly skin cancer checks and eye exams for all employees.

e. Mandatory use of quality 100% UV protection sunglasses with side protection which does not obscure peripheral vision.

2. All lifeguard agencies are encouraged to support their employees in obtaining qualified physician evaluation of any suspicious skin lesions, treatment of such lesions, and employment modification as necessary.

3. All lifeguards and lifeguard organizations should be at the forefront of public education on the dangers of sun exposure and skin cancer. They should be instructive in the avoidance of sun damage including the use of clothing, sunscreen, hats and sunglasses and promote these principles by example.

References

1. The United States Lifesaving Association Manual of Open Water Lifesaving (ISBN #08359-4919-2)

2. Proceedings of the International Life Saving Federation International Medical-Rescue Conference, September 1997, San Diego, California

3. Surf Life Saving Australia Policy Statements

4. Public Health Hazards to Lifeguards from Sun Exposure, Special Report from the Centers for Disease Control and Prevention (CDC)

September 26 1998

Children

Climatic Heat Stress and the Exercising Child (RE9845)

American Academy of Pediatrics (AAP), Committee on Sports Medicine

Web site: www.aap.org/policy/9845.html

ABSTRACT. For morphologic and physiologic reasons, exercising children do not adapt as effectively as adults when exposed to a high climatic heat stress. This may affect their performance and well-being, as well as increase the risk for heat-related illness. This policy statement summarizes approaches for the prevention of the detrimental effects of children's activity in hot and humid climates, including the prevention of exercise-induced dehydration.

© July 2000

American Academy of Pediatrics

Volume 106, Number 01, pp158-159

Excessive Physical Training in Children and Adolescents

International Federation of Sports Medicine (FIMS)

Web site: www.fims.org

It is generally accepted that physical fitness is important for optimal development in children and adolescents. For this reason, physical fitness programs for youth should be recommended and encouraged (1, 2).

Medical and public health authorities should view the physical fitness of youth as being within their sphere of competence and responsibility. Children have a natural need to measure their maturing strength, skill, speed, and endurance against each other. Free play, exercise, and games provide a natural way for children and youth to gain an appropriate level of fitness.

A great increase has occurred during recent years in the number of children and adolescents participating in organized sports. Competitive sport contributes to the physical, emotional, and intellectual development of children and adolescents. Experience in sport can build self-confidence and encourage social behavior (3). For all these reasons, children's competitive sport must be considered in a positive light.

The quantitative and qualitative training effort devoted to prospective careers in top level competitive sport entails a great many biological and pedagogical influences. The reason for devoting increasing amounts of time to sports training is that optimal performance can be achieved only after a long period of development. To excel in sports today, the young athlete is forced to train longer and harder and to start at an earlier age. A distinction needs to be made between sports which demand non-specific training over a wide activity range and those in which training for competition must begin early enough to master high skill and to achieve top level performance.

For many reasons which will be presented, this intensified training has no physiological or educational justification. Moreover, it frequently leads to extremely great physical and mental stress during training and competition.

High-level competitive sport in childhood not only entails biological limits for performance but also carries risks of a psychological and social developmental nature. Intensive preparation for high-level sports competitions may occasionally create dropouts and / or psychologically injured children. Such sport competition may be so organized (by adults) that there is little or no room for social relationships and social development.

Content and methods of training must be appropriate to children. Diversity of movement and all-around physical conditioning should have priority as specialization comes later. Training environments must be organized accordingly (3).

A conscientious medical examination must be performed which guarantees that only children without health risk are admitted to competitive sport. In addition, counseling should be provided regarding the various possibilities for sports participation and for medical supervision during training. In some children where the medical supervision is inadequate or the training methods and sport are inappropriate to the age group, damage to health can occur. Such situations warrant the serious attention of all professional personnel involved in the sports programs.

An increasing number of overuse injuries is registered in children engaged in organized sports. These injuries are the result of frequent overloading causing microtrauma to tissues of the upper to lower extremity overstressed by this training (4,5,6). Children are more susceptible to overuse injuries than adults because of the presence of growing tissue and growth cartilage as well as the growth process itself which may induce muscular imbalances around the joints and increase the risk of injuries (4,6). Biomechanical studies have suggested that growth cartilage is more susceptible to stress in children than in adults. Repetitive microtrauma are often caused by overuse and may be associated with overtraining. Etiological factors include the increase in the amount of or intensity of training, inappropriate training methods, and poor equipment (7). Experienced coaches know that, during periods of rapid growth, the intensity of training should be reduced and specific compensatory exercise programs introduced in order to prevent injuries and compensate the muscular imbalances. The theoretical grounds outlined above indicate that growth itself is a risk factor in overuse injuries and that there is a need for vigilance with the prepubescent and pubescent athlete.

It is well known that tolerable levels of exercise seem to stimulate normal physical growth. In healthy young individuals, the positive growth stimulating effects of physical activity outweigh any potential negative effects and negate the growth-related risk factors. However, it is likely that, when physical loading becomes excessive, the beneficial effects on the skeletal system are lost and training becomes traumatic and disturbs normal growth (6, 8). Data concerning the influences of intensive physical exercise and training on the circulatory system are not numerous. The American Academy of Pediatrics warns of the tendency for weight lifting to result in an elevated blood pressure and that the lifting of very heavy weights can cause epiphysial damage in preadolescents (10).

The different levels of performance within a given age group are often the result of different levels of maturity rather than a difference in skill. The level of performance in this reason, the classification on the basis of chronological age is not satisfactory during adolescence. Other systems based on estimation of secondary sexual development should be used (14,15). Very little has been known until now

about the influence of repetitive excessive physical stress on the development of various organs and systems in children and adolescents.

It should be possible in this situation to apply the experience of many years of occupational medicine. In many countries, frequent repetition of stereotype work movements and excessive loading are forbidden by law for children and adolescents. In the codes of work-laws are included many limitations on the loads to be employed. In the same way, the number of repetitions of the same work-movement is limited. It would be useful to elaborate similar prescriptions in sport training, especially in children (16).

Parents, teachers, and coaches must be made sensitive to the psychological processes and stresses experienced by the child involved in competitive sport. The sum of the motor abilities, the personal abilities, and the social needs of the child are to be stimulated through sport. Only when children can attribute this to themselves and become self-motivated can top performance in sports be facilitated. The child must be able to maintain diverse social contacts not only in training but also outside of sport. Social isolation because of a special position in sport must be avoided (3). To impair these principles is unacceptable under the pretext of great success or talent. When children are young (or at least under the age of about ten), they fail to recognize that the outcome of a game is determined by both ability and effort. Therefore, winning and losing in sport is not particularly informative to children in relation to their abilities. It is only when children are aged 12 to 13 years of age that they begin to recognize that outcomes are determined jointly by effort and ability (8).

On the basis of the considerations described above, the International Federation of Sports Medicine presents the following recommendations:

1. Prior to participation in a competitive sport program, each participant should undergo a detailed medical examination which guarantees, on the one hand, that only children without

health risks are admitted to competitive sport and, on the other hand, provides an opportunity for advice regarding the various possible sports and training. Thorough and regular medical supervision is necessary, especially to prevent overuse and overgrowth injuries, which are more frequent in young adults.

2. The coach has a pedagogical responsibility for the present and future of the children entrusted to him/her beyond the purely athletic task. He / she must have knowledge of the special biological, physical, and social problems related to the development of the child and be able to apply this knowledge in coaching.

3. The child's individuality and opportunities for further development must be identified by the coach and regarded as major criteria governing his / her organization of training programs. Responsibility for the child's overall development must take precedence over training and competition requirements.

4. If "child coaching" is subjected to medical and pedagogical control as indicated above, it can afford valuable developmental opportunities for the children involved. However, if it takes the form of training for maximum performance at any price, it is to be roundly condemned on ethical and medical grounds. Nor is there any doubt that what has been presented here in relation to children also applies to a large extent to adolescents.

5. Children should be exposed to a wide variety of sporting activities to ensure that they identify the games which best meet their needs, interests, body build, and physical capacities. This tends to increase their success and enjoyment of sport and reduces the number of "dropouts." Early specialization should be discouraged.

6. Participants, particularly in collision sports, should be classified according to maturity, body size, skill, and gender, not only on a chronological age basis.

7. The rules and duration of games should be appropriate to the age of the participants while the training sessions should be relatively short and well-planned. The planned session maximizes activity and skills instruction and minimizes the risk on injury.

8. Competitive weightlifting and power lifting should not be recommended before the completion of puberty.

9. Excessively long distance competitive running events are not recommended for children prior to maturation.

References

1. American College of Sports Medicine. Opinion Statement on Physical Fitness in Children and Youth. *Medicine and Science in Sports and Exercise* 20:422-423, 1988.

2. Mácek, M. Vávra, J. FIMS Position Statement on Training and Competition in Children. *Journal of Sports Medicine and Physical Fitness* 20:135-138, 1980.

3. Council of Europe, Committee for the Development of Sport. *Sport for Children.* 1983, CDDS (83) Inf. 4.

4. Micheli, L J. Sports injuries in children. *Annales Nestlé* 44:20-27, 1986.

5. Personne, J. Commandré, F. Gounelle de Pontanel, H. Surles risques de l'entrainement sportif intensif précoce. *Bulletin Academie Nationale de Médecine* 167:207-214, 1983.

6. Micheli, L J. Overuse injuries in children's sports: the growth factor. *Orthopedic Clinics of North America* 14:337-359, 1983.

7. Codmmandré, F, Gagnerie F, Zakarian, M. The child, the spine and sport. *Journal of Sports Medicine and Physical Fitness* 28:11-19, 1988.

8. Caine, D J, Lindner, K J. Overuse injuries of growing bones. The young female gymnast at risk. *The Physician and Sportsmedicine* 13:51-65, 1985.

9. Roberts, G C. Children in competition. *Motor Skill* 4:37-50, 1980.

10. American Academy of Pediatrics. Weight training and weight lifting: information for the pediatrician. *The Physician and Sportsmedicine* 11:157-162, 1983.

11. Plas, F. *Guide de Cardiologie du Sport.* Paris, Baillére Ed., 1976,

12. Cumming, G R, Garant, T, Boryzyk, L. Correlation of performance in track and field events with bone age. *Journal of Pediatrics* 80:970-973, 1972.

13. Hollmann, W, Bouchard, C. Untersuchungen über die Beziehungen zwischen chronologischem und biologischem Alter zu spiroergometrischen Meßgrößen, Herzvolumen, anthropometrischen Daten and Skelettmuskelkraft bei 8-bis 18-jährigen Jungen. *Zeitschrift für Kreislaufforschung* 59:160-172, 1970.

November 1990

Elderly people

Physical Activity and Health in the Elderly

Brazilian Society of Sports Medicine and Brazilian Society of Geriatrics and Gerontology

Introduction

This publication represents the joint and official position statement of the Brazilian Society of Sports Medicine and Brazilian Society of Geriatrics and Gerontology about physical activity and health in elderly subjects. The purpose of this document is to make public current concepts concerning this issue in a practical and objective way, aiming to increase physical activity recommendation given by health professionals who deal with older people. The reader interested in more detailed information on this issues are recommended to consult the references listed at the end of this document.

Rationale

Life expectancy of the modern man has been increasing in last years, mostly as a consequence of the discover of several new medications that allowed a better control and more efficient treatment of chronic-degenerative and infectious diseases and also secondary to development of more efficient and sophisticated diagnostic and surgical techniques. The natural consequence was the increase of human's life average that today is placed around 66 years (20 years more than in 1950). Currently it is estimated that for every ten individuals, one is above 60 years of age. In developing countries people who are above this age are considered as elderly by the World Health Organization.

Population aging is a worldwide phenomenon that can also be seen in Brazil. According to data of the IBGE (Brazilian Institute of Geography and Statistics), by the year 2030 Brazil will be the sixth greatest world population of aged people in absolute numbers. The dis-eases linked to aging lead to a dramatic increase of health costs besides severe social consequences and deep impact in the economy of the countries. The majority of evidences show that the best way to improve and promote health in the elderly is to prevent its common medical problems. These interventions must be aimed specially at the prevention of cardiovascular diseases (CVD) considered the main cause of death in older people. On the other hand, a sedentary life-style, incapacity and dependence are the greatest health adversities related to aging. The main causes of incapacity are chronic diseases, including cerebrovascular accident sequelae, bone fractures, rheumatic diseases and CVD, among others.

The National Center of Statistics for Health estimates that about 84% of people aged 65 or above are dependent on others to carry out their daily activities.

It is estimated that in 2020 there will be seen an increase from 84 to 167% on the amount of older people suffering of moderate or serious incapacity. However, the implementation of preventive strategies, like practicing physical activity (PA) regularly and developing rehabilitation programs, should promote functional capacity improvement and minimize or prevent the appearance of such incapacity.

Physiology of Aging

Aging is a continuous process, during which occurs a progressive decline in all physiologic processes. Keeping an active and healthy lifestyle one should delay the morphologic and functional deterioration that occurs with age. Figure 9.1 on page 196 shows schematically the vicious cycle of aging.

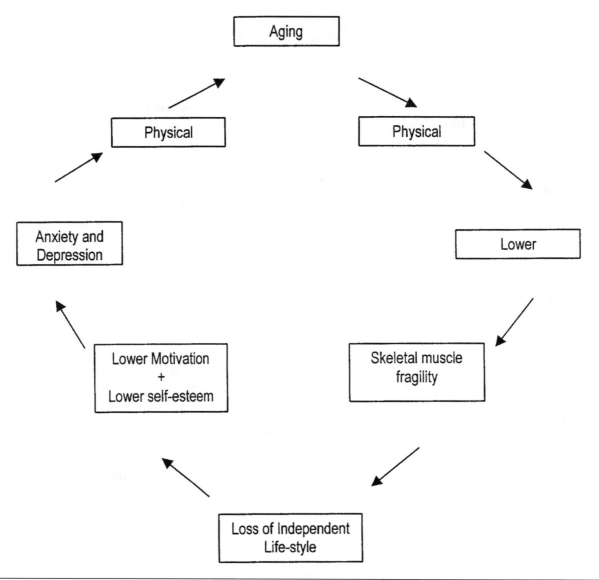

Figure 9.1 The vicious cycle of aging.

Cardiovascular Changes of Aging

The increase in life expectancy improved the knowledge concerning physiological changes that occur in the cardiovascular system and skeletal muscle. However, it remains difficult to determine the narrow border between normal aging and pathological alterations.

Aging is associated with cardiac structural alterations that tend to be individualized. It is noticeable between the ages of 30 and 90 years an increase of cardiac muscle mass of the order from 1 to 1.5 g/year. Left ventricular (LV) walls as well as septum show a slight increase in thickness even in the absence of CVD, keeping nor-

mal echocardiographic indices. These alterations are related to a greater rigidity of the aorta, determining an increase in the impedance to the emptying of LV, with consequent increase of the afterload. Besides, there is collagen deposition, mainly in the LV posterior wall. Myocardial collagen infiltration increases heart rigidity. The systolic function remains unchanged, but there is a reduction of the LV compliance with impairment of the diastolic function, determining an increase in the time for ventricular relaxation. It is probable that those findings are related to the reduction of the re-uptake of calcium by the sarcoplasmatic reticulum.

With aging, the autonomic nervous system modulation (adrenergic and vagal) of cardiac function diminishes, leading to a decline in the response to adrenergic stimulation on the senescent heart. The reduced beta-adrenergic response (lesser neural activation and reduction of beta-adrenergic receptors density) leads to a lower chronotropism, inotropism and arterial vasodilation. As a consequence, during exercise there is a reduction of the maximum heart rate (HR) and of maximum stroke volume (responsible for 50% of maximal oxygen consumption reduction consequent to aging).

The arteries suffer changes in their elasticity and compliance. The ventricular emptying in a less compliant aorta favors the increase of the systolic arterial pressure, while the increase of total peripheral vascular resistance determines a gradual increment of the mean arterial pressure. The aortic walls become thicker as a consequence of collagen and mucopolissacarids infiltration and calcium deposition, with loss of continuity of elastic layers. The pulse wave velocity is increased, reflecting vascular compliance reduction. The peripheral circulation suffers morphologic and functional alterations, such as the reduction of capillary/muscle fiber ratio, smaller capillary diameter and changes in the endothelial function. Specifically, it occurs a reduction in nitric oxide release and lower endothelial dependent vasodilator response, even though smooth muscle response to direct vasodilators remains unchanged.

These cardiovascular limitations lead to a reduction of maximum cardiac output that produces a reduction in the maximal oxygen consumption (VO_2max) of 0.4 to 0.5 ml $\{kg^{-1}\{min^{-1}\{year^{-1}$ (i.e., 1% per year in the adult). Although genetic characteristics may influence the rate of VO_2max decline, the maintenance of regular physical activity can slow this reduction to 50 percent.

Skeletal Muscle Alterations in Aged People

In humans, neuromuscular system reaches its full maturation between 20 to 30 years of age. Between the third and forth decades maximal force remains unchanged or with no significant reductions. Around 60 years, a reduction of muscular maximal strength between 30 and 40% begins, that means a loss of strength of about 6% per decade from 35 to 50 years of age and of 10% per decade for individuals older than that.

A reduction of bone mass also occurs in older people, more frequently in women. When it occurs in higher levels this characterizes osteoporosis that can predispose the occurrence of bone fractures.

After the age of 35 there are natural changes of articular cartilage that associated with biomechanic alterations acquired or not, provokes several degenerations that can lead to locomotive function and flexibility reduction, carrying increased risk of injuries.

Effects of Physical Activity in Aged People

Regular physical activity is recommended to maintain and/or to improve the bone mineral density and to prevent bone mass loss. However, physical exercise must not be considered as a substitute of hormonal therapy. The association between drug treatment and physical activity is an excellent way to prevent bone fractures.

Physical activity improves muscular force and mass as well as articular flexibility, especially in individuals above 50 years of age. Older people's trainability (the capacity of physiological adaptation to exercise) does not differ from that of youngers.

Physical activity is an outstanding health device in all ages, especially in the elderly and brings several physiological and psychological adaptations, such as:

- increase of VO_2max
- better peripheral vascular benefits
- increase of muscular mass
- better control of glycemia
- favorable changes in lipid profile
- reduction of body weight
- better control of resting blood pressure

- improvements of pulmonary function
- improving in balance and deambulation
- lower dependence for accomplishment of daily activities
- improvements of self-esteem and self-confidence
- significant improvement of the quality of life

Regular physical activity decreases the incidence of falls, risk of fractures and mortality in subjects with Parkinson's disease. For greater benefits, physical activity in those patients must include balance training exercises, walking and resistance exercises.

Physical activity has been indicated also for other neurological illnesses, such as multiple sclerosis and Alzheimer disease.

In aged people, regular physical activity, particularly weight-bearing and resistance exercises, promotes greater bone calcium fixation, assisting in prevention and treatment of osteoporosis. Physical activity also increases muscular strength and endurance, balance, and flexibility, consequently reducing fall incidence, bone fractures and its complications. Older people suffering of osteoarthrosis can also and must practice regular physical activity, as long as it is adapted to their condition.

Pre-participation Medical Evaluation

Although a pre-participation medical evaluation is a basic need, the unavailability must not hinder the adoption of an active life-style. Alternative evaluations go from simple questionnaires until sophisticated examinations. The main objectives of clinical examination are: identification of former and current illnesses, evaluation of nutritional status, medicine use, orthopedic limitations and current level of physical activity.

Amongst the complementary laboratory tests, the most important is the exercise stress test which main objectives are: determination of exercise tolerance and detection of exercise-induced myocardial ischemia. The basic reason for performing exercise stress test in older

people, even in asymptomatic ones lacking coronary disease risk factors, is that above 55 years of age the risk of coronary artery disease (CAD) exceeds 10%, giving a great diagnostic value to this test, that is, a negative result reduces the risk of CAD to 2%, while a positive result raises this risk to 90%. The exercise stress test can include measurement of pulmonary ventilation and expired gases (ergospirometry or cardiopulmonary exercise test) that allows the direct measure of VO_2max, determination of ventilatory threshold and better identification of exercise intolerance.

The ideal pre-participation evaluation must still include muscular strength and flexibility tests, postural analysis and determination of body composition. The overall objective of these tests is to develop an individualized prescription, offering a higher improvement in quality of life when one is involved with recreational activities and optimizing performance when practice of a specific sport modality is intended.

Exercise Prescription

When one considers exercise prescription for aged individuals, it must be considered – as in other ages – the different components of physical fitness: aerobic conditioning, muscle endurance and strength, body composition and flexibility. The later assures mobility and agility maintenance, keeping independence and improving quality of life of aged people.

A physical activity program for aged groups must aim to break the vicious cycle of aging (refer to figure 1), improving aerobic conditioning and diminishing the deleterious effects of a sedentary life-style. It must also maximize social interaction, reducing anxiety and depression, common problems seen in older people.

As seen in other medical interventions, regular physical activity must follow some guidelines, in order to assure the best risk/benefit relationship. The main parameters to be observed for an adequate prescription are: modality, duration, frequency, intensity and mode of progression. However, it is important to emphasize that exercise planning must be individualized, using the pre-participation evaluation results and considering the co-morbidities.

Exercise modality choice must primarily take into account individual preferences and capabilities of aged people. After the pre-participation evaluation is completed, one or more modalities can be restricted in consequence of the diseases found in the individual. Leisure and socialization must be incorporated in a successful program. In order to accomplish this, the activities should, as frequent as possible, be made in groups and be varied.

Some years ago, aerobic exercise prescription stated that they should be done from 3 to 5 times a week, lasting 20 to 30 minutes, with intensity going from light to moderate. Alternatively to this formal prescription, a significant reduction of general and cardiovascular mortality can be observed if one accumulates 2.000 kcal or more of weekly energy expenditure. This energy expenditure can be reached through formal activities (for example: walking, swimming, hydrogymnastics) and also through daily and leisure activities, like stair climbing, accomplishing domestic tasks, gardening, dancing, etc.

More recent studies suggest that activities of intensity above 4.5 metabolic equivalents (METs) provide an additional reduction of the general and cardiovascular mortality of approximately 10%. Thus, changing from an inactive state to light activities bring benefits. However, for those who already practice physical activity regularly, higher intensities are capable to increase even more those benefits.

However, in some aged individuals, their low functional capacity does not allow ideal exercise prescription. For those, an initial adaptation phase is required, in which intensity and duration will be determined in levels below those commonly used.

Physical activity must be initiated by a warm-up phase, range of motion exercises and stretching, along with the main activity at light intensities. Warm-up is an important phase as it reduces risk of injuries and increases blood flow to skeletal muscles. Progressive slow-down is equally important in preventing post-exercise hypotension. This complication can be more intense in the aged, as their hemodynamic adjustments are frequently slower and the use of cardiovascular acting drugs is common.

The intensity of aerobic phase can be determined using percentages of VO_2max or of maximal HR measured directly in an exercise stress test or estimated by some equations. Cardiovascular acting drugs can modify the relationship between HR and exercise intensity. In this case, rating of perceived exertion scales can be used (Borg scale), an excellent alternative for any subject. Generally a moderate intensity is recommended, from 40 to 75% of VO_2max or from 55 to 85% of the HR maximal, what in general corresponds to 3 to 5 or 12 to 13 on Borg scales depending on which scale is used (0-10 or 6-20, respectively). It should be emphasized that high intensity sessions are associated with low rates of adherence secondary to muscular discomfort, especially at the initial phase.

The duration of activity can vary from 30 to 90 minutes, keeping an inverse relationship with the intensity. The so called "frail aged" and individuals in initial phases of an exercise program can benefit themselves from short duration sessions (five to ten minutes) carried out in two or more periods along the day.

Ideally, exercise should be performed in most of—if possible in all—the days of the week, in order to reach more easily the necessary energy expenditure to attain health benefits.

Safety is essential in the initial phase of an appropriate exercise program. Thus, educating practitioners about exercise principles and stimulating self-monitoring is important. Also, efforts should be done to make the exercise a habit as natural as, for example, taking care of one's personal hygiene.

For muscular strength and endurance training, large muscle groups should be involved. Two to three series of six to twelve bouts increase muscle strength and endurance. These series should be performed two to three times/week, at an intensity equivalent to 60% of one maximal repetition.

Stretching exercises should be done avoiding ballistic movements. Progressive movements until a light discomfort is reached are adequate, and must take part of aerobic and strength sessions. In order to lessen the risk of injuries a higher level of care should be taken on movements' execution.

Safety is essential, not only from a cardiovascular perspective but also related to the locomotor system. It is important to consider aged people's lower ability of adapting to temperature extremes and impaired control of hydration. Adequate information about clothes, footwear and hydration during the activity must be given. Also, it is important to assure well-illuminated and ventilated environments, and to avoid sliding surfaces.

Finally, physical activity programs must be stimulated for aged individuals, even by government or private institutions since they consist in an excellent health-promoting tool. These programs already exist in some Brazilian cities. No other segment of the population acquires more benefits with regular physical activity than the elderly.

Practical Recommendations

Some recommendations must be observed in order to assure a correct and safe exercise practice.

- Exercise only if there is a physical well-being.
- Wear appropriate clothes and shoes.
- Avoid smoking and taking sedatives.
- Do not exercise after prolonged fasting. Prefer carbohydrates before exercise.
- Respect individual limitation, suspending exercise if discomfort or pain occurs.
- Avoid extremes of humidity and temperature.
- Begin activities slowly and progressively to allow adaptation.
- Assure proper hydration before, during, and after physical activities.

Conclusions

1. Regular physical activity improves quality of life and longevity of elderly people.
2. A physical activity program for aged people must be preceded by a medical evaluation and must also respect the different components of physical fitness, including aerobic, muscular strength, stretching and balance exercises.
3. Government at all levels, medical and scientific institutions, non-governmental organizations and the media must widespread the concept that physical activity is fundamental for health promotion of aged people and must also develop objective actions in order to make possible regular physical activity to this particular population.

Bibliography

1. American College of Sports Medicine Position Stand on Osteoporosis and Exercise. *Med Sci Sports Exerc* 1995;27: i-vii.
2. American College of Sports Medicine. ACSM Position stand on exercise and physical activity for older adults. *Med Sci Sports Exerc* 1998;30:992-1008.
3. Blair SN, Kohl III HW, Paffenbarger Jr RS, Clark DG, Cooper KH, Gibbons LW. Physical fitness and all-cause mortality - a prospective study of healthy men and women. *JAMA* 1989;2395-401.
4. Carvalho T, Nóbrega ACL, Lazzoli JK, Magni JRT, Rezende L, Drummond FA, et al. Posição oficial da Sociedade Brasileira de Medicina do Esporte: atividade física e saúde. *Rev Bras Med Esporte* 1996;2:79-81.
5. Fiatarone MA, Marks EC, Ryan ND, Meredith CN, Lipsitz LA, Evans WJ. High-intensity strength training in nonagenarians: effects on skeletal muscle. *JAMA* 1990;263:3029-34.
6. Fletcher GF, Balady G, Blair SN,

Blumenthal J, Caspersen C, Chaitman B, et al. Statement on exercise: benefits and recommendations for physical activity programs for all americans - a statement for health professionals by the Committee on Exercise and Cardiac Rehabilitation of the Council on Clinical Cardiology, American Heart Association. *Circulation* 1996;94:857-62.

7. Lee I-M, Hsieh C-C, Paffenbarger Jr RS. Exercise intensity and longevity in men - the Harvard Alumni Health Study. *JAMA* 1995;273:1179-84.

8. Paffenbarger Jr RS, Hyde RT, Wing AL, Hsieh CC. Physical activity, all-cause mortality, and longevity of college alumni. *N Engl J Med* 1986;314:605-13.

9. Pate RR, Pratt M, Blair SN, Haskell WL, Macera CA, Bouchard C. Physical activity and public health - a recommendation from the Centers for Disease Control and Prevention and the American College of Sports Medicine. *JAMA* 1995;273:402-7.

10. Pollock ML, Mengelkoch L, Graves J, Lowenthal D, Limacher M, Foster C et al. Twenty-year follow-up of aerobic power and body composition of older track athletes. *J Appl Physiol* 1997;82:1508-16.

11. Spirduso WW. Physical fitness, aging and psychomotor speed: a review. *J Gerontol* 1980;35:850-65.

12. WHO Expert Committee. Report of a rehabilitation after cardiovascular diseases, with special emphasis on developing countries. Geneva: *Bulletin of the World Health Organization* 1993.

November 1995

Originally published in *Revista Brasileira de Medicina do Esporte 1999; 5(6): 207-11.*

Female Athletes

Women's Division

The National Junior College Athletic Association (NJCAA)

It is the basic belief of the Women's Division of the NJCAA that the athletic program for the woman compliments the existing programs offered by the NJCAA. The Women's Program is an integral part of the total educational process, which fosters sound educational goals concurrent with those of the member institutions.

Because of the uniqueness of the Community/Junior College, it is important to provide an organization which provides equal representation through the twenty-four elected regional directors for each division. The Women's Division of the NJCAA provides programs which afford opportunities for the participation of all community colleges. Through the existing structure of the NJCAA, representatives of both the Men's and Women's Division work together to develop and maintain eligibility rules, which will be applied equally to all athletes, both male and female.

For those Community Colleges seeking an affiliation for their women's athletic program, the NJCAA offers an organization that can meet the individual needs of all students because it provides national competition for all eligible member schools through regional affiliation.

It is important to emphasize that the Women's Division is dedicated to meeting the needs of all women athletes, providing them with the highest caliber of national competition in a wide range of sports.

From its inception, the Women's Division of the National Junior College Athletic Association has fostered among its goals the encouragement, promotion and advancement of all Women's Athletic Programs in the junior college. In order to insure progress in meeting these objectives and goals, women of compe-

tency and experience, as well as those whose backgrounds have been limited, should not be excluded from leadership roles. As a group, we are strongly opposed to any and all measures which would remove or exclude capable, qualified and/or interested women from assuming those leadership positions relating to Women's Athletics. It is a specific concern that the Women's Regional Directors position be held by a woman.

We would strongly urge all regions of the NJCAA to provide for access to an input from women within their respective regions at each regional meeting relating to the business and conduct of the Women's Division. In those regions where a few women currently serve in any leadership capacity, we would urge that a conscientious, active and ongoing effort be made to identify, attract and develop the leadership potential of women throughout that region.

It is through these efforts that we hope to expand leadership opportunities, promote conscientious awareness, stimulate further interest on the part of women in the NJCAA, and to recognize the significant contributions women can make in the leadership and administration of women's athletics.

The NJCAA believes in the value of equitable participation and treatment of men and women in intercollegiate athletics and through its structure, programs, legislation and policies will promote these values. The NJCAA will act to encourage its member institutions to assure equity in the quantity and quality of participation in women's athletics through its programs. The NJCAA stands with other athletic organizations in believing, at an institutional level, gender equity in intercollegiate athletics describes an environment in which fair and equitable distribution of overall athletic opportunities, benefits and resources is available to women and men and in which student-athletes, coaches and athletic administrators are not subject to gender based discrimination.

An athletic program can be considered equitable when the participants in both the men's and women's sports programs would accept as fair and equitable the overall program of the other gender. No individual should be discriminated against on the basis of gender, institutionally or regionally or nationally in intercollegiate athletics.

The Female Athlete Triad

International Federation of Sports Medicine (FIMS): A statement for health professionals from the Scientific Commission

Web site: www.fims.org

Introduction

It is generally accepted that regular physical activity is important for health in females and males. For this reason, physical fitness programs for women should be recommended and encouraged all over the world (22). The gender-specific physiological, anatomical, psychological, and social aspects of the female athlete, however, need specific consideration in all levels of women sport.

Since the death of gymnast Christy Henrich from anorexia in 1994 at the age of 22 and a weight of 64 pounds or 29 kg, athletes, parents, coaches, medical personnel, judges, sport federations and sport governing bodies have become more aware of the medical and psychological conditions that can afflict young women participating in competition sport 41)" (35, 41). Of particular concern is the **"Female Athlete Triad"** of **Disordered Eating, Amenorrhea and Osteoporosis**.

Definitions And Basics Of Eating Disorders, Menstrual Dysfunction And Osteoporosis

The **"Female Athlete Triad"** was described in 1992 by the Women's Task Force of the American College of Sports Medicine (53). It refers to the inter-relatedness of three discrete medical entities that can occur in the female athlete population: disordered eating, menstrual dysfunction and premature osteoporosis. Individuals with one of the triad disorders are at risk and should be screened for the others.

Eating Disorders and Disordered Eating

Eating disorders encompasses a number of abnormal eating patterns, including **Anorexia Nervosa** and **Bulimia Nervosa**. The latter two psychological conditions have strict criteria, as defined by the American Psychiatric Association (3). These must **all** be satisfied in order to make the diagnosis.

Anorexia Nervosa

- Refusal to maintain body weight at or above a minimally normal weight for age and height (e.g. weight loss leading to maintenance of body weight less than 85 % of that expected; or failure to make expected weight gain during period of growth, leading to body weight less than 85 % of that expected).
- Intense fear of gaining weight or becoming fat, even though underweight.

- Disturbance in the way in which one's body weight or shape is experienced, undue influence of body weight or shape on self-evaluation, or denial of the seriousness of the current low body weight.
- In post-menarchal females, amenorrhea, i.e. the absence of at least three consecutive menstrual cycles.

Specify type

- **Restricting type:** During the episode of anorexia nervosa, the person does not regularly engage in binge eating or purging behaviour (i.e., self-induced vomiting or the misuse of laxatives or diuretics).
- **Binge eating/purging type:** During this episode of anorexia nervosa, the person regularly engages in binge eating or purging behaviour (as defined above).

Bulimia Nervosa

- Recurrent episodes of binge eating, characterized by both of the following:

   1. Eating in a discrete period of time (e.g., within any 2-hour period) an amount of food that is definitely larger than most people would eat during a similar period of time and under similar circumstances.
   2. A sense of lack of control over eating during the episode (e.g. a feeling that one cannot stop eating or control what or how much one is eating).

- Recurrent inappropriate compensatory behaviour in order to prevent weight gain, such as self-induced vomiting; misuse of laxatives, diuretics, enemas, or other medications; fasting; or excessive exercise.
- The binge eating and inappropriate compensatory behaviours both occur, on average, at least twice a week for 3 months.
- Self-evaluation is unduly influenced by body shape and weight.
- The disturbance does not occur exclusively during episodes of anorexia nervosa.

Specify type

- **Purging type:** The person regularly engages in self-induced vomiting or the misuse of laxatives or diuretics.
- **Nonpurging type:** The person uses other inappropriate compensatory behavior, such as fasting or excessive exercise, but does not regularly engage in self-induced vomiting or misuse of laxatives or diuretics.

A separate category of **Eating Disorders Not Otherwise Specified (EDNOS)** covers the wider variety of conditions that do not conform completely to the above definitions of anorexia and bulimia. It is important to recognize, however, that there is a spectrum of **disordered eating**, ranging from preoccupation with food, body size, shape and composition, to the more severe **eating disorders**. At any point along the continuum, there can be serious health implications. Nutritional deficiency, i.e. insufficient caloric intake for the amount of training and competition can result in an energy deficit, which in turn can lead to the other triad conditions: amenorrhea and osteoporosis.

Prevalence of eating disorders among athletes

Female athletes have a higher risk for the development of eating disorders compared to male athletes (47). Anorexia nervosa, bulimia nervosa and eating disorders not otherwise specified occur more often in female and male athletes compared to non-athletes (47, 48). Furthermore, eating disorders occur more often in female athletes of esthetical sports and sports with weight-classes, compared to sports where weight is not thought to be important for a good result.

Factors associated with eating disorders in athletes

Eating disorders may have many causes. Due to the additional stresses in the surroundings of athletes, top level sport women seem to be more susceptible to the development of eating disorders compared to female non-athletes 50)" (48, 50). The factors associated with eating disorders in athletes include:

- **Caloric deficiency:** A sudden increase in training volume might induce a caloric deficit. This deficit might be associated with biological and social consequences and end up in eating disorders (47).

- **Beginning of sport-specific training before puberty:** Athletes with eating disorders started their career at an earlier age compared to athletes without eating disorders (47). If an athlete starts a sport-specific training before puberty, growth spurt and body development might lead to a body shape that is not ideal for the selected sport. This discrepancy might end in the attempt to change body shape by food restriction.

- **Traumatical experiences:** Traumatical experiences for athletes may be the loss or changing of a trainer or an injury or illness, that do not allow normal training. This might lead to weight gain and, in some cases, to an irrational fear of getting fat, and subsequently in dieting behavior in order to compensate reduction of energy expenditure (50). Other traumatical experiences that are associated with the development of eating disorders in athletes are longer lasting phases of diets, a casual comment (on body shape etc.), moving away from home, failure at school or work, problems with the partner or family, death of a friend, and sexual misuse by the trainer.

- **Compulsion to weight reduction and weight fluctuations:** There is increasing awareness of the influence of body composition on athletic performance. In some activities an increase in body weight can decrease performance. However, pressure to decrease body weight or body fat percentage to unrealistic levels contribute to the development of disordered eating practices. Excessive weight loss can lead to loss of fat mass, dehydration, and a decrease in performance (36). Compulsion to weight reduction is an often mentioned possible cause for eating problems in athletes.

However, the problem is not the compulsion to weight reduction per se, but the personal situation and the way of communication in which an athlete is talked to loose weight, and whether he or she is guided or not. Furthermore, athletes often have to loose weight in a short time period. The consequences are phases of diets and weight fluctuations, which are very probably associated with the risk of developing eating disorders (7, 47). Very probably, trainers alone might not cause eating disorders in athletes, although the problem might be set off or intensified by unsuitable training in vulnerable persons. The role of the trainer has to be seen as part of the whole situation.

- **Attraction of sport to persons being susceptible to eating disorders:** Beside food restriction, excessive physical activity is one mean to loose weight in persons suffering from eating disorders. Therefore, one might speculate, that persons with a predisposition to eating disorders are found in sports to a higher extent than in the normal population. This might be true for a normal physical activity level. If the only motivation for an athlete for sporting is to loose weight, however, this athlete very probably will not reach the top level. Therefore, a higher prevalence of persons already suffering from eating disorders, is probably seen in recreational rather than in top level sport (48).

Consequences of eating disorders for health

Eating disorders may lead to severe health problems in athletes and non-athletes. Rate of mortality is about 6 % in anorexia nervosa (34). There are many harmful effects of poor eating behaviors, including a decrease in metabolic rate, depletion of muscle glycogen stores, loss of muscle mass, hypoglycemia and dehydration. These can render the athlete more susceptible to fatigue and musculoskeletal injuries due to impaired coordination and decreased concentration. Electrolyte imbalance may lead to serious and potentially fatal cardiac arrythmias. There are changes in the endocrine and thermoregulatory systems. Bulimics in particular may suffer from severe gastrointestinal disorders. An increase in size of parotid glands, and erosion of dental enamel may also result from recurrent vomiting of acidic stomach contents. The long lasting effects of eating disorders are not clear in detail. They include, however, the effects of estrogen deficiency, like skeletal demineralization, osteopenia and premature osteoporosis.

Delayed Menarche And Menstrual Dysfunction

Commonly, menstrual cycles are described as **eumenorrheic, oligomenorrheic** and **amenorrheic**, based on the occurrence of menstrual bleeding. The term **eumenorrheic** refer to cycles that occur at intervals of approximately 28 days, with the 10th and 90th percentile of 22 and 36 days respectively, for women between the ages of 20 to 40 years (52). The term **oligomenorrhea** is used to indicate menstrual cycles that occur inconsistently. Menstrual bleeding occurs at intervals greater than 36 days, or 3 to 6 periods a year. **Amenorrhea** is a clinical symptom that indicates a disruption of the reproductive cycle with probable anovulation and refers to the absence of menstruation. In **primary amenorrhea**, a girl had no menarche (first menstrual bleeding) by the age of 16, or has not developed any secondary sexual characteristics such as breasts and pubic hair by the age of 14. **Secondary amenorrhea** refers to the cessation of menses after menarche, specifically the absence of menses for 3 consecutive months, or less than 3 periods a year (9).

The variability of the length of the menstrual cycle is only one factor in characterizing its normalcy. One must also consider hormonal levels that change according to follicular and luteal development. Three aberrations are identified: the short luteal phase, luteal phase insufficiency, and anovulation (9). The short luteal phase is characterized by a shortened menstrual cycle length (21 days and less), with hormonal pattern similar to a normal cycle. Luteal phase insufficiency is an ovulatory cycle, with deficient corpus luteum function and deficient progesterone production. Anovulation is a cycle without ovulation, though withdrawal bleeding may occur due to declining estrogen levels. These three aberrations in menses can be easily missed if only menstrual history data are available to the researcher (4).

Prevalence of menstrual dysfunction in athletes—delayed menarche

The average age of menarche is about 12.8 and 13.0 years in North American and European girls, respectively, with a wide range of normal variation. In female athletes, it was previously thought that training prior to menarche might delay menarche, but more rigid analysis of the data has attempted to refute this theory (44). This remains, however, a controversial area. Retrospective studies have shown that by the age of 14, only 20 % of gymnasts had reached menarche, compared with 40 % of distance runners, 70 % of anorexics, and 95 % of the normal population (5). Other investigators have also documented a higher age of menarche (ranging from 14.3 to 16.2 years) in gymnasts relative to non-athletic controls (6, 10, 20, 40). Some experts maintain that these sports attract females who are genetically thin with a boyish stature and preprogrammed delay in puberty. Many gymnasts come from families with late maturation, where short stature is in part familial. Nevertheless, a decrease in training level or intensity, as occurs in the case of injury, will frequently precipitate a growth spurt and subsequent menarche in the prepubertal athlete, or resumption of cycles in an athlete with secondary amenorrhea. A 5 year prospective study found a delay in age of menarche in gymnasts (14.5 years) compared to a control group (13.2 years), suggesting that physical training of more than 10 - 20 hours per week may be detrimental (28). Though a negative calorie balance and not the number of hours could be the cause. There is currently debate about the risks of impaired growth and development, and a fear that elite gymnasts, with their restrictive eating habits and intensive training practices, may not reach their genetically programmed adult height (50). Therefore, some authors have suggested that training should decrease during puberty (33). More research, however, is needed in this area.

Amenorrhea and oligomenorrhea

The prevalence of **secondary amenorrhea** and **oligomenorrhea** varies widely due to the lack of standard definitions for these symptoms. In the general adult population the prevalence of menstrual irregularities is estimated to be from 2–5 %. Surveys of adult athletes show 1–79 (2, 36). These variations reflect methodological problems, like lacking of standard definitions, differences in age, sport modality, level of activity and performance, training prior to menarche, and others (11).

Short luteal phase and anovulation

Recent works have suggested that many of the so-called eumenorrheic athletes, i.e., those with regular menstrual cycles are actually suffering from hidden menstrual dysfunction such as anovulatory cycles or luteal phase insufficiencies. The exact prevalence of these less obvious forms of menstrual dysfunction is not known, as these athletes consider themselves perfectly regular. Short luteal phase and anovulation might represent a mild form of the athletic reproductive system dysfunction that can lead to amenorrhea under greater stress (27).

Factors associated with menstrual dysfunction in athletes

The factors associated with menstrual dysfunction in athletes may be divided into three major categories: genetic, environmental, and reproductive maturity (11).

- **Genetic factors:** The high correlations that exists in menarcheal age between mothers and daughters in non-athletes seems to be less pronounced in athletes. In active females, there are other variables that are better predictors of menarcheal age such as leanness and intense prepubertal activity (45).

- **Reproductive maturity:** Amenorrheic athletes have a higher prevalence of prior menstrual irregularities that athletes with regular cycles. These athletes seem to have an a prior tendency to menstrual dysfunction, and exercise alone is not a causative factor. Therefore, menstrual dysfunction and athletic training are not cause-effect relationships but might rather be signs of hypothalamic-pituitary-gonadal axis maturation (27).

- **Environmental factors:** Among the factors that are associated with menstrual cycle disturbances in athletes are energy and nutrient balance, sport modality, performance level, body weight and composition, eating disorders, and mental stress.

- **Energy and nutrient balance:** Energy availability is defined as nutritional energy intake minus energy expenditure in sport and other daily activities. Dietary restriction reduces LH pulse frequency in women (21). In animals, amenorrhea induced by exercise can be reversed by increased feeding without a reduction in the exercise regimen (30). Some athletes with a high energy expenditure have a relatively low energy intake and are therefore under a discrete but chronic energetical deficit (18). Furthermore, normalization of menstruation was observed in athletes who reduced training or increased caloric intake (16, 17). Altogether low energy intake seems to be the most important factor for the induction of menstrual cycle irregularities in athletes.

- **Sport modality:** Athletic activities requiring thin bodies, such as ballet dancing, long-distance running, and gymnastics, and sports with weight classes tend to have a much higher prevalence of menstrual cycle irregularities and a later age of menarche, which might be due to the athletes pathological eating behavior and negative energy balance (46, 47, 48).

- **Level of performance:** The better performing athletes tend to have higher prevalence of menstrual irregularities (42). The better the performance level, the higher is the daily energy expenditure especially in endurance sports, and the higher the risk of an energetical deficit.

- **Body weight and composition**: In early studies, low body weight and low body fat was thought to be causal for the development of menstrual cycle irregularities in athletes (23, 24). Other authors, however, denied this hypothesis but favored other factors as possible causes (31). Nowadays is it generally believed that low body fat rather is a symptom of an energetical deficit rather than the main cause for menstrual irregularities in athletes, although body fat is an important endocrine organ for the conversion of androgens to estrogens (31, 48).

- **Eating disorders**: Anorectic patients suffer from amenorrhea due to low caloric intake. Fifty percent of bulimic women have menstrual cycle irregularities (49). Therefore, eating disorders very probably play an important causal role in the development of menstrual cycle irregularities in athletes (48).

- **Mental stress**: It is difficult to define and measure mental stress in athletes. In spite of these difficulties, it is generally believed that many athletes are subjected to constant psychological stress during training and competition. Stress mastering, however, shows a wide inter-personal variability. It is well established that mental stress plays an important role in the induction of hypothalamic dysfunction, including the GnRH pulse generator. Therefore, the individual stress reaction in one single athletes might be causally related to menstrual irregularities (11, 48).

Pathogenesis of menstrual dysfunction in athletes

The exact pathophysiological mechanisms leading to menstrual dysfunction in athletes are still unclear in detail. Causes of menstrual cycle disturbances may include dysfunction at the level of the hypothalamus, pituitary, ovaries or uterus. Exercise-associated amenorrhea is a diagnosis of exclusion. It is important to exclude other medical causes, including pregnancy (39). Normal initiation and maintenance of menstruation requires integration and function of all organs. The hypothalamus produces gonadotropin releasing hormone (GnRH) in a regular pulsatile pattern. This has a direct effect on secretion of luteinizing hormone (LH) and follicle-stimulating hormone (FSH) from the pituitary gland, which subsequently stimulate ovary estrogen production and ovulation. After ovulation, both estrogen (estradiol) and progesterone are produced in high quantities by cells in the ovary (1).

Excessive exercise and/or emotional stress can affect many hormones including neurohormones like dopamine, serotonine, melatonin, endorphins, and catecholamines. Endogenous opioids, the hormones of the "runner's high", can suppress the frequency and amplitude of GnRH pulses. Melatonin and dopamine can decrease GnRH secretion. The chronic stimulation of the adrenal axis under physical and/or mental stress also has an inhibitory action on GnRH pulsatiliy (27). An imbalance between energy expenditure due to the demands of the sport, and caloric intake can cause the body to perceive inadequate net energy stores to support development of a fetus. The reproductive system effectively "shuts down" as a self-protective mechanism (32).

Consequences of menstrual irregularities for health

Amenorrhea is neither desirable nor a "normal" result of physical training. It is a symptom of an underlying problem that requires medical evaluation within the first three month of occurrence. Exercise associated amenorrhea is a diagnosis of exclusion, and all other possible causes of amenorrhea must be excluded by a thorough medical evaluation (36). Low estrogen levels may have many consequences for the female organism. Ovulation and reversal of amenorrhea are unpredictable in amenorrheic women. Because ovulation precedes menstruation, all sexually active amenorrheic women should be tested for pregnancy as part of their medical evaluation and receive contraception counseling (36). Amenorrhea, once felt to be a benign, reversible condition, has been linked to premature loss of bone mineral density since

1984 (13). In order to assure to calcium balance, amenorrheic athletes should be encouraged to ingest at least 1500 mg of elemental calcium per day (36, 48). Beside the effects on the skeleton, menstrual dysfunction has some other complications for health. Data indicate that the beneficial effects of habitual physical activity on serum lipoprotein profiles are reversed by exercise-induced hypoestrogenic amenorrhea (11). Furthermore, the risk of endometrial hyperplasia and adenocarcinoma due to a chronic, unopposed estrogen level, which might occur in luteal phase deficiency, has been raised, but so far not been reported (8). The effects of chronically reduced estrogen levels on performance are not clear so far. However, as estrogen appears to enhance lipid oxidation and lessen glycogen depletion, a hypoestrogenic state in an athletic female might have effects on performance (8).

Osteoporosis

Definition

Osteoporosis is defined as "a systemic skeletal disease characterized by low bone mass and microarchitectural deterioration of bone tissue, with a consequent increase in bone fragility and susceptibility to fracture risk" (26).

The following diagnostic criteria have been established (26):

1. **Normal**: Bone mineral density (BMD) is no more than 1 standard variation (sd) below the mean of young adults.

2. **Osteopenia**: BMD between 1 and 2.5 sd below the mean of young adults.

3. **Osteoporosis**: BMD more than 2.5 sd below the mean of young adults.

4. **Severe osteoporosis**: BMD more than 2.5 sd below the mean of young adults plus one or more fragility fractures.

Peak bone mass

Peak bone mass or maximal bone density is reached at the third decade and possibly even earlier, with a gradual decline until menopause when more rapid bone loss occurs. At least 60 to 70 % of peak bone mass is laid down during the adolescent growth spurt. This critical "window of opportunity" for children must not be missed. Inadequate training regimens in combination with other negative factors like eating problems during childhood can delay menarche and the onset of puberty. Growth can be stunted, and as a consequence optimal bone density may not be realized.

Factors affecting bone in athletes with menstrual dysfunction

Estrogens and progesterone are important endocrine factors for maintenance of bone health by influencing remodeling processes (19, 37). Therefore, each factor associated with menstrual dysfunction in athletes might be directly or indirectly related to loss of bone mineral density. The principle causes of premenopausal osteoporosis in athletic women are menstrual cycle irregularities according to the associated hypoestrogenemia (14, 36). Other causes include inappropriate nutritional calcium intake and vitamin D deficiency.

Bone mineral density in athletes with eating disorders and menstrual dysfunction

Hypoestrogenism in female athletes is associated with reduced bone mass and increased rates of bone loss. This loss is similar to bone loss in postmenopausal women or in women with a pathological hypoestrogenic condition such as premature ovarian failure (36). In earlier studies on female athletes with menstrual dysfunction, decreased BMD was reported only for the lumbar spine. Newer studies, however, indicate the deficit appears to be generalized throughout the skeleton (36). Whether bone loss is observed at all regional sites may depend in part on the extend of mechanical loading at specific sites in various sports (43).

Loss of BMD in athletes with menstrual cycle disturbances may be irreversible, as no changes or only slight gains in BMD could be achieved with a return of normal menstrual cycles, and/or hormonal replacement therapy (15, 25).

The combination of disordered eating practices and low calcium intake combined with menstrual dysfunction may exacerbate bone loss. Not all amenorrheic athletes, however, have low bone mass. Their skeletal status depends upon the length and severity of their menstrual irregularity, as well as factors that influence their BMD prior to the onset of amenorrhea: the type of skeletal loading during activity, their nutritional status, and a genetic component (12, 36). A recent study could demonstrate that weight-bearing exercise can prevent or attenuate bone loss at specific skeletal sites in normal weight bulimic patients, but not in anorectics (49).

Other consequences for the skeleton

As a consequence to the decline in BMD, athletes with menstrual dysfunction have an increased susceptibility to stress fractures, and other musculoskeletal injuries during the competitive years (29). However, amenorrheic athletes might have a pathological mental drive to do their sport, and therefore might ignore minor injuries unless they exaggerate. In these athletes, a higher prevalence of injuries is rather a consequence of overtraining than of low BMD (38).

Diagnostic Clues

Eating disorders and disordered eating

As a trainer has close contact to his/her athlete, changes in behavior and physical symptoms should easily be recognized. However, symptoms of disordered eating in competition athletes are often ignored, not seen or realized. One explanation is a lack of knowledge about this problem. Most persons with eating disorders do not realize their health problems by themselves. They only see that something is going wrong when they get injured or loose performance (48). Athletes suffering from bulimia nervosa often have a normal or nearly normal body weight and are therefore difficult to be diagnosed. Therefore, trainers, parents, and the people around the athlete should be able to see and realize the symptoms of disordered eating patterns.

Signs and symptoms of disordered eating may include weight loss, a decrease in athletic ability and skill, a preoccupation with calories, fat intake and weight, and increasing self-criticism. The athlete may have wide fluctuations in her weight, and avoid eating in the presence of others. Other suspicious behavior may include frequent visits to the bathroom after meals, laxative packages in lockers, and excessive physical activity over and above what is required for training.

Delayed puberty and menstrual dysfunction

The diagnosis of exercise-associated menstrual disorders is still one of exclusion and it is important to first rule out other common causes of amenorrhea. Menstrual dysfunction is obvious by the time frank amenorrhea occurs. Earlier disturbances of the hypothalamic pituitary axis, however, often initially go unrecognized. In moderation, ovulatory symptoms such as breast tenderness, food cravings, fluid retention and mood changes in the week or so before menstruation, signal that all of the interdependent hormonal systems are working correctly. If the athlete does not have any of these symptoms, she may be suffering from short luteal phase or anovulatory cycles, despite the presence of "regular" menstrual bleeding.

A full history should be taken with special emphasis on type of activity and competitive level, energy output, nutrition, eating behavior, changes in weight, and fractures history. Signs and symptoms of androgen excess, galactorrhea, and hot flushes should be looked for. Physical and pelvic examinations and measurements of blood concentrations of prolactin, thyroid function tests, FSH, LH, testosterone, DHEA-S, E_2, and ßHCG should be done. A progestin challenge test might be indicated to induce withdrawl bleeding (11).

Osteoporosis

Osteoporosis does not become evident on radiographs until approximately 20–30 % of bone density is lost. As definition of osteoporosis or osteopenia is based on bone mineral density, measurement of BMD is the standard method for the determination of a beginning osteopenia or more severe osteoporosis. Newer techniques of measuring BMD, specifically dual energy x-ray absorptiometry (DXA) can identify individuals with low BMD and, if done serially, can assess those who are rapidly loosing bone and monitor their response to therapy (36). In athletes with eating disorders or menstrual irregularities, who are at risk for osteoporosis or osteopenia, measurement of BMD should be performed as early as possible in order to start intervention and therapy immediately. Decreased bone density should especially be suspected in women presenting with recurrent stress fractures, or fractures associated with minimal trauma.

Intervention And Treatment Of The Triad Disorders

Sensitivity and a respect for confidentiality are required when trying to help an athlete with disordered eating and other related health problems. The best time to intervene is as soon as the problem is suspected. A "caring confrontation" involves showing concern for the health, well-being, and feelings of the individual involved, without being judgemental about the behavior.

Treatment of these disorders depends on the specific medical presentation. There should be a set mechanism for referral, and a multidisciplinary team approach, including evaluation by a trained mental health professional. Amenorrhea should ideally be diagnosed and managed within 3 to 6 months, to avoid compromising bone density. A slight reduction in the amount of training, or an improvement in nutrition and/or body weight may be sufficient to allow menstrual cycles to resume. Athletes with the triad disorders should consume at least 1500 mg of elemental calcium daily. Hormonal replacement in the form of supplemental estrogen or birth control pill may be required for hypoestrogenic amenorrhea that does not respond to other therapy. If necessary, this therapy may be safely used in adolescents over the age of 16, or three years post puberty (2).

Preventive Measures

Prevention of the triad disorders and the accompanying medical problems remains the most efficacious and cost-effective treatment. Efforts in this area fall under the basic domains of **education** and **enforcement**.

Education

It is critical to develop a positive sporting environment that does not encourage eating disorders. Educational materials and/or seminars for athletes, parents, coaches, trainers and administrators should focus on the physiologic and psychological effects of disordered eating, amenorrhea and osteoporosis. The media, specifically that which target the high risk groups, can be utilized in a positive way to spread accurate information about healthy training methods, as well as the potential for development of the triad disorders.

Athletes should be educated early on in their career or season. There should be positive peer pressure to maintain good nutrition. An adequate support network at all levels should be developed. A nutritionist can supervise dieting if it is needed, and provide professional advice on sound, effective and safe nutritional practices. An effective referral mechanism should be in place, and should also include the availability of individual psychiatric counselling.

It is critical to have well-established coaching and/or training standards. Certification of coaches must include education regarding the Female Athlete Triad, normal child development, and safe training practices. Standards of conduct should be strictly enforced through the various licensing agencies. Coaches must be taught to recognize athletes with disordered eating patterns, and to promote sensitivity to weight issues. The setting of goals for body weight, and body fat percentage, the linking of performance to weight loss, and practices such as public weighing should be discouraged. Coaches and parents should promote healthy eating and training behaviors, with the emphasis on athletic performance and the development of lean body mass. They should reinforce specific achievements, rather than weight loss. A range of age-appropriate acceptable weights and body composition can be determined with the help of scientists such as exercise physiologists.

Parents should also be educated about normal child growth and development. Girls between 6 and 10 years of age should gain, on average, approximately 5 to 7.5 cm (2 to 3 inches) per year and about 2.5 to 3.5 kg (5 to 8 pounds) per year. Parents are advised to monitor the environment of the gymnasium or sport hall where their daughter trains. An administrative policy of "open practices" will facilitate this. Parents must be careful of over-involvement to avoid "achievement by proxy" (51).

Physicians and scientists who can address lay and professional audiences should be identified, and given opportunities to educate these groups about health risks of the Triad disorders. Specific clinical guidelines will help primary care and team physicians to prevent, identify and treat the Triad disorders. Medical specialty groups and researchers need to address and develop preventative measures, including pre-participation screening protocols.

Important initiatives have already been undertaken by many different groups and organizations throughout the world, but much work still remains to be done.

Enforcement

Some risk sports, like gymnastics itself requires a review of rules and judging practices that may encourage unhealthy behavior. Athleticism and skill, rather than an athlete's appearance should be emphasized. Rule changes need to be initiated at the international level, and strictly enforced.

The **Fédération Internationale de Gymnastics (FIG)** has recently moved to increase the age requirement for senior international competition from 15 to 16 years, effective January 1, 1997. Junior international age eligibility was also increased from 12 to 13 years. The hope is that this may help to limit the amount

and intensity of prepubertal training, and to create a more realistic ideal body image for gymnasts. Alternatively, this new rule may only create further problems. Accepting a gymnast for competition at an international level one year later may cause an even greater effort to delay puberty through intense dieting and training practices. Exclusion of underweight gymnasts according to age or height could be another alternative, though, exclusion criteria have not been defined.

Conclusions

Finally, societal influences to "be thin" and "to win at any cost", should be somehow moderated. Sport for women should be promoted for the physical, social and psychological benefits that it can offer to participants of all ages and at all levels.

Literature

1. Adashi E. Y. The ovarian life cycle. In: Textbook of Endocrinology. J. D. Wilson, D. W. Foster (eds.) Philadelphia: Saunders, 1992, pp. 181-237.

2. American Academy of Pediatrics: Committee on Sports Medicine. Amenorrhea in adolescent athletes. Pediatrics 84:394-5, 1989.

3. Diagnostic and Statistical Manual of Mental Disorders, DSM-IV. In: Diagnostic and Statistical Manual of Mental Disorders, DSM-IV. American Psychiatric Association (ed.) Washington D.C.: 1994.

4. Arendt E. A. Osteoporosis in the athletic female: Amenorrhea and amenorrheic osteoporosis. In: The Athletic female. A. J. Pearl (ed.) Champaign: Human Kinetics, 1993, pp. 41-59.

5. Bale, P., Doust, J., & Dawson, D. (1996): Gymnasts, distance runners, anorexics, body composition and menstrual status. *J Sports Med Phys Fitness* 36, 49-53.

6. Baxter-Jones, A. D. G., Helms, P., Baines-Preece, J., & Preece, M. (1994): Menarche in intensively trained gymnasts, swimmers

and tennis players. *Ann Human Biol* 21, 407-415.

7. Brownell K. D., S. N. Steen, and J. H. Wilmore. Weight regulation practices in athletes: analysis of metabolic and health effects. *Med Sci Sports Exerc* 19:546-56, 1987.

8. Bunt J. C. Metabolic actions of estradiol: significance for acute and chronic exercise responses. *Med Sci Sports Exerc* 22:286-90, 1990.

9. Carr B. R. Disorders of the ovary and female reproductive tract. In: Textbook of Endocrinology J. D. Wilson, D. W. Foster (eds.) Philadelphia: Saunders, 1992, pp. 733-798.

10. Claessen, A. L., Malina, R. M., & Lefevre, J. (1992): Growth and menarchal status of elite female gymnasts. *Med Sci Sports Exerc* 24, 755-763.

11. Constantini M. W. and M. P. Warren. Physical activity, fitness, and reproductive health in women: clinical observations. In: Physical activity, fitness, and health. C. Bouchard, R. J. Shephard, and T. Stephens (eds.) Champaign: Human Kinetics, 1992, pp. 955-966.

12. Dequeker, J., Nus, J., Verstraeten, A., Guesens, P., & Gevers, G. (1987): Genetic determination of bone mineral content at the spine and radius: a twin study. *Bone* 8, 207-209.

13. Drinkwater B. L., K. Nilson, C. H. Chesnut 3d, W. J. Bremner, S. Shainholtz, and M. B. Southworth. Bone mineral content of amenorrheic and eumenorrheic athletes. *N Engl J Med* 311:277-81, 1984.

14. Drinkwater B. L., K. Nilson, C. H. Chesnut 3d, W. J. Bremner, S. Shainholtz, and M. B. Southworth. Bone mineral content of amenorrheic and eumenorrheic athletes. *N Engl J Med* 311:277-81, 1984.

15. Drinkwater, B. L., Nilson, K., Ott, S., & Chesnut, C. H. (1986): Bone mineral density after resumption of menses in amenorrheic athletes. *JAMA* 256, 380-382.

16. Dueck C. A., M. M. Manore, and K. S. Matt. Role of energy balance in athletic menstrual dysfunction. *Int J Sport Nutr* 6:165-90, 1996.

17. Dueck C. A., K. S. Matt, M. M. Manore, and J. S. Skinner. Treatment of athletic amenorrhea with a diet and training intervention program. *Int J Sport Nutr* 6:24-40, 1996.

18. Edwards J. E., A. K. Lindeman, A. E. Mikesky, and J. M. Stager. Energy balance in highly trained female endurance runners. *Med Sci Sports Exerc* 25:1398-404, 1993.

19. Einhorn T. A. The bone organ system: form and function. In: Osteoporosis R. Marcus, D. Feldman, and J. Kelsey (eds.) San Diego: Academic Press, 1996, pp. 3-22.

20. Fehling P. C., L. Alekel, J. Clasey, A. Rector, and R. J. Stillman. A comparison of bone mineral densities among female athletes in impact loading and active loading sports. *Bone* 17:205-10, 1995.

21. Fichter M. M. and K. M. Pirke. Hypothalamic pituitary function in starving healthy subjects. In: The psychobiology of anorexia nervosa. K. M. Pirke, D. Ploog (eds.) Berlin: Springer, 1988, pp. 124-135.

22. FIMS and WHO. Joint position statement on public policy from FIMS and WHO on "Physical Activity for Health". FIMS, 1995.

23. Frisch R. E. Pubertal adipose tissue: is it necessary for normal sexual maturation? Evidence from the rat and human female. *Fed Proc* 39:2395-400, 1980.

24. Frisch R. E. Body fat, puberty and fertility. *Biol Rev Camb Philos Soc* 59:161-88, 1984.

25. Hergenroeder A. C. Bone mineralization, hypothalamic amenorrhea, and sex steroid therapy in female adolescents and young adults. *J Pediatr* 126:683-9, 1995.

26. Kanis, J. A., Melton, I. I. I. J., Christiansen, C., Johnston, C. C., & Kaltaev, N. (1994): The diagnosis of osteoporosis. *J Bone Miner Res* 9, 1137-1141.

27. Keizer, H. A., & Rogol, A. D. (1990): Physical exercise and menstrual cycle alterations. What are the mechanisms? *Sports Med* 10, 218.

28. Lindholm, C., Hagenfeldt, K., & Ringertz, B.-M. (1994): Pubertal development in elite juvenile gymnasts: effects of physical training. *Acta Obstet Gynecol Scand* 73, 269-273.

29. Lloyd T., S. J. Triantafyllou, E. R. Baker et al. Women athletes with menstrual irregularity have increased musculoskeletal injuries [published erratum appears in *Med Sci Sports Exerc* 1987 Aug;19(4):421] *Med Sci Sports Exerc* 18:374-9, 1986.

30. Loucks A. B. Physical activity, fitness, and female reproductive morbidity. In: Physical activity, fitness, and health. C. Bouchard, R. J. Shephard, and T. Stephens (eds.) Champaign: Human Kinetics, 1992, pp. 943-954.

31. Loucks A. B. and S. M. Horvath. Athletic amenorrhea: a review. *Med Sci Sports Exerc* 17:56-72, 1985.

32. Loucks A. B., J. Vaitukaitis, J. L. Cameron et al. The reproductive system and exercise in women. *Med Sci Sports Exerc* 24:S288-93, 1992.

33. Mansfield, M. J., & Emans, S. J. (1993): Growth in female gymnasts: Should training decrease during puberty? *J Pediatr* 1993 122, 237-240.

34. Neumärker, K. J. (1997): Mortality and sudden death in anorexia nervosa. *Int J Eat Disord* 21, 205-212.

35. OConnor P. J., R. D. Lewis, and A. Boyd. Health concerns of artistic women gymnasts. *Sports Med* 21:321-5, 1996.

36. Otis C. L., B. Drinkwater, M. Johnson, A. Loucks, and J. Wilmore. American College of Sports Medicine position stand. The Female Athlete Triad [see comments] *Med Sci Sports Exerc* 29:i-ix, 1997.

37. Oursler M. J., M. Kassem, R. Turner, B. L. Riggs, and T. C. Spelsberg. Regulation of bone cell function by gonadal steroids. In: Osteoporosis R. Marcus, D. Feldman, and J. Kelsey (eds.) San Diego: Academic Press, 1996, pp. 237-260.

38. Prior J. C., Y. M. Vigna, and D. W. McKay. Reproduction for the athletic woman. New understandings of physiology and management. *Sports Med* 14:190-9, 1992.

39. Putukian M. The female triad. Eating disorders, amenorrhea, and osteoporosis. *Med Clin North Am* 78:345-56, 1994.

40. Robinson T. L., C. Snow Harter, D. R. Taaffe, D. Gillis, J. Shaw, and R. Marcus. Gymnasts exhibit higher bone mass than runners despite similar prevalence of amenorrhea and oligomenorrhea. *J Bone Miner Res* 10:26-35, 1995.

41. Ryan, J. (1995) Little Girls in Pretty Boxes: The Making and Breaking of Elite Gymnasts and Figure Skaters., Warner Books, New York.

42. Schwartz, B., Cumming, D. C., Riordan, E., Selye, M., Yen, S. S. C., & Rebar, R. W. (1981): Exercise associated amenorrhea: A distinct entity? *Am J Obstet Gynecol* 141, 662-670.

43. Slemenda, C. W., & Johnson, C. C. (1993): High intensity activities in young women: site specific bone mass effects among female figure skaters. *Bone Mineral* 20, 125-132.

44. Staeger, J. M., Wigglesworth, J. K., & Hatler, L. K. (1990): Interpreting the relationship between age of menarche and prepubertal training. Med Sci Sports Exerc 22, 54-58.

45. Stager, J. M., & Hatler, L. K. (1988): Menarche in athletes: The influence of genetics and prepubertal training. *Med Sci Sports Exerc* 20, 369-373.

46. Sundgot Borgen J. Nutrient intake of female elite athletes suffering from eating disorders. *Int J Sport Nutr* 3:431-42, 1993.

47. Sundgot Borgen J. Risk and trigger factors for the development of eating disor-

ders in female elite athletes. *Med Sci Sports Exerc* 26:414-9, 1994.

48. Sundgot-Borgen, J. (1998): The triad of eating disorders, amenorrhea and osteoporosis. Isostar Sport Nutrition Foundation. 7, 3-8.

49. Sundgot Borgen J., R. Bahr, J. A. Falch, and L. S. Schneider. Normal bone mass in bulimic women. *J Clin Endocrinol Metab* 83:3144-9, 1998.

50. Theintz G., F. Ladame, H. Howald, U. Weiss, T. Torresani, and P. C. Sizonenko. [The child, growth and high-level sports] Schweiz Z Med Traumatol :7-15, 1994.

51. Tofler, I. R., Katz-Stryer, B., Micheli, L. J., & Herman, L. R. (1996): Physical and emotional problems of elite female gymnasts. *N Eng J Med* 1996 335, 281-283.

52. Vollmann, R. F. (1977) The Menstrual Cycle., Saunders, Philadelphia.

53. Yeager K. K., R. Agostini, A. Nattiv, and B. Drinkwater. The female athlete triad: disordered eating, amenorrhea, osteoporosis. *Med Sci Sports Exerc* 25:775-7, 1993.

The Female Athlete Triad

> ### American College of Sports Medicine (ACSM)

Summary

The Femal Athlete Triad is a syndrome occurring in physically active girls and women. Its interrelated components are disordered eating, amenorrhea, and osteoporosis. Pressure placed on young women to achieve or maintain unrealistically low body weight underlies development of the triad. Adolescents and women training in sports in which low body weight is emphasized for athletic activity or appearance are at greatest risk. Girls and women with one component of the triad should be screened for the others.

Alone or in combination, female athlete triad disorders can decrease physical performance and cause morbidity and mortality. More research is needed on its causes, prevalence, treatment, and consequences. All individuals working with physically active girls and women should be educated about the female athlete triad and develop plans to prevent, recognize, treat, and reduce its risks.

1995

Med. Sci. Sports Exerc., Vol. 29, No. 5, pp i-ix, 1997.

Impaired People

Impaired Persons, Participation in Sports and Physical Activities

American Academy of Family Physicians (AAFP)

The AAFP adopts the World Health Organization's definition of "impaired" to replace the word "handicapped": "Any loss or abnormality of psychological, physiological or anatomical structure or function" (World Health Organization, 1980)

The AAFP encourages participation of impaired persons in sports and physical activities to the full extent of their abilities in the appropriate setting.

The AAFP recognizes that a program of regular exercise for impaired persons contributes to improved health, rehabilitation, a sense of self-worth and improved productivity.

The AAFP recognizes that appropriate supervision, facilities and accessibility should be integral parts of any sports and physical activities for impaired individuals.

1996

AAFP Reference Manual

Support of Sports and Recreational Programs for Physically Disabled People

American Academy of Orthopaedic Surgeons (AAOS)

Web site: www.aaos.org/wordhtml/papers position/recprog.htm

The American Academy of Orthopaedic Surgeons strongly supports the expressed interests of people with physical disabilities of all ages who want to participate in sports and recreational programs.

Participation in such activities can be fulfilling, increase physical fitness, and enhance personal image. Having the ability to set and achieve goals and the capability to deal with success and failure in the competitive arena are important accomplishments.

The American Academy of Orthopaedic Surgeons believes there should be continued attempts to organize efforts among existing sports and recreational groups to foster communication and improve programs.

Sports and recreational programs for people with physical disabilities, as they exist today, have developed largely through the efforts of a multitude of organizations and individuals, both lay and professional. The full potential of these efforts has not yet been fully realized because no central organizing body exists.

Recreational programs have originated in the home, school, community, and camp. Sports competitions for people with physical disabilities exist at the local, state, national, and international levels within separate organizations whose activities may focus on a specific kind of disability. There is presently no central organizing body that coordinates these efforts.

The American Academy of Orthopaedic Surgeons urges further coordination of efforts to increase the availability of sports and recreation programs for people with physical disabilities. The American Academy of Orthopaedic Surgeons suggests there is a need for public education on the subject.

There are almost 9 million injuries annually that require medical attention, and more than 300,000 of those injuries caused either permanent partial or permanent total disability. In addition, there is a significant number of people with either congenital or non-traumatic acquired disability. Spurred by the pioneer efforts of the original wheelchair athletes, these millions of people have developed a deep interest in recreational and competitive sports activities. When they decide to participate however, they often face additional handicaps. Special education and physical education teachers, counselors, administrators, some physicians and the general public often are unaware of available resources and the potential of people with physical disabilities.

Sports and recreation activities for people with physical disabilities are beneficial provided the necessary precautions are taken. However, some people with physical disabilities do have special considerations, including insensitive skin, joint deformities, difficulties in balance and coordination, and temperature regulation. Most sports and recreational activities can be adapted for them. Physicians involved with disabled athletes have a role to play in assessing the medical needs limitations. Medical precautions should be appropriate without needless restrictions.

The American Academy of Orthopaedic Surgeons recognizes a need for ongoing research among groups involved in athletic programs for people with physical disabilities.

The American Academy of Orthopaedic Surgeons is committed to the further advancement of sports and recreational activities for people with physical disabilities. The American Academy of Orthopaedic Surgeons recognizes the need for continued research to enhance the ability of people with disabilities to participate in both competitive and recreational sports.

For additional information, contact the Public and Media Relations Department, Joanne L. Swanson at (847) 384-4142 or email: swanson@aaos.org; or Paula Poda at (847) 384-4139 or email: poda@aaos.org.

Older Adults

Exercise and Physical Activity for Older Adults

American College of Sports Medicine (ACSM)

Summary

By the year 2030, the number of individuals 65 yr and over will reach 70 million in the United States alone; persons 85 yr and older will be the fastest growing segment of the population. As more individuals live longer, it is imperative to determine the extent and mechanisms by which exercise and physical activity can improve health, functional capacity, quality of life, and independence in this population. Aging is a complex process involving many variables (e.g., genetics, lifestyle factors, chronic diseases) that interact with one another, greatly influencing the manner in which we age. Participation in regular physical activity (both aerobic and strength exercises) elicits a number of favorable responses that contribute to healthy aging. Much has been learned recently regarding the adaptability of various biological systems, as well as the ways that regular exercise can influence them.

1998

Med. Sci. Sports. Exerc., Vol. 30, No. 6, pp 992-1008, 1998.

Pregnant Athletes

Exercise and Pregnancy

Canadian Academy of Sports Medicine (CASM)

The Canadian Academy of Sport Medicine (CASM) has developed guidelines for safe exercise during low risk pregnancy based on a review of the scientific literature. This position statement was authored by representatives of the subcommittee of the CASM, Women's Issues in Sport Medicine and the Canadian Society for Exercise Physiology. The Chairperson was Dr. Lisa Stevenson.

Introduction

The current data suggest that a moderate level of exercise on a regular basis during a low risk pregnancy has minimal risk for the fetus and beneficial metabolic and cardiorespiratory effects for the exercising pregnant woman.

The guidelines listed in the PARmed-X for pregnancy document (appendix A) are now well established as a safe level of exercise for healthy medically prescreened and monitored pregnant women. The results of several studies using the guidelines for medical screening and exercise prescription provide strong scientific support for the use of the guidelines. It is our recommendation that the PARmed-X be utilized as the basis of safe and practical exercise prescription in pregnancy.

Guidelines published in the 1980's were conservative, lacked scientific support and were based mainly on common sense (1). More recent guidelines are still conservative and somewhat nonspecific (2). In this position paper, the first section will present a review of the current scientific knowledge on the risks and benefits of exercise and pregnancy. This information was extracted from the large volume of research done to date on this subject including; medline searches, conference proceedings, expert knowledge and pertinent review articles.

The second section will give specific recommendations on the prescription of exercise in pregnancy. It will also introduce the PARmed-X for Pregnancy. This is a form developed by the Canadian Society for Exercise Physiology (CSEP) to aid physicians counseling pregnant women who would like to exercise. It is the recommendation of this position statement that the PARmed-X for Pregnancy be utilized as the basis of safe and practical exercise prescription in pregnancy.

Theoretical Concerns of Research Methodology

Previous studies and consequent conclusions have been limited in their applicability and validity by the lack of scientific rigor that has been applied to research in the area of exercise and pregnancy. Limitations include:

- Expectant mothers cannot be exposed to exhaustion for fear of maternal and fetal safety.
- It is very difficult to separate the physiological effects of pregnancy from the effects of exercise.
- Many of the studies do not describe specific exercise prescriptions; including the type of exercise, or, the intensity, duration and frequency of the exercise.
- It is difficult to make generalizations on research as much of the research to date has been on healthy, nonsmoking, Caucasian, previously fit women with low risk pregnancies.
- Little research exists on the effects of exercise on women at risk for an adverse pregnancy outcome.

- Many of the concerns surrounding exercise and pregnancy were raised from adverse outcomes noted in animal studies.

- Many of the animal studies were performed on unfit pregnant species pushed to exhaustion, while human studies involved more physically fit pregnant women exercising at more moderate levels.

Summary of Physiological Research

Exercise Induced Hyperthermia

It has been shown in pregnant animal studies that increases in core body temperature above 39°C in the first trimester can result in an increased incidence of neural tube defects (12, 13). Few studies have examined maternal heat exposure induced by exercise as opposed that induced by sauna, hot tub and fevers (13). No prospective studies to date have found any association between increased maternal temperature induced by exercise and congenital malformations (14,15). The human data suggest that women allowed to self pace their level of exercise during pregnancy do not produce a sufficient elevation of core body temperature to be detrimental to the fetus (12).

Due to the lack of sufficient data to support or refute the risk of hyperthermia in pregnancy, one should continue to use caution particularly in the first trimester.

Exercise, Blood Flow Redistribution and Birth Weight

In the nonpregnant state, splanchnic blood flow may decrease up to 50% of resting values at moderate exercise intensities and drop a further 30% with prolonged high intensity exercise (11). Since uterine blood flow is part of the splanchnic circulation, the concern is that during exercise the blood flow with its supply of glucose and oxygen will be shunted away from the placenta and the developing fetus to the exercising muscles. Ultimately, the concern is that fetal malnutrition will lead to a decrease in birth weight and intrauterine growth restriction. There is controversy regarding the actual

effect of exercise on blood flow redistribution and birth weight with some studies citing no change or a slight increase and others reporting lower birth weights (4, 6, 16, 17, 18, 19 20). Some researchers concluded that exercise did restrict storage of fetal fat near the end of pregnancy, but it had no significant effect on the other parameters of fetal growth (18).

These studies confirm that guidelines are necessary for maternal exercise because the threshold for exercise, above which problems may occur, is not well defined.

Exercise and fetal stress

Wolfe et al. (10) presented a review on fetal responses to maternal exercise where conflicting data regarding fetal heart rate responses to maternal exercise was identified. It has been shown that the most common response to exercise is a rise of approximately 10 beats per minute in fetal heart rate during exercise, which returns to baseline 10 to 20 minutes after exercise is over (3, 16). The magnitude of the rise and fall depends on the intensity and duration of the maternal exercise. Researchers found no evidence of fetal distress during exercise and in fact demonstrated a decrease in the incidence of meconium staining, abnormal fetal heart rate patterns, cord entanglement and low apgar scores during labour and delivery in the exercising groups (17,19).

These studies confirm that guidelines are necessary for maternal exercise because their is still some controversy regarding the threshold for exercise and fetal stress. There is growing evidence to support the benefits of exercise include a reduction in fetal stress.

Exercise and Early Miscarriage

There is no information on the safety of beginning a regular exercise program in the period just prior to conception or very early in the first trimester. There are very few studies that have investigated the effect of continuing regular exercise in the first trimester however, a prospective study of 158 previously fit women who continued to exercise at a level above current guidelines during their pregnancies found no significant difference in the rate of spontaneous abortion, congenital abnormalities or implantation problems (21).

Women who have been previously inactive are not advised to initiate an exercise program during the first trimester. Those women who have been previously exercising may continue but not increase their intensity or frequency during the first trimester.

Exercise and Labour

To date, there have been no studies that have shown an increased risk of preterm labor, or, an increased incidence of premature rupture of membranes in exercising pregnant women, not already at risk for these conditions (16, 17, 19). Most studies suggest that exercise has no effect on the length of labor (6, 16). Some studies have shown that less medical intervention, for example, oxytocin, forceps and cesarean section, is required in women who exercised throughout their pregnancy (17, 19).

Exercise is not detrimental to labour and may even produce benefits of less medical intervention.

Exercise and Maternal Injury

As pregnancy progresses and maternal body mass increases, there is an increase in the hormonal levels that aid in the relaxation and mobilization of the pelvic, sacroiliac and sacrococcygeal joints (22) . All of these changes can alter the balance, co-ordination and exercise tolerance of a pregnant woman and could, in theory, make her vulnerable to joint injury. However, there has been no reported increase in injury rate when exercising in pregnancy (11). There has actually been an observed decrease in the incidence of musculoskeletal complaints by women exercising during pregnancy (3, 17).

To date there are no specific reports of exercise-associated injuries to support the concern of exercise leading to maternal injury but, until more data are available, it is probably prudent to still advise some care and caution (24).

Acute Exercise and Maternal Responses

Heart rate changes during pregnancy are well-documented. It is well known that resting heart rate increases abruptly in early pregnancy followed by a moderate increase with advancing gestational age (28-30). Heart rate responses to standard submaximal exercise (e.g. stationary cycling) follow the same pattern as resting heart rate. Rating of perceived exertion (RPE) during standard submaximal exercise (e.g. stationary cycling) is not altered significantly by pregnancy status or with advancing gestational age, but is increased during weight bearing activities such as walking, jogging or running (27, 33).

The modified heart rate target zones included in the PARmed-X for Pregnancy document reflect the documented physiological changes that occur in pregnancy. The Rate of Perceived Exertion is considered a reliable index of exercise intensity for pregnant women.

Maternal Physical Conditioning Responses

Recent studies have established that physical conditioning during the second and third trimesters improves maternal aerobic fitness (16, 26, 27). Such exercise is also reported to reduce heart rate, the ventilatory equivalent for oxygen and the rate of perceived exertion (RPE) during submaximal exercise (16, 26, 27) increase the ventilatory "anaerobic" threshold and may help to preserve the ability to metabolize carbohydrate and produce lactate during strenuous exertion (26). Training-induced reductions in heart rate are observed during standard submaximal exercise, with training-induced changes becoming more evident with increasing exercise intensity.

It appears that gestational factors that increase heart rate in pregnancy override the normal training stimulus to reduce heart rate in the resting state. Training effects are achieved due to the physiological changes of pregnancy and become more evident with increasing exercise intensity.

Possible Benefits of Exercise During Pregnancy

- May decreases the incidence of depression and anxiety and increases self esteem (3, 5)
- May decreased recuperation time from labour postpartum (3)
- May be a safe therapeutic approach to the prevention and treatment of gestational diabetes (3, 40)
- Active women may have a lower incidence of pregnancy induced hypertension (41)
- Active women report fewer physical symptoms of pregnancy ie. nausea, heartburn, leg cramps, insomnia etc. (17)

Summary of Clinical Recommendations

Parts A and B of the PARmed-X for pregnancy are completed by the patient to determine if any underlying general medical problems, and/ or previous or current pregnancy complications exist. Part B also identifies the patient's current fitness status, future exercise goals, and lifestyle factors, all of which will influence the exercise prescription. In Part C the list of absolute and relative maternal contraindications to exercise in pregnancy is presented. If absolute contraindications are identified, the risk to the fetus and to the mother far outweighs any of the exercise related benefits identified. If relative contraindications are identified, in these situations, the safety of exercise must be assessed on an individual basis with careful medical surveillance.

Frequency

- Women who exercised on a regular basis prior to pregnancy may maintain their routine during the first trimester and follow the ParMed-X guidelines as the pregnancy progresses.
- Women who did not exercise on a regular basis should not start to exercise until the second trimester.
- Most authorities agree that regular exercise is better than sporadic exercise. It is recommended to begin at a frequency of 3 times per week, progressing to a maximum of 4-5 times per week depending on the level of maternal fitness (2, 22).
- The number of sessions per week is also dependent on the duration and intensity of the exercise sessions. A good rule of thumb is not to exercise strenuously more than two days in a row.

Intensity

- The safe upper limit for an exercising target heart rate in pregnancy is controversial.
- The PARmed-X provides a safe and practical target heart rate range based on maternal age and level of fitness (6, 16, 22, 25).
- Rating of perceived exertion (RPE) is probably the least affected by gestational adaptations.
- Borg's 15-point (6-20) RPE scale has been recommended to maintain a target range up to 12 to 14 (moderate to somewhat hard intensity) throughout pregnancy.
- The talk test can also provide a good measure of intensity. It is defined as the intensity where an exercising mother can easily carry on a verbal conversation.

Time

- It is recommended to begin cardiovascular exercise for 15 minutes.
- The duration of exercise may be increased slowly, usually two minutes per week until a maximum of 30 minutes is achieved at the target heart rate.
- There should also be a good warm-up and an adequate cool down.

Type

- Avoid any exposure to hyperbaric, hyperthermic, humid or hypoxic environmental conditions.
- For a woman who was inactive prior to her pregnancy, nonweightbearing activities are ideal, such as cycling, swimming and aquafit.

- Less strenuous but continuous aerobic activities such as walking and low impact aerobics are also recommended.

Muscular Conditioning

- Muscular conditioning is generally considered safe if precautions are met as outlined on page 3 of the PARmed-X.

- In particular advise the woman to avoid breath holding during resistance training, as well as exercising in the supine position after the fourth month of pregnancy.

- Abdominal exercises are not recommended if a diastasis recti develops.

Pregnancy Monitoring

Monitoring: The pregnant woman

- The exercising mother should be instructed on the importance of drinking water before, during and after exercise to prevent dehydration.

- She should monitor the colour of her urine and insure that it remains clear to a light yellow, indicating sufficient hydration (25, 42).

- She can also measure her acute weight loss after an exercise session and this should not exceed 1 kg (43).

Monitoring: The physician

- Monitoring an exercising pregnant woman must include regular visits as outlined in the standard provincial prenatal guidelines.

- These include assessment of sufficient weight gain, increasing symphysis fundal heights according to gestation, and ultrasound monitoring as required to assess fetal well-being.

References and Reading List

1. American College of Obstetricians and Gynecologists. *Exercise during pregnancy and the postnatal period.* Washington, DC: American College of Obstetricians and Gynecologists, 1985.

2. American College of Obstetricians and Gynecologists. *Exercise during pregnancy and the postnatal period.* Technical Bulletin No. 189. Washington, DC: American College of Obstetricians and Gynecologists, 1994.

3. Wolfe, LA, Hall, P, Webb, KA, Goodman, L, Monga, M and McGraith, MJ. Presciption of Aerobic Exercise During Pregnancy. *Sports Medicine* 1989; 8(5): 273-301.

4. Hatch, MC, Shu, XO, McLean, DE, et al. Maternal Exercise during Pregnancy, Physical Fitness, and Fetal Growth. *American Journal of Epidemiology* 1993; 137(10): 1105-1114.

5. Clapp, JF, Rokey, R, Treadway, JL, Carpenter, MW, Artal, RM and Warrnes, C. Exercise in Pregnancy. *Medicine and Science in Sports and Exercise* 1992; 24 (6 supplement): S294-S300.

6. Lokey, EA, Tran, ZV, Wells, CL, Myers, BC and Tran, AC. Effects of physical exercise on pregnancy outcomes: a meta-analytic review. *Medicine and Science in Sports and Exercise* 1991; 23(11): 1234-1239.

7. Stevenson, L. Exercise in pregnancy; Part 1: Update on pathophysiology. *Canadian Family Physician* 1997; 43: 97-104.

8. Stevenson, L. Exercise in pregnancy ; Part 2: Recommendations for individuals. *Canadian Family Physician* 1997; 43: 107-111.

9. Wolfe, LA, Ohtake, PJ, Mottola, MF and McGrath, MJ. Physiological interactions between pregnancy and aerobic exercise. *Exercise Sports Science Reviews* 1989; 17: 295-351.

10. Wolfe, L, Brenner, IKM and Mottola, MF. Maternal exercise, fetal well-being and pregnancy outcome. *Exercise Sports Science Reviews* 1994b; 22: 145-194.

11. Clapp, JF. Exercise in Pregnancy: Good, Bad, or Indifferent? In: Lee RV, Cotton DB, Barron W, et al. (eds): *Current Obstetric Medicine.* Vol 2. Chicago: Mosby-Year Book, Inc., 1993: 25-49.

12. McMurray, RG, Mottola, MF, Wolfe, LA, Artal, R, Millar, L and Pivarnik, JM. Recent Advances in Understanding Maternal and Fetal Responses to Exercise. *Medicine and Science in Sports and Exercise* 1993; 25(12): 1305-1321.

13. McMurray, RG and Katz, VL. Thermoregulation in Pregnancy. *Sports Medicine* 1990; 10(3): 146-158.

14. Clarren, SK, Smith, DW, Harvey, MAS, Ward, RH and Myrianthopoulos, NC. Hyperthermia-a prospective evaluation of a possible teratogenic agent in man. *The Journal of Pediatrics* 1979; 95(1): 81-82.

15. Jones, RL, Botti, JJ, Anderson, WM and Bennett, NL. Thermoregulation During Aerobic Exercise in Pregnancy. *Obstet. Gynecol.* 1985; 65(3): 340-345.

16. Webb, KA, Wolfe, LA and McGrath, MJ. Effects of acute and chronic maternal exercise on fetal heart rate. *J. Appl. Physiol.* 1994; 77(5): 2207-13.

17. Sternfeld, B, Quesenberry, JR, Eskenazi, B and Newman, LA. Exercise during pregnancy and pregnancy outcome. *Medicine and Science in Sports and Exercise* 1995; 27(5): 634-640.

18. Clapp, JF and Capeless, EL. Neonatal morphometrics following endurance exercise during pregnancy. *American Journal of Obstetrics and Gynecology* 1990; 163: 1805-1811.

19. Clapp, J. The course and outcome of labor following endurance exercise during pregnancy. *American Journal of Obstetrics and Gynecology* 1990; 163: 1799-1805.

20. Bell, RJ, Palma, SM and Lumley, JM. The effect of vigorous exercise during pregnancy on birth-weight. *Aust NZ J Obstet Gynaecol* 1995; 35(1): 46-51.

21. Clapp, J. Exercise and Fetal Health. *Journal of Developmental Physiology* 1991; 15: 9-14.

22. Paisley, JE and Mellion, MB. Exercise during Pregnancy. *American Family Physician* 1988; 38(5): 143-50.

23. Ostgaard, HC, Zetherstrom, G, Roos-Hansson, E and Svanberg, B. Reduction of back and posterior pelvic pain in pregnancy. *Spine* 1994; 19(8): 894-900.

24. Mittelmark RA, Wiswell RA and Drinkwater BL, eds. *Exercise in Pregnancy.* Second Edition. Baltimore, Maryland: Williams and Wilkins, 1991.

25. Wolfe, LA and Mottola, MF. Aerobic exercise in pregnancy: An update. *Journal of Applied Physiology* 1993; 18(2): 119-147.

26. Wolfe, LA, Walker, RMC, Bonen, A and McGrath, MJ. Effects of pregnancy and chronic exercise on repiratory responses to graded exercise. *Journal of Applied Physiology* 1994a; 76: 1928-34.

27. Ohtake, PJ and Wolfe, LA. Physical conditioning attenuates respiratory responses to exercise in late gestation. *Medicine Science Sports Exercise* (in review).

28. Clapp, JF. Maternal heart rate in pregnancy. *American Journal of Obstetrics and Gynecology* 1985; 152: 659-660.

29. Clapp, JF, Seaward, BL, Sleamaker, RL and Miser, J. Maternal physiologic adaptations to early human pregnancy. *American Journal of Obstetrics and Gynecology* 1988; 159: 1456-1460.

30. Capeless, EL and Clapp, JF. Cardiovascular changes in early phase of pregnancy. *American Journal of Obstetrics and Gynecology* 1989; 161: 1449-1453.

31. Lotgering, FK, Struijk, PC, Van Doom, MK and Wallenberg, HCS. Errors in predicting maximal oxygen consumption in pregnant women. *Journal of Applied Physiology* 1992; 72: 562-567.

32. Sady, SP, Carpenter, MW, Thompson, PD, Sady, MA, Haydon, B and Coustan, DR. Cardiovascular response to cycle exercise during and after pregnancy. *Journal of Applied Physiology* 1989; 66: 336-341.

33. Pivarnik, JM, Lee, W and Miller, JF. Physiological and perceptual responses to cycle and treadmill exercise during preg-

nancy. *Medicine Science Sports Exercise* 1991; 23: 470-475.

34. Pernoll, ML, Metcalfe, J, Kovack, PA, Wachtel, R and Durham, MJ. Ventilation at rest and exercise in pregnancy and postpartum. *Respiratory Physiology* 1975; 25: 295-310.

35. Lotgering, FK, Struijk, PC, Van Doom, MK, Spinnewijn, WEM and Wallenberg, HCS. Anaerobic threshold and respiratory compensation in pregnant women. *Journal of Applied Physiology* 1995; 78: 1772-1777.

36. McMurray, RG, Katz, VL, Berry, MJ and Cefalo, RC. The effect of pregnancy on metabolic responses during rest, immersion and aerobic exercise in the water. American Journal of *Obstetrics and Gynecology* 1988; 158: 481-486.

37. Clapp, JF and Little, KD. Effect of recreational exercise on pregnancy weight gain and subcutaneous fat deposition. *Medicine and Science in Sports and Exercise* 1995; 27: 170-177.

38. Greer, FA and Wolfe, LA. Chronic exercise effects on subcutaneous adiposity in pregnancy. *Medicine Science Sports Exercise* 1994; 26: S119.

39. George, KP, Wolfe, LA, Burggraf, GW, Haliburton, SL and Norman, R. Aerobic training effects on resting hemodynamics during pregnancy. *Medicine Science Sports and Exercise* 1990; 22: S27.

40. Artal, R. Exercise during pregnancy. *Clinics in Sports Medicine* 1992; 11: 363-377.

41. Marcoux, *J. Epidemiol. Comm. Health* 1989; 43: 147-52.

42. White, J. Exercising for Two. *The Physician and Sportsmedicine* 1992; 20: 179-186.

43. Clapp, J. A clinical approach to exercise during pregnancy. *Clinics in Sports Medicine* 1994; 13: 443-459.

44. Clapp, JF. Exercise in pregnancy : a brief clinical review. *Fetal Medicine Review* 1990; 2: 89-101.

July 1998

Wrestlers

Weight Loss in Wrestlers

American College of Sports Medicine (ACSM)

Summary

ACSM Position Stand on Weight Loss in Wrestlers. Despite a growing body of evidence admonishing the behavior, weight cutting (rapid weight reduction) remains prevalent among wrestlers. Weight cutting has significant adverse consequences that may affect competitive performance, physical health, and normal growth and development. To enhance the education experience and reduce the health risks for the participants, the ACSM recommends measures to educate coaches and wrestlers toward sound nutrition and weight control behaviors, to curtail "weight cutting," and to enact rules that limit weight loss.

1996

Med. Sci. Sports Exerc., Vol. 28, No. 2, pp ix-xii, 1996.

10

Ergogenic Aids and Other Substances

Alcohol

The Use of Alcohol in Sports

American College of Sports Medicine
Web site: www.acsm.org

Based upon a comprehensive analysis of the available research relative to the effects of alcohol upon human physical performance, it is the position of the American College of Sports Medicine that:

1. The acute ingestion of alcohol can exert a deleterious effect upon a wide variety of psychomotor skills such as reaction time, hand-eye coordination, accuracy, balance, and complex coordination.

2. Acute ingestion of alcohol will not substantially influence metabolic or physiological functions essential to physical performance such as energy metabolism, maximal oxygen consumption (VO_2max), heart rate, stroke volume, cardiac output, muscle blood flow, arteriovenous oxygen difference, or respiratory dynamics. Alcohol consumption may impair body temperature regulation during prolonged exercise in a cold environment.

3. Acute alcohol ingestion will not improve and may decrease strength, power, local muscular endurance, speed, and cardiovascular endurance.

4. Alcohol is the most abused drug in the United States and is a major contributing factor to accidents and their consequences. Also, it has been documented widely that prolonged excessive alcohol consumption can elicit pathological changes in the liver, heart, brain, and muscle, which can lead to disability and death.

5. Serious and continuing efforts should be made to educate athletes, coaches, health and physical educators, physicians, trainers, the sports media, and the general public regarding the effects of acute alcohol ingestion upon human physical performance and on the potential acute and chronic problems of excessive alcohol consumption.

Research Background for the Position Stand

This position stand is concerned primarily with the effects of acute alcohol ingestion upon physical performance and is based upon a comprehensive review of the pertinent international literature. When one interprets these results, several precautions should be kept in mind. First, there are varying reactions to alcohol ingestion, not only among individuals, but also within an individual depending upon the circumstances. Second, it is virtually impossible to conduct double-blind placebo research with alcohol because subjects can always tell when alcohol has been consumed. Nevertheless, the results cited below provide us with some valid general conclusions relative to the effects of alcohol on physical performance. In most of the research studies, a small dose consisted of 1.5-2.0 ounces (45-60 ml) of alcohol, equivalent to a blood alcohol level (BAL) of 0.04-0.05 in the average-size male. A moderate dose was equivalent to 3-4 ounces (90-120 ml), or a BAL of about 0.10. Few studies employed a large dose, with a BAL of 0.15.

1. Athletes may consume alcohol to improve psychological function, but it is psychomotor performance that deteriorates most. A consistent finding is the impairment of information processing. In sports involving rapid reactions to changing stimuli, performance will be affected most adversely. Research has shown that small to moderate amounts of alcohol will impair reaction time (8,25,26,34-36,42) hand-eye

coordination (8,9,14,40), accuracy (36,39), balance (3), and complex coordination or gross motor skills (4,8,22,36,41). Thus, while Coopersmith (10) suggests that alcohol may improve self-confidence, the available research reveals a deterioration in psychomotor performance.

2. Many studies have been conducted relative to the effects of acute alcohol ingestion upon metabolic and physiological functions important to physical performance. Alcohol ingestion exerts no beneficial influence relative to energy sources for exercise. Muscle glycogen at rest was significantly lower after alcohol consumption, compared to control (30). However, in exercise at 50% maximal oxygen uptake (VO_2max), total glycogen depletion in the leg muscles was not affected by alcohol (30). Moreover, Juhlin-Dannfelt et al. (29) have shown that although alcohol does not impair lipolysis or free fatty acid (FFA) utilization during exercise, it may decrease splanchnic glucose output, decrease the potential contribution from liver gluconeogenesis, elicit a greater decline in blood glucose levels leading to hypoglycemia, and decrease the leg muscle uptake of glucose during the latter stages of a 3-h run. Other studies (17,19) have supported the theory concerning the hypoglycemic effect of alcohol during both moderate and prolonged exhaustive exercise in a cold environment. These studies also noted a significant loss of body heat and a resultant drop in body temperature and suggested that alcohol may impair temperature regulation. These changes may impair endurance capacity.

In one study (5), alcohol has been shown to increase oxygen uptake significantly during submaximal work and simultaneously to decrease mechanical efficiency, but this finding has not been confirmed by others (6,15,33,44). Alcohol appears to have no effect on maximal or near-maximal VO_2 (5-7,44).

The effects of alcohol on cardiovascular-respiratory parameters associated with oxygen uptake are variable at submaximal exercise intensities and are negligible at maximal levels.

Alcohol has been shown by some investigators to increase submaximal exercise heart rate (5,20,23) and cardiac output (5), but these heart rate findings have not been confirmed by others (6,15,33,36,44). Alcohol had no effect on stroke volume (5), pulmonary ventilation (5,15), or muscle blood flow (16,30) at submaximal levels of exercise, but did decrease peripheral vascular resistance (5). During maximal exercise, alcohol ingestion elicited no significant effect upon heart rate (5-7), stroke volume and cardiac output, arteriovenous oxygen difference, mean arterial pressure, and peripheral vascular resistance, or peak lactate (5), but did significantly reduce tidal volume resulting in a lowered pulmonary ventilation (5).

In summary, alcohol appears to have little or no beneficial effect on the metabolic and physiological responses to exercise. Further, in those studies reporting significant effects, the change appears to be detrimental to performance.

3. The effects of alcohol on tests of fitness components are variable. It has been shown that alcohol ingestion may decrease dynamic muscular strength (24), isometric grip strength (36), dynamometer strength (37), power (20), and ergographic muscular output (28). Other studies (13,20,24,27,43) reported no effect of alcohol upon muscular strength. Local muscular endurance was also unaffected by alcohol ingestion (43). Small doses of alcohol exerted no effect upon bicycle ergometer exercise tasks simulating a 100-m dash or a 1500-m run, but larger doses had a deleterious effect (2). Other research has shown that alcohol has no significant effect upon physical performance capacity (15,16), exercise time at maximal levels (5), or exercise time to exhaustion (7).

Thus, alcohol ingestion will not improve muscular work capacity and may lead to decreased performance levels.

4. Alcohol is the most abused drug in the United States (11). There are an estimated 10 million adult problem drinkers and an additional 3.3 million in the 14–17 age range. Alcohol is significantly involved in all types of accidents—motor vehicle, home, industrial,

and recreational. Most significantly, half of all traffic fatalities and one-third of all traffic injuries are alcohol related. Although alcohol abuse is associated with pathological conditions such as generalized skeletal myopathy, cardiomyopathy, pharyngeal and esophageal cancer, and brain damage, its most prominent effect is liver damage (11,31,32).

5. Because alcohol has not been shown to help improve physical performance capacity, but may lead to decreased ability in certain events, it is important for all those associated with the conduct of sports to educate athletes against its use in conjunction with athletic contests. Moreover, the other dangers inherent in alcohol abuse mandate that concomitantly we educate our youth to make intelligent choices regarding alcohol consumption. Anstie's rule, or limit (1), may be used as a reasonable guideline to moderate, safe drinking for adults (12). In essence, no more than 0.5 ounces of pure alcohol per 23 kg body weight should be consumed in any one day. This would be the equivalent of three bottles of 4.5% beer, three 4-ounce glasses of 14% wine, or three ounces of 50% whiskey for a 68-kg person.

References

1. Anstie, F.E. *On the Uses of Wine in Health and Disease.* London: MacMillan, 1811, pp. 5-6.

2. Asmussen, E. and O. Boje. The effects of alcohol and some drugs on the capacity for work. *Acta Physiol. Scand.* 15: 109-118, 1948.

3. Begbie, G. The effects of alcohol and of varying amounts of visual information on a balancing test. *Ergonomics* 9:325-333, 1966.

4. Belgrave, B., K. Bird, Cl. Chesher, D. Jackson, K. Lubbe, G. Starmer. and R. Teo. The effect of cannabidiol. alone and in combination with ethanol, on human performance. *Psyche pharmacology* 64:243-246, 1919.

5. Blomqvist, G., B. Saltin, and J. Mitchell. Acute effects of ethanol ingestion on the response to submaximal and maximal exercise in man. *Circulation* 42:463-410, 1970.

6. Bobo, W. Effects of alcohol upon maximum oxygen uptake, lung ventilation, and heart rate. *Res. Q.* 43:1-6, 1972.

7. Bind, V. Effect of alcohol on cardiorespiratory function. In: *Abstracts: Research Papers of 1979 AAHPER Convention*, Washington, DC AAHPER, 1979, p. 24.

8. Carpenter, J. Effects of alcohol on some psychological processes. *Q.J. Stud. Alcohol* 23:274-314, 1962.

9. Collins, W., D. Schroeder, R. Gilson, and F. Guedry. Effects of alcohol ingestion on tracking performance during angular acceleration. *J. Appl.* Psychol. 55:559-563, 1971.

10. Coppersmith, S. The effects of alcohol on reaction to affective stimuli. *Q.J. Stud. Alcohol* 25:459-475, 1964.

11. Department of Health, Education, and Welfare. Third special report to the U.S. Congress on alcohol and health. *NIAAA & formation and Feature Service.* DHEW Publication No. (ADM) 78-151, November 30, 1978, pp. 1-4.

12. *Dorland's Illustrated Medical Dictionary.* 24th Edition. Philadelphia: W.B. Saunders, 1974, p. 1370.

13. Enzer, N., E. Simonson, and G. Ballard. The effect of small doses of alcohol on the central nervous system. *Am. J Clin. Pathol.* 14:333-341, 1944.

14. Forney, R., F. Hughes, and W. Greatbatch. Measurement of attentive motor performance after alcohol. *Percept. Mot. Skills* 19:151-154, 1964.

15. Garlind, T., L. Godberg, K. Graf, E. Perman, T. Strandell, and G. Strom. Effect of ethanol on circulatory, metabolic, and neurohumoral function during muscular work in man. *Acta Pharmacol. et Toxicol.* 17:106-114. 1960.

16. Graf, K. and G. Strom. Effect of ethanol ingestion on arm blood flow in healthy

young men at rest and during work. *Acta Pharmacol. et Toxicol.* 17:115-120. 1960.

17. Graham, T. Thermal and glycemic reponses during mild exercise in +5 to – 1°C environments following alcohol ingestion. *Aviat. Space Environ. Med.* 25:517-522, 1981.

18. Graham, T. and J. Dalton. Effect of alcohol on man's response to mild physical activity in a cold environment. *Aviat. Space Environ. Med.* 51:793-796, 1980.

19. Haight, J. and W. Keatinge. Failure of thermoregulation in the cold during hypoglycemia induced by exercise and ethanol. *J Physiol. (Lond.)* 229:87-978, 1973.

20. Hebbelinck. M. The effects of a moderate dose of alcohol on a series of functions of physical performance in man. *Arch. Int. Pharmacod.* 120:402-405, 1959.

21. Hebellinck, M. The effect of a moderate dose of ethyl alcohol on human respiratory gas exchange during rest and muscular exercise. *Arch. Int. Pharmacod.* 126:214-2 18, 1960.

22. Hebbelinck, M. *Spierarbeid en Ethylalkohol.* Brussels: Arsica Uitgaven, N.V., 1961, pp. 81-84.

23. Hebbelinck, M. The effects of a small dose of ethyl alcohol on certain basic components of human physical performance. The effect on cardiac rate during muscular work. *Arch. Int. Pharmacod.* 140:61-67, 1962.

24. Hebbelinck, M. The effects of a small dose of ethyl alcohol on certain basic components of human physical performance. *Arch.* Int. Pharmacod. 143:247-257, 1963.

25. Huntley, M. Effects of alcohol, uncertainty and novelty upon response selection. *Psychopharmacologia* 39:259-266, 1974.

26. Huntley, M. Influences of alcohol and S-R uncertainty upon spatial localization time. Psychopharmacologia 27:131-140, 1972.

27. Ikai, M. and A. Steinhaus. Some factors

modifying the expression of human strength. *J Appl. Physiol.* 16:157-161, 196l.

28. Jellinek, E. Effect of small amounts of alcohol on psychological functions. In Yale University Center for Alcohol Studies. *Alcohol, Science and Society.* New Haven, CT, Yale University, 1954, pp. 83-94.

29. Juhlin-Dannfelt, A.G. Ahlborg, L. Hagenfeldt, L. Jorfeldt, and P. Felig. Influence of ethanol on splanchnic and skeletal muscle suhstrate turnover during prolonged exercise in man. *Am. J Physiol.* 233:E195-E202, 1977.

30. Juhlin-Dannfelt, A.L. Jorfeldt, L. Hagenfeldt, and B. Hulten. Influence of ethanol on non-esterified fatty acid and carbohydrate metabolism during exercise in man. *Clin. Soc. Mol. Med.* 53:205-214, 1977.

31. Lieber, C.S. Liver injury and adaptation in alcoholism. *N. Engl. J Med.* 288:356-362, 1973.

32. Lieber, C.S. The metabolism of alcohol. *Sci. Am.* 234 (March):25-33, 1976.

33. Mazess, R., E. Picon-Reategui, and R. Thomas. Effects of alcohol and altitude on man during rest and work. *Aerospace Med.* 39:403-406, 1968.

34. Moskowitz, H. and M. Burns. Effect of alcohol on the psychological refractory period. Q. J Stud. *Alcohol* 32:782-790, 1971.

35. Moskowitz, H. and S. Roth. Effect of alcohol on response latency in object naming. Q. J *Stud. Alcohol* 32:969-975, 1971.

36. Nelson, D. Effects of ethyl alcohol on the performance of selected gross motor tests. *Res. Q.* 30:3 12-320, 1959.

37. Pihkanen, T. Neurological and physiological studies on distilled and brewed beverages. *Ann. Med. Exp. Biol. Fenn.* 35:Suppl. 9, 1-152, 1957.

38. Riff, D., A. Jain, and H. Williams. Alcohol and speed-accuracy tradeoff, *Hum. Factors* 21:433-443, 1979.

39. Rundell, 0. and H. Williams. Alcohol and speed-accuracy tradeoff. *Hum. Factors* 21:433-443, 1979.

40. Sidell, F. and J. Pless. Ethyl alcohol blood levels and performance decrements alter oral administration to man. *Psychopharmacoiogia* 19:246-261, 1971.

41. Tang, P. and R. Rosenstein. Influence of alcohol and Dramamine, alone and in combination, on psychomotor performance. *Aerospace Med.* 39:818-821, 1967.

42. Tharp, V., O. Rundell, B. Lester, and H. Williams. Alcohol and information processing. *Psychopharmacologia* 40:33-52, 1974.

43. Williams, M.H. Effect of selected doses of alcohol on fatigue parameters of the forearm flexor muscles. *Res. Q.* 40:832-840, 1969.

44. Williams, M.H. Effect of small and moderate doses of alcohol on exercise heart rate and oxygen consumption. *Res. Q.* 43:94-104, 1972.

1982

Med. Sci. Sports Exerc., Vol. 14, No. 6, pp ix-xi, 1982.

Blood Doping

The Use of Blood Doping as an Ergogenic Aid

American College of Sports Medicine (ACSM)

Web site: www.acsm.org

Summary

American College of Sports Medicine Position Stand on the Use of Blood Doping as an Ergogenic Aid. *Med. Sci. Sports Exerc.*, Vol. 28, No. 3, pp I-viii, 1996. Blood doping has been achieved by either infusing red blood cells or by administering the drug erythropoietin to artificially increase red blood cell mass. Blood doping can improve an athlete's ability to perform submaximal and maximal endurance exercise. In addition, blood doping can help reduce physiologic strain during exercise in the heat and perhaps at altitude. Conversely, blood doping is associated with risks that can be serious and impair athletic performance. These known risks are amplified by improper medical controls, as well as the interaction between dehydration with exercise and environmental stress. Finally, the medical risks associated with blood doping have been estimated from carefully controlled research studies, and the medically unsupervised use of blood doping will increase these risks. It is the position of the American College of Sports Medicine that any blood doping procedure used in an attempt to improve athletic performance is unethical, unfair, and exposes the athlete to unwarranted and potentially serious health risks.

1996

Med. Sci. Sports Exerc., Vol. 28, No. 3, pp i-viii, 1996.

Creatine

The Effects of Creatine and/or Phosphocreatine as Ergogenic Aids

FISA Sports Medicine Commission

Creatine is a natural compound that is produced in the kidney, liver, and pancreas. It is also found in meat and fish and if these food are eaten regularly the consumer will take in approximately Ig of creatine per day. The total creatine turnover from use and resupply amounts to approximately 2g daily.

Creatine is stored primarily in skeletal muscle and its phosphorylated form, phosphocreatine, plays an essential role in the resynthesis of adenosine triphosphate (ATP), our most immediate energy source for muscle contraction. Previous studies have reported that a daily oral intake of creatine monohydrate, an odorless, tasteless white powder that is a synthesized form of phosphocreatine, of 20-30g per day significantly increased intramuscular concentrations of creatine. Review of recent studies investigating the ergogenic effects of creatine suggest that increased performances occurred only in repeated (not single) high intensity short-term exercise bouts with short recovery periods between bouts of exercise. However, these results were not consistently found and revealed quite large variations among subjects probably due to individual differences of initial or pre-exercise intramuscular concentrations of creatine. No performance-enhancing effect has been shown in endurance events, including rowing.

There is both anecdotal and objective data to indicate that creatine supplementation at or above recommended dosages can lead to side effects which can reduce performance. Rapid weight gains have bee observed (1-3 kg) primarily due to water retention and this could potentially be a major problem for lightweight rowers who are attempting to lose or maintain weight. There have also been reports from team doctors of a substantial number of musculo-tendinous problems and injuries following use of creatine. Although there have been some reports of kidney and liver problems associated with creatine supplementation, these reports are not documented or verified. It is important to note that no performance studies have been conducted where the long-term effects of creatine use on the health and well being of the athlete have been investigated.

At present creatine or creatine phosphate are not among the banned or restricted substances of the IOC doping list. The knowledge concerning creatine supplementation and it effects is at a point where the knowledge of anabolic-androgenic steroids and their effects was 25 years ago. As a result our Commission recommends caution when using creatine supplementation. We do not recommend the use of creatine in rowing especially the supplementation in children, adolescents, and junior rowers.

June 1998

Doping

The fight against doping:
An Ethical Issue / A Health Issue

Federation Internationale De Gymnastique

Since the beginning of time, man has striven to improve his physical and intellectual performances by means of drugs and medication. His reasons vary from a desire to improve sexual capacity to the awakening of the fighting spirit to the preparation for examinations. Sports are not exempt from such practice.

It would seem that the term 'doping' derives its meaning from the African "DOP", the name of a kind of liquor used by certain tribes as a stimulant inducing a state of trance during religious ceremonies. The word 'doping' appears in an English dictionary in 1889, defined as a mixture of opium and analgesics administered to racehorses. Doping is not an invention of modern times.

At the World Conference on Sports Doping in Lausanne, February 4, 1999, doping was defined as "the use of a device (substance or method) that is potentially dangerous to an athlete's heath and/or is able to improve his or her performance, or the presence of a substance or the use of a method listed in the list annexed to the Olympic Movement's Anti-doping Code."

The Olympic Movement's Anti-doping Code "applies to all athletes, coaches and official instructors as well as to medical and paramedical personnel working with or treating athletes who participate or are preparing to participate in sports competitions that fall into the Olympic Movement framework."

The FIG not only entirely supports this statement, but also endorses it by claiming it as its own principle in the fight against doping. On a practical level, two major elements must be extracted from this definition, motivating our fight: **doping is contrary to sports ethics,** it is a way of cheating that distorts all aspects of a given performance and **doping entails risks that can injure an athlete's overall heath.** These risks may be obvious and acknowledged or they may be pernicious with consequences becoming apparent only years following the act.

If doping is an historical reality, then it is also a current issue in our society, and no sport is out of its reach. Some sports are more affected than others, but vigilance is the answer for everyone who wishes to stop the spreading of this phenomenon. The actual dimensions of doping are difficult to zero in on since only regular doping controls at competitions, and increasingly outside of competitions, allow for a realistic evaluation.

The press is generally imprecise and only covers certain individual cases at the risk of generalising the problem. On the other hand, certain practices are not denounced and fought against strongly enough. Rumours are not an objective basis for judging and, as athletes rarely confess by their own will, the silence that follows implies tacit complicity, which is often the rule of the game.

Doping motives often relate directly to financial, political, athletic and professional stakes as well as media pressure, the search for stardom, over-loaded calendars and increasingly difficult performances and records. All of this is, of course, encouraged by our society centred on the consumption of "medication".

Doping is not a privilege of high level sports and competition, it extends to all levels of practice and to all ages, from adolescence to sports veterans.

Where is doping in terms of gymnastics?

Of course, there are no products available to improve our perception of space or our automatic functioning, no products enabling us to go from a double to a triple somersault. Yet it is easy to imagine that certain gymnasts or coaches, incompetent and with poor intentions, may seek out products for the increasing of physical and muscular strength and weight loss (body fat). Such measures would fail to take into account that modern gymnastics is not a matter of pure strength, but of speed and momentum, and that products favouring such morphological changes all entail side effects that are not only harmful to one's general health, but that disturb the practice of gymnastics itself.

For the moment, it would seem that our gymnasts are showing a good amount of wisdom. Controls executed systematically for over 10 years at all FIG competitions, and at those of the Continental Unions, have never revealed the presence of "major" doping products in the urine. The few existing cases were the results of minor stimulants with a low toxic level that, for the most part, failed to demonstrate a concrete desire to engage in doping on the part of the athlete. Sanctions were moderate (1 to 6 month(s) of suspension).

With this said, let us avoid all triumphalism and remain ever vigilant. We believe that the laboratories the FIG uses for analysis (IOC accredited) are extremely effective, but can only discover substances present in the urine at the time of control. This means that athletes may use doping products outside of competitions to "improve" or "facilitate", according to them, preparation during training sessions.

To remain in accordance with IOC requirements, the FIG must quickly **develop out of competition controls** to be executed at any time of the year and within any FIG Affiliated Federation.

Different Categories of Doping Substances

The list of prohibited substances developed by the FIG Medical Commission duplicates that of the IOC. The FIG has added Cannabis (or Marijuana) to its list, a substance that the IOC determined relative to each international federation. Current FIG regulations apply to all FIG competitions, as well as those organised by its Continental Unions, and to all out of competition controls.

Normally, these substances act as medication intended for specific illnesses that have been competently diagnosed, but have been abusively directed towards improving sports performance. Furthermore, incoherent parties who know nothing of potential effects and dangers usually administer them in massive doses for prolonged and repetitive treatments.

Thus, there is the risk of exceeding physiological limits, of addiction and of pathological effects that are often serious, sometimes fatal and that have a short or long term duration.

Prohibited Classes Of Substances

1. Amphetamines and Other Stimulants. These include amphetamines, caffeine, cocaine, Ephedrin, Penfluramine, etc. Desired effects include learning stimulation (central nervous system), cardiac-respiratory stimulation, the reduction of fatigue, increase in the fighting spirit.

   Dangers and side effects are significant. Administration of these substances entails considerable risks such as an increase in blood pressure, body temperature and heart rate. Ultimate physical reserves may be tapped, resulting in total exhaustion or even death. Regular intake is accompanied by a decrease in desired effects, requiring an increase in dosage. Consequences include insomnia, anorexia, toxicity, drug addiction, depression and suicidal tendency.

   In addition, gymnasts risk feverishness, excitation and the loss of mastery.

2. Pain Reducing Narcotics and Other Pain Reducers Called Narcotic Analgesics. These substances include Cannabis, diverse opiates, Morphine, Heroin, Pentazocine, etc. They are administered to those practising disciplines that often incur pain. In small doses, they have eu-

phoric and analgesic effects that reduce inhibition. In relation to stimulants, they are supposed to improve performance by reducing indications of pain. Side effects include mood swings, aggressiveness, trouble with coordination and consciousness, digestive, and more importantly respiratory, disturbances. Narcotics can lead to addiction or toxicity.

In addition, gymnasts risk disorientation in space perception, reduction of "reflexes" and watchfulness.

3. Cortisone and Other Basic Corticosteroids (prohibited when administered orrally, rectally or by intravenous or intramuscular injection). These are betamethasone, cortivazol, hydrocortisone, prednisone, triamcinolone, etc. Desired effects include euphoria, the stimulation of determination and analgesic effects. Dangers are manifold-. hydromineral and glucidic imbalance (diabetes), gastrointestinal disorders, osteoporosis, muscular atrophy, acute tendency to infection, ocular disturbances, hypertension and neuropsychiatric disorders.

4. Testosterone and Other Anabolic Steroids. These are Clostebol, Dehydrotestosterone, Metandienone, Nandrolone, Stanozolol, Androstenediol, Testosterone, etc. Desired effects include muscular development, an increase in training capacity, the stimulation of determination, aggressiveness and an increase in the fatigue threshold.

The unsupervised intake of anabolic steroids produces numerous toxic effects on the liver, prostate, cardiovascular system, cholesterol level, hormonal balance and the psyche. It can cause acne, water retention (oedema), libido disorders, sterility and a high risk for injuries and ruptures to ligaments and tendons.

Virilism has been found in women along with voice change, hirsutism, reduction in breast size and disturbances in the menstrual cycle. Cancer has been indicated. Anabolic steroids can stunt growth in young people.

Despite such major risks, gymnasts may be tempted to use such drugs to develop their muscles. On a **quantitative** level, the muscle mass will certainly develop, but without the **quality** necessary for the mechanical stress that characterises gymnastics.

5. Peptide Hormones - Mimetics and analogues. These are Corticotropin (ACTH), Erythropoietin(EPO), Chorionic Gonadotropin (HCG), Somatotropin (GH), etc. Desired effects include:

For **ACTH,** effects of Cortisone and Corticosteroids.

For **GH,** growth increase and muscle mass development with the reduction of body fat.

As beneficial as currently used synthetic GH effects may be on patients suffering from specific growth disorders, they are nonetheless extremely dangerous to the healthy individual, causing diabetes, bone development disorders (Pachyacria), neurovascular and even immunological disorders.

Erythropoietin (EPO) triggers red blood cell production, oxygen carriers in the blood, satisfying the high demand of oxygen during exertion. **EPO** can cause hypertension, thrombosis, pulmonary and cerebral embolism and even death.

Gymnastics requires very little metabolic endurance, making it purely stupid to use this substance in our sport.

6. Diuretics and Concealed Substances. These are Amiloride, Furosemide, Probenecid, Spironolactone, Triameterene, etc. Desired effects include rapid weight loss, the dilution of urine prior to doping controls and for some, the concealment of the elimination of certain drugs. By violently dehydrating the body, diuretics cause an imbalance in minerals and a thickening of the blood that can result in dehydration, acute hypertension, kidney injury and muscle cramps.

These substances may be tempting, especially for young female gymnasts wishing to lose weight, but the nearly constant onslaught of disorders listed above should persuade them otherwise.

Classes Of Substances Permitted In Certain Circumstances

1. Beta-blockers (if notification before competition). These are Acebutol, Atenolol, Labetalol, Metoprolol, Propranolol, Setalol, etc.

   They are generally used in the treatment of hypertension. Those practising certain sports use them for their anti-stress effect, improvement of psychomotor coordination and decrease in heart rate. They do, however, come with dangerous side effects including a drop in blood pressure, digestive disturbances, headaches, vertigo, fatigue, insomnia, hypoglycaemia, and heart rate disorders.

   The use of these substances will only bring about deterioration in a gymnast's physical performance.

2. Glucocorticosteroids. Local injections—local cream (if notification before the competition)

3. Local Anaesthetics (if notification before the competition). These are Mepivacaine, Bupivacaine, Lidocaine, Procaine, Tetracaine, etc.

   Desired effects are the local suppression or subduing of pain. Effects may include anaphylactic allergic reactions.

4. Beta 2 Agonists. Only by inhalation (if notification before the competition) and only Salbutamol- Salmeterol - Terbutalline.

5. Other Substances. Alcohol. Certain federations report quantitative alcohol levels (Modern Pentathlon, Shooting). The FIG has not indicated a precise level, but advocates great moderation or even abstinence.

Annex

Prohibited doping methods must be added to the list of prohibited doping substances or restrictions per each country, international federation or other bodies such as the IOC, the European Council, etc. These are blood doping (autologous transfusion), pharmaceutical, chemical, genetic, biological or physical manipulation.

Anti-doping Controls. An anti-doping control consists in taking a gymnast's urine sample (divided into two flasks, A and B) by which testing is carried out to determine the presence of prohibited substances in the urine. It is very possible that in the near future these controls will be carried out by the taking of a blood sample.

The FIG decides when and where a control will take place, whether during a competition or out of competition and where its own competitions are concerned. In certain countries governments, anti-doping agencies or Olympic Committees may request a control at certain competitions, in accordance with the laws of each respective country.

The individual in charge of the control must be authorised by the FIG upon proposal by the local organising committee. The official FIG physician supervises sampling. According to regulations, the designated athlete, either by the drawing of lots or due to his or her competition results (mainly medal-holders) will receive notification to be countersigned following the procedure. The gymnast must appear in the control hall within an hour. During this time, he or she remains under constant surveillance by an official from the control hall. Sanctions will be given should the gymnast refuse. Urine samples will be sent to an IOC and FIG approved laboratory.

Sanctions. Should the laboratory analysis reveal prohibited substances in flask A, the FIG will inform the athlete by way of his or her national federation and communicate the possibility of an expert analysis of the second flask (flask B). Should the gymnast refuse the testing of flask B and thereby confirm the intake of a prohibited substance, or should test results of flask B come out positive, then the FIG will apply the sanctions foreseen in its regulations, after taking into account the gymnast's defence.

FIG sanctions are listed in the official regulations. They consist of different levels based on whether the substance is labelled "major" or "minor". They may be increased or decreased, depending on the aggravating or extenuating circumstances mentioned by the gymnast.

Sanctions entail both a period of suspension, during which the gymnast is forbidden to compete, and, if the substance was taken during a competition, the possible nullification of results and the withdrawal of medals.

A gymnast may appeal to the IOC Arbitral Sports Court in Lausanne. Sanctions apply to all competitions organised in all FIG affiliate countries.

Moreover, the FIG reserves the right to intervene in situations relating to all Affiliated Federations failing to respect anti-doping regulations.

How tempting it is to artificially go beyond one's physical capacities and limits! But turning to a "magical potion" will never lead to victory, certainly not on a long-term basis. The pressure put on athletes is getting ever stronger. "Farther, higher, stronger", such is the slogan. Nevertheless, performances that are a result of doping will never be true performances, victories will never be true victories and the bottom line is that addiction is heavy. Of course, sanctions are one aspect, but everyone knows that modern gladiators who turned to doping are condemned to suffer life-long effects, not to mention those who are dead.

Gymnastics has so much to offer. It allows for an understanding of one's physical capacities, but also of one's limits. The system is constructed to allow for high-level sports performances without the need for doping. **The system is constructed so as to eliminate the need or "interest" in a doping substance for gymnastic performance.** Nearly all of these substances incur extremely dangerous effects on one's health. All voluntary or involuntary doping is contrary to sports ethics and to the principle of fair play.

Personalised training and perseverance, a balanced diet, sufficient rest, good psychological balance and rigorous and regular medical assistance are the only conditions that lead to success.

June 2000

Statement on Doping in Sport

International Federation of Sports Medicine (FIMS)

Web site: www.fims.org

Doping in sport is the deliberate or inadvertent use by an athlete of a substance or method banned by the International Olympic Committee (IOC). FIMS supports the prohibition of doping to protect athletes from:

1. the unfair advantage which may be gained by those athletes who use banned substances or methods to enhance performance.

2. the possible harmful side effects which some substances or methods can produce.

In addition to the ethical and health consequences surrounding doping, recognition is made of potential legal implications. The distribution of many banned substances (e.g., anabolic steroids), if not for a medically justified reason, is illegal in many countries. Encouraging or assisting athletes to use such substances or methods is unethical and, therefore, equally forbidden.

Note: This statement may be reproduced and distributed with the sole requirement that it be identified clearly as a Position Statement of the International Federation of Sports Medicine.

Erythropoietin

Use of Erythropoietin (EPO) as an Ergogenic Aid

FISA Sports Medicine Commission

Erythropoietin (EPO) is a naturally occurring hormone produced by the kidneys. This hormone elevates red blood cell (RBC) production as a normal response to a decrease in oxygen in the blood. The major stimuli for the release of EPO are increasing volume of exercise training, exposure to altitude, and severe hemorrhaging. Human EPO has now been synthesized in the laboratory. Theoretically, if administered to endurance athletes, EPO should have the same effects as reinfusion of RBC (blood doping) with the sole purpose of increasing the blood's oxygen-carrying capacity. Use of EPO along with blood doping are currently listed on the IOC Medical Code banned list of peptide hormones and procedures respectively.

Only limited research has been conducted using EPO as a possible ergogenic aid, it appears to mimic the effects of blood doping by improving endurance performance. However, these studies were conducted only in the laboratory and there has been no conclusive evidence that EPO supplementation has the same effect in actual competition.

The lack of knowledge of the possible short- and long-term detrimental effects of this hormone are unknown at this time and the results of its use is far less predictable than those of blood doping. Some deaths among highly competitive road cyclists in the early 1990's were suggested to be associated with EPO use but these reports were not documented or verified. Decisions concerning the appropriate and safe quantity and quality of EPO to be used, how it enters the body, and the timing of its use have not been based on good science. Following the introduction of EPO there is no evidence to indicate how much RBC production will occur. Individual responses to hormones and drugs show wide variations. The major health concern is the possible significant increase in blood viscosity (thick or heavy blood) which could result in abnormal clotting of blood and increase vascular resistance to an extent where even a healthy exercise-trained heart may be damaged in its attempts to develop force to overcome increased resistance of blood flow.

The Sports Medicine Commission of FISA unanimously supports the IOC ban of EPO and cautions its use among rowing athletes. The proposed ergogenic effects of EPO are not worth the risk of serious cardiovascular problems.

June 1998

Steroids

Anabolic Steroids to Enhance Athletic Performance

American Academy of Orthopaedic Surgeons (AAOS)

Web site: www.aaos.org/wordhtml/papers position/steroids.htm

The American Academy of Orthopaedic Surgeons recognizes that although anabolic steroids may enhance athletic performance by increasing both the size and strength of athletes, their use can cause serious harmful physiological, pathological, and psychological effects.

The American Academy of Orthopaedic Surgeons believes that anabolic steroids should not be used to enhance performance or appearance, and that they be banned from use in all sports programs. We recommend that sports-governing bodies make every effort to deter and to detect their use. When feasible, the relevant sports medicine bodies should implement aggressive drug testing programs to detect their use and impose harsh penalties for those athletes who use them and those individuals or institutions who facilitate their use.

The Code of Ethics for Orthopaedic Surgeons specifically addresses this issue. It provides in Paragraph VII.B: "...It is unethical to prescribe controlled substances when they are not medically indicated. It is also unethical to prescribe substances for the sole purpose of enhancing athletic performance."

Use of anabolic steroids has been associated with the following adverse effects: increased risk of benign and malignant tumors of the liver, testes, and prostate; increased risk of serious cardiovascular disease; impaired reproductive functioning in males and females which may be irreversible; tendon weakening and potential ruptures; irreversible closure of bone growth centers in adolescents; menstrual irregularity; and psychological dependence which may lead to withdrawal symptoms and depression upon the cessation of use. Major personality changes may occur, manifested by increasing aggressiveness and intensity which may lead to intense anti-social or psychotic behavior.

The use of performance-enhancing substances by athletes represents a most serious violation of ethical standards of organized sports activities at all levels, and should not be tolerated.

Recent legislation classifies anabolic steroids as controlled substances, and imposes restrictions on their distribution and use. The Academy strongly supports law enforcement agencies in their efforts to enforce existing legislation to control the distribution and use of anabolic steroids.

December 1991

American Academy of Orthopaedic Surgeons

Document Number: 1102

Substance Use

Substance Use and Abuse

The National Junior College Athletic Association (NJCAA)

The National Junior College Athletic Association (NJCAA) is the governing body of inter-collegiate athletics for two-year colleges. As such, its programs are designed to meet the unique needs of a diverse group of student-athletes who come from both traditional and non-traditional backgrounds and whose purpose in selecting a junior college may be as varied as their experiences before attending college.

Given this perspective, the NJCAA accepts its responsibility by seeking to provide a competitive environment that is free from drug and substance use and abuse in any form for the purpose of facilitating or enhancing athletic performance by any athlete engaged in competition that is either sponsored or sanctioned by the NJCAA.

It is the position of the NJCAA that it will serve as a resource and referral agency for any athlete, coach, or administrator who wishes to secure information relative to the effects, consequences and potential avenues of treatment for substance abuse; to coordinate the efforts of coaches and athletic administrators in their efforts to serve as educational liaisons for those student-athletes wishing to further their athletic careers at four-year institutions that are subject to drug testing procedures; and to continue to endorse and encourage efforts on the part of member institutions to educate their athletes to the implications of drug usage in their lives beyond athletics.

It is a fundamental belief of the NJCAA that athletic participation is a privilege and that those athletes who use illegal performance-enhancing and/or recreational drugs substantively violate that privilege. In response to any violations of this nature that occur and are detected in NJCAA-sponsored or sanctioned events, continuation of rights and privileges of participation by the individual or the institution will be reviewed or revoked, as appropriate.

The NJCAA requires of its member institutions the following:

1. Development and implementation of a drug and alcohol (to include tobacco) awareness education program for all members of inter-collegiate athletic department staffs and student-athletes.

2. Development and distribution of an institutional policy statement relative to the use and abuse of alcohol, tobacco, drugs, and other controlled substances. This policy statement should address participation and the expectations of the member institution for each intercollegiate athletic department staff member's and student-athlete's standard of behavior.

3. Development and implementation of a plan for referral, treatment, rehabilitation for all members of intercollegiate athletic department staffs and student-athletes with drug and/or alcohol-related problems.

4. By using various resources of individual institutions in response to institutional needs and demands, investigate the feasibility of a complete and comprehensive drug use and abuse screening program.

Statement on NCAA Drug-Testing Exceptions Procedure

> ### National Collegiate Athletic Association

The NCAA list of banned-drug classes (NCAA Bylaw 31.2.3.1) is comprised of substances that are generally reported to be performance enhancing and/or potentially harmful to the health and safety of the student-athlete.

The NCAA recognizes that some banned substances are used for legitimate medical purposes. Accordingly, the NCAA allows exception to be made for those student-athletes with a documented medical history demonstrating the need for regular use of such a drug.

Exceptions may be granted for substances included in the following classes of banned drugs: stimulants, beta blockers, diuretics and peptide hormones. (Bylaw 31.2.3.1)

Procedure for Exceptions

1. Alternative nonbanned medications for the treatment of various conditions exist and should be considered before an exception is pursued.

2. In the event that the student-athlete and the physician (in coordination with sports-medicine staff at the student-athlete's institution) agree that no alternative to the use of the banned substance is available, the decision may be made to continue the use of the banned substance (i.e., stimulant, beta blocker, diuretic or peptide hormone).

3. The institution should maintain in the student-athlete's medical record on campus a letter from the prescribing physician that documents that the student-athlete has a medical history demonstrating the need for regular use of such a drug. The letter should contain information as to the diagnosis (including appropriate verification), medical history and dosage information.

4. A student-athlete's medical records or physicians' letters should not be sent to the NCAA unless requested by the NCAA. Also, the use of the substance need not be reported at the time of an NCAA drug testing.

5. In the event that a student-athlete is tested by the NCAA and tests positive for a substance for which the institution desires an exception, normal procedures for reporting positive test results will be followed (See NCAA Drug-Testing Protocol Section No. 8.0.) and the institution, through its director of athletics, may request an exception by submitting to the NCAA the Exceptions Procedure physician's letter and any other medical documentation it wishes to have considered.

6. Requests for exceptions will be reviewed by the chair of the drug-testing and drug-education subcommittee of the NCAA Committee on Competitive Safeguards and Medical Aspects of Sports or his/her designate.

7. The NCAA will inform the director of athletics regarding the outcome of the exception request. In the event that the exception is not granted, the institution may appeal this action according to Section 8.0. of the drug-testing protocol.

8. The eligibility of the involved student-athlete will be maintained during the period of time the exception is being reviewed by the drug subcommittee.

9. Institutions may contact the NCAA regarding this procedure.

Sources

1. NCAA Drug Testing Program, 1999-2000.

2. Athletic Drug Reference, 1999.

3. The National Collegiate Athletic Association August 1999

4. FDU

NCAA Drug-Testing Programs Drugs and Procedures Subject to Restrictions

National Collegiate Athletic Association (NCAA)

The use of the following drugs and/or procedures is subject to certain restrictions and may or may not be permissible, depending on limitations expressed in these guidelines and/or quantities of these substances used.

(a) Blood Doping. The practice of blood doping (the intravenous injection of whole blood, packed red blood cells or blood substitutes) is prohibited and any evidence confirming use will be cause for action consistent with that taken for a positive drug test.

(b) Local Anesthetics. The Executive Committee will permit the limited use of local anesthetics under the following conditions:

1. That procaine, xylocaine, carbocaine or any other local anesthetic may be used, but not cocaine;

2. That only local or topical injections can be used (i.e., intravenous injections are not permitted), and

3. That use is medically justified only when permitting the athlete to continue the competition without potential risk to his or her health.

(c) Manipulation of Urine Samples. The Executive Committee bans the use of substances and methods that alter the integrity and/or validity of urine samples provided during NCAA drug testing.

Examples of banned methods are catheterization, urine substitution, and/or tampering or modification of renal excretion by the use of diuretics, probenecid, bromantan or related compounds, and epitestosterone administration.

(d) Beta 2 Agonists. The use of beta 2 agonists is permitted by inhalation only.

(e) Additional Analysis. Drug screening for select nonbanned substances may be conducted for nonpunitive purposes.

CHAPTER

11

Policies

Athletic Trainers

Athletic Trainers for High School Athletes

American Academy of Family Physicians (AAFP)

The AAFP encourages that high schools have a National Athletic Trainers Association (NATA)-certified or additionally registered/licensed athletic trainer as an integral part of the high school athletic program.

1989; 1995 (revised)

AAFP Reference Manual

Cardiomyopathy

Recommendations for Medical Evaluation and Sports Participation in Athletes With a Family History of Sudden Cardiac Death

International Federation of Sports Medicine (FIMS): Scientific Commission

Web site: www.fims.org

Hypertrophic Cardiomyopathy (HCM)

HCM is a primary and usually familial cardiac disease for which several disease-causing mutations in genes encoding proteins of the sarcomere have been identified. HCM presents heterogeneous morphologic alterations and clinical course. The characteristic of this disorder is a hypertrophied and non-dilated left ventricle; in the absence of other conditions that could produce the magnitude of hypertrophy present.

The following information was considered regarding this disease:

1. HCM is the most common structural cardiac abnormality associated with sudden death in young athletes.

2. Certain genetic mutations, such as Arg403Gln and cardiac troponin T mutations, are associated with a particularly adverse prognosis.

3. Occurrence of sudden death in the family is a marker of high risk for all affected members.

4. The risk for sudden death increases in youth until the third decade. After that age, the likelihood of sudden death decreases.

5. Morphologic features of HCM may not be present (and identifiable by echocardiography) until adolescence, and diagnosis may not be certain in children. The probability of correct diagnosis increases in advanced youth and adult age.

6. Genetic analysis of families where the gene mutation(s) is identified may diagnose with certainty the affected family members.

7. The prognostic value of genetic mutations in young asymptomatic carriers with mild (or absent) phenotypic expression of the disease is still uncertain, however.

Recommendations for Diagnostic Evaluation

1. Candidates with relatives (parents, siblings, grandparents, uncles, aunts, and cousins) who have been diagnosed with HCM should undergo a cardiovascular examination that includes at least a 12-lead ECG and 2D-echocardiography.

2. When these diagnostic tests suggest the diagnosis of HCM, a comprehensive cardiac evaluation (including exercise stress test, 24-hour ECG Holter monitoring) is recommended.

3. Genetic analysis is recommended when the mutation(s) responsible for the familial HCM is known.

Recommendations for Participation in Athletic Activities

1. Candidates with unequivocal diagnosis of HCM who are < 35 years of age should avoid strenuous training and athletic competition. They should not participate in any competitive athletic activities, with the possible exception of the low-intensity physical activities (Class IA). Candidates should not participate in competitive athletic activities, based on the

likelihood that intense athletic training and competition increase the risk of sudden death in these patients.

2. Candidates with unequivocal diagnosis of HCM who are > 35 year of age and have no risk factors (e.g., family history of sudden death, syncope, sustained or non-sustained ventricular tachycardia, marked left ventricular hypertrophy, left ventricular outflow gradient >50 mmHg, exercise-induced ischemia or hypotension, and carriers of certain high-risk genes) may reasonably be considered at low risk for sudden cardiac death. In selected subjects, participation in mild to moderate athletic activities (Classes IA, IB, and IIA) may be allowed, as long as periodic evaluations are done at least once a year.

3. Candidates with HCM diagnosed among relatives, but who do not have evidence of HCM based on a 12-lead ECG and 2D-echocardiography, should be restricted from competitive athletic activities during adolescence until full body growth is reached. When familial genetic mutation is known, genetic testing is recommended to exclude the presence of the disease. In the absence of this analysis, presence of HCM should be periodically (yearly) checked until complete body growth is reached. After that, candidates who do not show evidence of HCM may participate in sport activities without restrictions, with the recommendation of periodic follow-up and testing.

4. If genetic analysis excludes the familial mutation responsible for HCM, the candidate should not be restricted from athletic activities.

References

1. Klues HG, Schiffers A, Maron BJ (1995). Phenotypic spectrum and patterns of left ventricular hypertrophy in hypertrophic cardiomyopathy: morphologic observations and significance as assessed by two-dimensional echocardiography in 600 patients. *J Am Coll Cardiol* 26: 1699-1708.

2. Lewis JF, Spirito P, Pelliccia A, et al. (1992). Usefulness of Doppler echocardiographic assessment of diastolic filling in the distinguishing "athlete's heart" hypertrophic cardiomyopathy. *Am J Cardiol* 68: 296-300.

3. Marian AJ, Roberts R (1995). Recent advances in the molecular genetics of hypertrophic cardiomyopathy. *Circulation* 92: 1336-47

4. Maron BJ (1997). Hypertrophic cardiomyopathy. *The Lancet* 350: 127-33.

5. Maron BJ, Pelliccia A, Spirito P (1995). Cardiac disease in young trained athletes: insights into methods for distinguishing athletes's heart from structural heart disease, with particular emphasis on hypertrophic cardomyopathy. *Circulation* 91: 1596-601.

6. Maron BJ, Spirito P, Wesley Y, Arce J (1986). Development and progression of left ventricular hypertrophy in children with hypertrophic cardiomyopathy. *N Engl J Med* 315: 610-614.

7. Pelliccia A, Maron BJ, Spartaro A, et al. (1991). The upper limit of physiologic cardiac hypertrophy in highly trained elite athletes. *N Engl J Med* 324: 295-301.

8. Rosenzweig A, Watkins H, Hwang D-S, Miri M, et al. (1991). Preclinical diagnosis of familial hypertrophic cardiomyopathy by genetic analysis of blood lymphocytes. *N Engl J Med* 325: 1753-1760.

Cardiorespiratory Fitness

The Recommended Quantity and Quality of Exercise for Developing and Maintaining Cardiorespiratory and Muscular Fitness, and Flexibility in Healthy Adults

American College of Sports Medicine (ACSM)

Web site: www.acsm.org

Summary

The combination of frequency, intensity, and duration of chronic exercise has been found to be effective for producing a training effect. The interaction of these factors provide the overload stimulus. In general, the lower the stimulus the lower the training effect, and the greater the stimulus the greater the effect. As a result of specificity of training and the need for maintaining muscular strength and endurance, and flexibility of the major muscle groups, a well-rounded training program including aerobic and resistance training, and flexibility exercises is recommended. Although age in itself is not a limiting factor to exercise training, a more gradual approach in applying the prescription at older ages seems prudent. It has also been shown that aerobic endurance training of fewer than 2 d·wk^{-1}, at less than 40-50% of VO$_2$R, and for less than 10 min^{-1} is generally not a sufficient stimulus for developing and maintaining fitness in healthy adults. Even so, many health benefits from physical activity can be achieved at lower intensities of exercise if frequency and duration of training are increased appropriately. In this regard, physical activity can be accumulated through the day in shorter bouts of 10-min durations.

In the interpretation of this position stand, it must be recognized that the recommendations should be used in the context of participant's needs, goals, and initial abilities. In this regard, a sliding scale as to the amount of time allotted and intensity of effort should be carefully gauged for the cardiorespiratory, muscular strength and endurance, and flexibility components of the program. An appropriate warm-up and cool-down period, which would include flexibility exercises, is also recommended. The important factor is to design a program for the individual to provide the proper amount of physical activity to attain maximal benefit at the lowest risk. Emphasis should be placed on factors that result in permanent lifestyle change and encourage a lifetime of physical activity.

1982

Med. Sci. Sports Exerc., Vol. 30, No. 6, pp. 975-991, 1998.

Communicable Diseases

Statement on Communicable Diseases

International Life Saving Federation (ILSF) Medical Commission

Web site: www.ilsf.org/medical
infection_control.html

Background

Lifeguards have always been aware of the need for basic hygiene in providing first aid, but several events over the past 40 years have greatly increased the risks of cross infection both to and from the lifeguard.

- Rescue breathing was introduced in most lifeguard services in about 1960.

- External CPR followed within a year or so.

- The use of training manikins subsequently became very popular and most training programs now require demonstration of proficiency using a manikin.

- Oxygen is now widely used and the equipment used requires decontamination.

- The description of the Acquired Immuno-deficiency Syndrome in 1981 in the New England Journal of Medicine hastened community and medical awareness of the need for emphasis on prevention of cross infection.

- Hepatitis B and C have become increasingly common and are now of very significant proportions. These diseases are also much more readily spread than HIV.

- Research has clarified the modes of transmission of these and other viruses.

- A vaccine suitable for mass immunisation against Hepatitis B became available in the late 1980's and has proven both safe and effective.

- The Centers for Disease Control and Prevention in Atlanta and most health agencies throughout the world now have formulated detailed policies for Health Care Workers. These policies are under continual review and are regularly updated.

- Lifeguards who are involved in rescue, resuscitation and first aid must use the same infection control guidelines as persons regarded as "Health Care Workers."

- Some lifeguards themselves may be carriers of potentially communicable diseases. In some cases they may be aware and in others, unaware.

Statement

While recognising the diverse cultural, religious, political, financial, legal and other considerations from country to country, the Medical Commission notes certain fundamentals which can be stated.

1. Lifeguards are comparable to Health Care Workers in having responsibility for and public expectation of professional standards in the administration of rescue, resuscitation and emergency medical aid.

2. All lifeguard organisations should have current comprehensive policies on infection control relevant to their particular areas of responsibility in their own country. This policy should conform with international standards and should be endorsed by a qualified medical authority.

3. The Commission strongly endorses the principle of universal body substance precautions as the ideal standard and this should be incorporated in the policies mentioned in paragraph #2 (above). These require all lifeguards

to assume that the blood and body substances of every person rescued or treated must be considered as potentially infective, independent of diagnosis or perceived risk. Universal body substance precautions should be used consistently when lifeguards are in contact with mucous membranes, broken skin and body substances including blood, urine, sputum, saliva and wound drainage. Of all body fluids, BLOOD is by far the most infective and therefore most dangerous.

4. All lifeguards should receive comprehensive instruction on relevant aspects of cross infection.

5. Whenever possible masks and gloves should be available for use in first aid and resuscitation.

6. All lifeguards are strongly advised to be immunised against Hepatitis B, whether there is legislation in their country or not. At present there is no vaccine available for Hepatitis C. Hepatitis A is a different disorder and immunisation should be considered for lifeguards in areas where the disorder is endemic or when travelling to such areas.

7. Lifeguards should be informed of their obligations and legal position should they know that they are carriers of a communicable disorder. This will vary from country to country and in some nations, from state to state. Furthermore, lifeguard organisations must be aware of their own legal position in the event of being informed that a lifeguard is a carrier of a communicable disease.

8. Any accidental exposure to body substances should be reported immediately so that appropriate action can be taken.

9. In particular, accidental needlestick injuries whether to a lifeguard or member of the public must be referred for urgent expert medical attention.

10. Decontamination of manikin parts and oxygen delivery equipment must be carried out according to the recommendations of the manufacturer or the responsible lifeguard authority.

11. The Centers for Disease Control and Prevention (CDC) in Atlanta, Georgia USA is recognised by the ILS Medical Commission and most health authorities internationally as being at the forefront of information and recommendations on infection control .

12. The website for the CDC is: www.cdc.gov. At the time this statement was published, the specific address of CDC information on Universal Precautions for Prevention of Transmission of HIV and Other Bloodborne Infections was: www.cdc.gov/ ncidod/hip/blood/universa.htm.

References

1. All information from the Centers for Disease Control and Prevention is highly recommended as totally reputable and up to date.

2. Communicable Disease Policy of Royal Lifesaving Society Australia

3. Communicable Disease Policy of Surf Life Saving Australia

September 1999

Defibrillator Use

Statement on Automatic External Defibrillation Use by Lifesavers and Lifeguards

International Life Saving Federation (ILSF) Medical Commission

Web site: www.ilsf.org/medical/AED.html

Background

Survival of cardiac arrest depends on a series of critical interventions. The term *chain of survival* has been used to describe this sequence. This chain has four interdependent links: early access, early basic cardiopulmonary resuscitation (CPR), early defibrillation, and early advanced cardiac life support. While all links are important, in cardiac arrest due to heart disease, early defibrillation is the most critical link in the *chain of survival*. (1,2)

Most victims who can be saved from cardiac arrest are in ventricular fibrillation (VF) or ventricular tachycardia (VT) rhythms. (8) Conversion of ventricular fibrillation to a normal heart rhythm requires defibrillation be administered within a few minutes of a cardiac arrest. The probability of successful defibrillation diminishes rapidly over time. (9)

To achieve the earliest possible defibrillation, many leading organizations in resuscitation have recommended that non medical individuals should be allowed and encouraged to use defibrillators. (1) There has been interest in the possibility of lifesavers and lifeguards receiving training in the use of AED to improve response times to early AED use in cases of sudden cardiac arrest on land, cardiac arrest in water and in some near-drowning cases. Experience and peer reviewed literature on defibrillation in near-drowning resuscitation by lifesavers and lifeguards is limited. There is no clear evidence of the value of early of defibrillation following near-drowning. Cost-benefit analysis for early defibrillation by lifeguard programs is absent. There will always be interesting discussion about the priority of early defibrillation by lifeguards in relation to other training and equipment needs of lifeguards and lifeguard programs.

Lifesavers and lifeguards have the unique challenge of providing rescue and resuscitation service in and around water. Drowning and near-drowning are hypoxic events with significant consequences. (3,4) The prevention of drowning deaths and near-drowning accidents must remain a principle function of lifesavers and lifeguards. When rescue is needed, speed to recognition and elevation of the head above the water are critical. This is easier, and quicker to achieve, in some environments (pools) than in other environments (open water or surf).

The speed of rescue and early initiation of the *chain of survival* will improve victim outcomes. (5) In cases of land based cardiac arrest and those near-drowning cases with rapid rescue and early effective resuscitation, VF and VT may be present and defibrillation may be helpful. (6,7)

To maximize successful outcomes after submersion, rescue prior to the hypoxic insults is ideal. In near-drowning cases with potentially good outcomes, early victim recognition, fast rescue, and early effective resuscitation are essential. Outcome studies after AED use by lifesavers and lifeguards are needed.

Statement

1. Outcomes from near-drowning and water related accidents can be tragic. The principal objective for lifesavers and lifeguards is to prevent near-drowning, drowning and water related accidents through education, supervision and rapid rescue response.

2. The principal consequence of near-drowning is hypoxia. The provision of lifesavers and

lifeguards with training and equipment for early recovery of victims from water is the highest priority.

3. All lifesavers and lifeguards should receive training in Basic Life Support (chain of survival, early access to EMS, Airway Management and CPR).

4. Early defibrillation in the management of cardiac arrest is effective in cases with VF and VT. When an arrest victim, in VF or VT, has early application of defibrillation, this is associated with conversion to sinus rhythm and to functional survival. VF and VT may be present in some near-drowning resuscitations when early recognition, speedy rescue and effective CPR with oxygen supplementation, has occurred. Early application of AED may be helpful in these cases.

5. Advanced Life Support skills (defibrillation, medication and intensive care) may be part of the community response to cardiac arrest. It is appropriate for some lifesaving and lifeguard services to investigate AED use. This review should include investigations of other community AED providers, AED response times, frequency of cardiac arrests, supervision and management of AED, AED license requirements, cost benefit analysis and outcome studies. Decisions about the availability, placement, training, and use of AED should be a community level decision based on the principles of the "Chain of Survival", local resources and community priorities.

6. Lifesavers and Lifeguards may play a role in the delivery of AED if this is consistent with the support and service priorities of that community.

7. If lifesavers or lifeguards will be delivering AED, they must receive appropriate training in the use of AED and the associated issues related to outcomes, stress and grief.

8. National, regional and local lifesaving and lifeguard organizations may choose to participate in the development of training policies for the use of AED by non-medical personnel, if and when communities choose to implement AED use by lifesavers or lifeguards. Lifesaver and Lifeguard services are part of a community risk management and response plan, an integral part of a wider population safety network.

9. Outcome studies of the application of AED by lifesavers and lifeguards in aquatic settings should be encouraged.

References

1. Kloeck W. et al, An Advisory Statement From the Advanced Life Support Working Group of the International Liaison Committee of Resuscitation (ILCOR): *Circulation* Vol 95, No 8 April 15 1997, pp. 2183-2184.

2. American Heart Association 1992 Guidelines for CPR and Emergency Cardiac Care, *JAMA*, Oct 28 1992, Vol 268, No 16, pp. 2171-2302.

3. Model, J H, Drowning *N Engl J Med*, 328, 253-256, 1993.

4. Model, J H, Graves, S A, and Kuck E J, Near-Drowning; Correlation of Level of Consciousness and Survival, *Can Anaesth Soc J*, 27, 211-215, 1980.

5. Orlowski J P, Drowning, Near-Drowning and Ice-Water Submersion, *Pediatric Clinics of North America*, Vol 34, No 1, Feb 1987.

6. Monolios N, Mackie I, Drowning and near-drowning on Australian beaches patrolled by life-savers: a 10 year study 1973-1983, *Med J of Australia*, 148(4), 165-171, Feb 15 1988.

7. Kuisma M, Suominen P, Korpela R, Paediatric out-of-hospital cardiac arrests—epidemiological and outcome, *Resuscitation* 30(2), 141-150, Oct 1995.

8. Weisfelt M, et al, American Heart Association Report on the Public Assess Defibrillation Conference, Dec 8-10, 1994, Automatic External Defibrillation Task Force. *Circulation* 92: 2740-2747 1995.

9. Herlitz J et al, Rhythm changes during resuscitation from ventricular fibrillation in relation to delay until defibrillation, number of shocks delivered and survival, *Resuscitation*, Vol 34, pg17-19, 1997.

The Use of Automatic External Defibrillators in YMCAs

YMCA of the USA Medical Advisory Committee:

Sudden cardiac arrest is a major cause of death in the United States. It claims an estimated 250,000 lives each year. Early use of cardio-pulmonary resuscitation (CPR) and rapid defibrillation are the two major contributors to the survival of adult victims of sudden cardiac arrest. As an organization dedicated to the health and safety of its constituents, many of whom participate in activities requiring physical exertion, YMCAs have long required staff to be certified in CPR in the event of a cardiac emergency in a YMCA activity. With the development of automatic external defibrillators (AEDs), YMCAs and other community organizations have access to a new tool which can significantly increase the survival rate of adult cardiac arrest victims.

AEDs that accurately analyze cardiac rhythms and, if appropriate, deliver an electric countershock were introduced in 1979. AEDs are widely used by trained emergency personnel and first- responders, and have proven accurate and effective. A logical extension of the AED concept is "public access defibrillation", the widespread use of AEDs by nonmedical, minimally trained personnel.

Recent technological breakthroughs have made AEDs easier to use and maintain, smaller and more lightweight, and lower in cost. The new generation of AEDs will make it more practical to train and equip a wide range of emergency first-responders in the community, including selected YMCA staff members. Safety is ensured by the built-in computers which allow the unit to recognize ventricular fibrillation (an arrhythmia that causes cardiac arrest), advise the operator that a shock is indicated, and deliver the shock as a safe level.

The American Heart Association has published a statement (1) endorsing the use of AEDs in public places, stating that "Automatic external defibrillation is one of the most promising methods for achieving rapid defibrillation. In public access defibrillation, the technology of defibrillation and training in its use are accessible to the community". It should be noted that the AHA recommends the use of AEDs only with persons over the age of eight.

The Medical Advisory Committee of the YMCA of the USA endorses the American Heart Association's position on the use of automatic external defibrillators, and suggests that YMCAs may want to consider having them available in their facilities and programs. Following are guidelines regarding the use of AEDs in the YMCA:

1. The AED equipment should be purchased from a manufacturer who has met FDA standards.

2. YMCA staff should be trained in the procedures and use of the AED. Supplying a training program in the use of the equipment is one of the benchmarks of a reputable vendor. Ongoing staff training on a yearly basis is recommended, either from the equipment manufacturer, the American Red Cross, or the National Safety Council.

3. In conjunction with their Medical Advisory Committee, YMCAs should establish and follow specific procedures for using the AED.

4. YMCAs should establish a regular maintenance and testing schedule for the AED equipment.

The price range for an FDA-approved AED in 1997 is $3,000 - $6,000. The American Heart Association recommends the following manufacturers who have met FDA standards for automatic external defibrillators:

Heartstream, 206-443-7630

Laerdal Medical Corporation, 800431-1055

Physio-Control Corporation, 800426-8047

SurVivalink, 800-991-5465

References

1. "Public Access Defibrillation", American Heart Association, June 1995

November 1997

Disclaimer: These recommendations were developed by the YMCA of the USA Medical Advisory Committee for the exclusive use by YMCAs in United States. As they were developed with the specific needs of the YMCAs in mind, they may not be applicable to other organizations. These recommendations are consistent with the mission and values of the YMCA.

Drowning: Use of Abdominal Thrusts

Statement on the Use of Abdominal Thrusts in Near Drowning

International Life Saving Federation (ILSF) Medical Commission

Web site: www.ilsf.org/medicalabdomen.html

Background

In January 1996 the Medical Commission of the International Life Saving Federation issued a statement on the use of abdominal thrusts in near drowning.

At a meeting of the Commission in San Diego in September 1997 the Statement was again discussed in the light of several papers presented at the preceding International Medical/ Rescue Conference.

The Commission decided to endorse the previous statement but with expanded explanation and list of references.

Statement

Near drowning victims present unique and challenging problems in airway management because of the nature of the episode. Since drowning is a process of asphyxiation, the victims are usually profoundly hypoxic. They have often swallowed large quantities of water and air; their stomachs frequently contain food and drink consumed just prior to entering the water.

This combination of hypoxia and a full stomach is the cause of the regurgitation that is very familiar to lifeguards and is an almost inevitable accompaniment of near drowning. This has been well-documented in the literature (1, 2).

Submersion victims may aspirate some fluid into their lungs but there is no evidence that this can or need be removed by any technique.

The priority for rescuers is to implement resuscitation at the earliest possible opportunity. In doing this, the maintenance of a clear air-

way and prevention of aspiration are of paramount importance.

The Medical Commission of the International Life Saving Federation has carefully considered the particular problems of upper airway management in near drowning. Techniques which have poor efficacy and purely anecdotal support are strongly discouraged. Abdominal thrusts (Heimlich Maneuver) to relieve airway obstruction have been carefully considered and the following conclusions drawn:

- In near drowning upper abdominal thrusts pose a great risk of precipitating gastro-oesophageal regurgitation and subsequent inhalation of stomach contents into the lungs.

- There is no clear medical rationale for its use and in particular it seems clear that the manoeuvre cannot expel sufficient water from the lower portions of the respiratory tree to aid in resuscitation.

- There are no well controlled blind studies to validate its value in near drowning.

- The use of abdominal thrusts as a first maneuver will merely serve to delay the institution of appropriate cardiopulmonary resuscitation which has been well proven to save life in this condition.

Therefore the Medical Commission of the International Life Saving Federation strongly recommends that in cases of near drowning the use of upper abdominal thrusts is contraindicated unless a solid foreign body (not water) is present in the upper airway and cannot be dislodged by other means. This would be demonstrated by inability to obtain adequate ventilation of the lungs in the course of basic resuscitation measures.

References

1. Manolios N & Mackie I, Drowning & near drowning on Australian beaches patrolled by lifesavers: 10 year study 1973-1983. *Med J Aust* Vol 148 February 15, 1988.

2. Modell J H, The Drowning Process and Lifeguard Intervention, *Proceedings of the International Medical Rescue Conference* San Diego, September 15-17, 1997.

3. Heimlich H J, Patrick E A: Using the Heimlich Maneuvre to Save Near-Drowning Victims. *Postgrad med*, 84: 62-27, 71-73, 1988.

4. Standards and Guidelines for Cardiopulmonary Resuscitation (CPR) and Emergency Cardiac Care (ECC). *JAMA*, 255: 2905-84., 1986.

5. Rozen P, Stoto M, Harley J, (eds): *The use of the Heimlich Maneuver in Near-Drowning*. Committee on the Treatment of Near-Drowning victims. Division of Health Promotion and Disease Prevention. Institute of Medicine, Washington, D.C., August 1994.

6. Orlowski J P: Vomiting as a Complication of the Heimlich Maneuver. *JAMA*, 258: 512-513, 1987.

7. Orlowski J P: Drowning, Near-drowning and ice-water submersions. *Pediatric Clinics of North America*. Vol 34 No 1 February 1987.

8. Heimlich H J: Subdiaphragmatic pressure to expel water from the lungs of drowning persons. *Ann Emerg Med* 10 (9): 476-480, 1981.

9. Orlowski J P: Heimlich maneuver for near-drowning questioned. *Ann Emerg Med* 11 (2): 111-113, 1982.

September 1998

Emergencies

AHA/ACSM Joint Statement: Recommendations for Cardiovascular Screening, Staffing, and Emergency Policies at Health/Fitness Facilities

American Heart Association (AHA)/American College of Sports Medicine (ACSM)

Summary

The promotion of physical activity is at the top of our national public health agenda. Although regular exercise reduces subsequent cardiovascular morbidity and mortality, the incidence of a cardiovascular event during exercise in patients with cardiac disease is estimated to be 10 times that of otherwise healthy persons. Adequate screening and evaluation are important to identify and counsel persons with underlying cardiovascular disease before they begin exercising at moderate to vigorous levels. This statement provides recommendations for *cardiovascular screening* of all persons (children, adolescents, and adults) before enrollment or participation in activities at health/fitness facilities. Staff qualifications and emergency policies related to cardiovascular safety are also discussed.

1998

Med. Sci. Sports Exerc. Vol. 30, No. 6, 1998.

Gender Verification

Sex Testing (Gender Verification) In Sport

Canadian Academy of Sport Medicine (CASM)

It is the position of the Canadian Academy of Sport Medicine that gender verification be eliminated from all sport competition.

For More Information

Telephone: 613-748-5851
FAX: 613-748-5792
Unit 14 - 1010 Polytek Street Gloucester, Ont. K1B 5N4

Specific Information about the Position Statement on Gender Verification: Dr. Pamela Doig General Information about CASM: Ms. Jacqueline Burke
Webmaster (for Web Page suggestions) : ishrier@med.mcgill.ca

January 1997

Sport Participation Assessment

Sport Preparticipation Assessment of Subjects Older Than 35 Years: Recommended Minimum Cardiological Evaluation

International Federation of Sports Medicine (FIMS)

Web site: www.fims.org

There is a general consensus in the medical community that everyone over the age of 35 years who wishes to participate in sport or fitness activities should undertake a medical examination. The aim of such an examination is

- to define the general state of health,
- to detect any defects which would contraindicate sports participation,
- to recognize and hence avoid situations which could cause cardiac complications.

The assessment should include a detailed cardiovascular history, a general physical examination, and a cardiological evaluation.

Nowadays, an increasing number of people of all ages exercise because of the known health benefits. However, some activities could be potentially harmful for individuals with undetected heart disease. The reported incidence of sudden death in sport is variable. Figures between 0.77 to 8.5/100,000/year have been quoted. The vast majority of these deaths are from ischemic heart disease. Hypothetically, some of these deaths could be prevented by an adequate program of evaluation but, in practice, it is not possible to universally implement these programs for several reasons:

1. the cost, in time and money, of the available techniques is high,
2. the efficiency of any complementary technique depends on available expertise and its diagnostic capacity, sensitivity, and specificity. (None of these techniques is 100% reliable),

3. frequently, potentially dangerous situations occur only on strenuous effort and/or under psychological stress, and
4. the use of these techniques in populations with a low prevalence of illness produces problems of diagnostic uncertainty. Also iatrogenic problems may result from sequential tests performed because of an abnormality.

It is, therefore, difficult to specify exactly the minimum requirements to be carried out prior to sports participation in these subjects, but the following information should be obtained:

1. a complete family and personal history to detect suspicious cardiac symptoms. Emphasis should be placed on breathlessness, fainting on effort, and pain. Prior to the medical examination, it is advisable for subjects to complete a questionnaire,
2. a careful physical examination,
3. a 12-lead resting electrocardiogram,
4. a maximal stress test to determine the adaptation to effort, the functional capacity and the incidence of arrhythmia, hypertension or ECG abnormalities, and
5. a chest x-ray.

If a murmur, hypertension, or an electrocardiograph abnormality is detected, further evaluation is mandatory. This includes an echocardiogram to rule out a structural heart defect as well as an assessment by a cardiologist. In cases where there is a minimally abnormal exercise test in an asymptomatic subject, one should be cautious about the interpretation. In such subjects, there is usually a low incidence of coronary heart disease. Risk factors should be considered. In doubtful cases (positive predictive value less than 90%), it is necessary to complete the investigation with a nuclear perfusion test (thallium, Tc99M). If any doubt remains, coronary angiography should be performed.

This statement may be reproduced and distributed with the sole requirement that it be identified clearly as a Position Statement of the International Federation of Sports Medicine.

PART IV

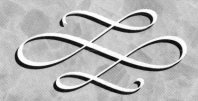

Educational
Information

CHAPTER 12

Sports Medicine Books

Publishers and Web Sites

ABBE Publishers Association of Washington, D.C.

American Academy of Orthopaedic Surgeons
www.aaos.org

American Academy of Pediatrics
www.aap.org

Aqua Quest Publications, Incorporated
http://aquaquest.com

Aspen Publishers
www.aspenpub.com

Blackwell Science, Incorporated
www.blackwell-science.com

BMJ Publishing Group
www.bmjpg.com

Book Tech, Incorporated

Butterworth-Heinemann
www.bh.com

Churchill Livingstone, Incorporated
www.harcourt-international.com

Clean Data, Incorporated
www.cleandata.com

Cramer Products, Incorporated
www.cramer

CRC Press LLC
www.crcpress.com

Crowood Press, Limited, The

Davis, F.A. Company
www.fadavis.com

Dekker, Marcel Incorporated
www.dekker.com

DIANE Publishing Company

Elsevier Science
www.elsevier.hl

Futura Publishing Company, Incorporated
www.futuraco.com

Hanley & Belfus, Incorporated
www2.hanleyandbelfus.com

Harcourt Brace & Company
www.harbrace.com

HarperCollins Publishers, Incorporated
www.harpercollins.com

Hogrefe & Huber Publishers
www.hhpub.com

Human Kinetics
www.humankinetics.com

Jones & Bartlett Publishers, Incorporated
www.jbpub.com

Lippincott-Williams & Wilkins
www.wwilkins.com

Macmillan Library Reference
http://mlr.com

McGraw-Hill Companies
www.mhhe.com

Mosby-Year Book, Incorporated
www.mosby.com

National Academy Press
www.nap.edu

Omnigraphics, Incorporated
www.omnigraphics.com

Oxford University Press, Incorporated
www.oup.co.uk

PRC Publishing
http://prcpub.com

Prentice Hall
www.prenhall.com

Preston Publications, Incorporated

Routledge
www.routledge-ny.com

Saunders, W.B. Company
www.wbsaunders.com

Singular Publishing Group, Incorporated
www.singpub.com

Skidmore-Roth Publishing, Incorporated
www.skidmore-roth.com

SLACK, Incorporated
www.slackinc.com

Sportsmed.com

Springer-Verlag New York, Incorporated
www.springer-ny.com

The Parthenon Publishing Group, Incorporated
www.parthpub.com

Thornes, Stanley Publishers, Incorporated

Whitston Publishing Company, Incorporated
www.whitston.com

Wiley, John & Sons, Incorporated
www.wiley.com

Books

1997 Year Book of Sports Medicine
Shephard, RJ
Mosby-Year Book, Incorporated 1998.

1998 Year Book of Sports Medicine
Shephard, RJ
Mosby-Year Book, Incorporated 1998.

1999 Year Book of Sports Medicine
Mosby-Year Book, Incorporated 1999.

2000 Year Book of Sports Medicine
Shephard, RJ
Mosby-Year Book Incorporated 2000.

2001 Year Book of Sports Medicine
Shephard, RJ
Mosby-Year Book, Incorporated 2001.

A Dictionary of Sports Injuries & Disorders
Potparic O, Gibson J
The Parthenon Publishing Group, Incorporated, 1996.

ABC of Sports Medicine
McLatchie G, Harries M, Williams C, King J (Editors)
BMJ Publishing Group 1995.

ACSM's Essentials of Sports Medicine
Sallis RE, Massimino F (Editors)
Mosby-Year Book, Incorporated 1996.

ACSM's Handbook for the Team Physician
Kibler WB (Editor)
Williams & Wilkins 1996.

Advances in Sports Cardiology
Pelliccia A, Caselli GA, Bellotti P
Springer-Verlag New York, Incorporated 1997.

Alcohol and Sport
Stainback RD
Human Kinetics 1997.

Allergic & Respiratory Disease in Sports Medicine
Weiler JM
Dekker, Marcel Incorporated 1997.

Amino Acids & Proteins for the Athlete
Di Pasquale MG
CRC Press LLC 1997.

Anabolic Steroids & Sports & Drug Testing, 1991-1997: An Annotated Bibliography
Paterson ER (Compiler)
Whitston Publishing Company, Incorporated 1998.

Anabolic Steroids in Sport and Exercise
Yesalis CE
Human Kinetics 1992.

Athletic Drug Reference '96
Fuentes RJ, Rosenberg JM, Davis A (Editors)
Clean Data, Incorporated 1996.

Athletic Injuries & Rehabilitation
Magee DJ
Saunders, W.B. Company 1996.

Athletic Taping
Sports Medicine Council of Britain
Davis, F.A. Company 1995.

Athletic Taping & Bracing
Perrin DH
Human Kinetics Publishers 1995.

Athletic Training for Student Assistants
Cartwright L, Pitney WA
Human Kinetics 1999.

Basic Sciences for Sports Medicine
Maughan RJ
Butterworth-Heinemann 1999.

Biomechanics of Musculoskeletal Injury
Whiting RF, Zernicke WC
Human Kinetics 1998.

Boxing & Medicine
Cantu RC (Editor)
Human Kinetics Publishers 1995.

Clinical & Event Sports Massage
Waslaski J
Other Stuff 1996.

Clinical Athletic Training
Konin J
SLACK, Incorporated 1996.

Clinical Experiences in Athletic Training: A Modular Approach
Knight KL
Human Kinetics Publishers 1998.

Clinical Orthopedic Assessment Guide, The
Loudon J, Bell SL, Johnston JM
Human Kinetics 1998.

Clinical Sports Medicine
Ullucci P, Edited by Robertson R
Skidmore-Roth Publishing, Incorporated 1998.

Complementary Sports Medicine
Maffetone P
Human Kinetics 1999.

Comprehensive Manual of Taping & Wrapping Techniques
Wright KE, Whitehill WR
Cramer Products, Incorporated 1996.

Concepts of Athletic Training
Pfeiffer RP, Mangus BC
Jones & Bartlett Publishers, Incorporated 1995.

Conservative Management of Sports Injuries
Hyde TE Jr, Gengenbach MS
Williams & Wilkins 1996.

Controversies in Orthopaedic Sports Medicine
Chan KM, Fu F, Maffuli N, Rolf C, Kurosaka M, Liu S
Human Kinetics 2000.

Cumulative Trauma Disorders
Cassvan A, Weiss LD, Weiss JM, Rook JL, Mullens SU
Butterworth-Heinemann 1997.

Diving Medicine for Scuba Divers
Edmonds C, McKenzie B, Thomas R
Aqua Quest Publications, Incorporated 1997.

Drug Testing in Sports
Black DL (Editor)
Preston Publications, Incorporated 1995.

Drugs in Sports
Mottram D
Routledge 1995.

Encyclopedia of Sports Science & Medicine
Zumerchik J
Macmillan Library Reference 1997.

Epidemiology of Sports Injuries
Caine DJ, Caine CG, Lindner KJ (Editors)
Human Kinetics Publishers 1996.

Essentials of Athletic Training
Arnheim DD
McGraw-Hill Companies, The 1998.

Evaluation of Orthopedic & Athletic Injuries
Starkey C, Ryan J
Davis, F. A. Company 1995.

Exercise in Rehabilitation Medicine
Frontera W, Slovik, DM, Dawson DM
Human Kinetics 1999.

Field Manual in Athletic Training
Anderson MK, Martin M
Williams & Wilkins 1998.

Foot Orthotics in Therapy & Sport
Hunter S, Dolan M, Davis JM
Human Kinetics Publishers 1995.

Fractures of the Distal Radius
Saffar P, Cooney WP (Editors)
Lippincott-Williams & Wilkins 1995.

Functional Evaluation & Outcomes in Sports & Orthopedic Physical Therapy
Brownstein B, Bronner S
Churchill Livingstone, Incorporated 1996.

Functional Rehabilitation of Sports & Musculoskeletal Injuries
Kibler WB, Staff RIC, Herring S, Press J
Aspen Publishers 1998.

Fundamentals of Sports Injury Management
Anderson MK, Hall SJ, Hitchings C
Williams & Wilkins 1997.

Fundamentals of Sports Injury Management Student Workbook
Martin M, Naderson KJ, Hall SJ
Williams & Wilkins 1997.

Handbook of Sports Epidemiology
Jordan B
C R C Press LLC 1999.

HIV Tracing & Transmission in People in Working, Sports & Professional Populations: Index of New Information
Dubrowski EL
ABBE Publishers Association of Washington, D.C. 1997.

HIV/AIDS in Sport
Sankaran G, Bonsall DR, Volkwein K
Human Kinetics 1998.

Imaging in Musculoskeletal & Sports Medicine
Halpern B
Blackwell Science, Incorporated 1997.

Injections in Orthopaedics & Sports Medicine
Saunders, Cameron
Saunders, W.B. Company 1997.

Injuries in Baseball
Andrews JR (Editor)
Lippincott-Williams & Wilkins 1998.

Instructions for Sports Medicine
Safran
Saunders, W.B. Company 1999.

Isokinetics in Human Performance
Brown LE
Human Kinetics 2000.

Legal Aspects of Sports Medicine
Herbert DL, Herbert WG
PRC Publishing 1995.

**Magnetic Resonance Imaging in
Orthopaedics & Sports Medicine**
Stoller DW
Lippincott-Williams & Wilkins 1996.

**Management of Bloodborne Infections in
Sport**
Zeigler TA
Human Kinetics Publishers 1996.

Manual of Athletic Taping
Sports Medicine Council of Brit
Davis, F. A. Company 1995.

Manual of Sports Medicine
Safran
Lippincott-Williams & Wilkins 1997.

Medical Problems in Athletes
Fields KB, Fricker PA
Blackwell Science, Incorporated 1997.

Office Sports Medicine
Mellion MB (Editor)
Hanley & Belfus, Incorporated 1995.

**On Field Evaluation & Treatment of Sport
Injuries**
Andrews JR
Mosby-Year Book, Incorporated 1997.

Orthopaedic Knowledge Update
Arendt EA, American Orthopaedic Society for
Surgeons 1999.

Orthopedic & Sports Physical Therapy
Malone TR
Mosby-Year Book, Incorporated 1996.

Oxford Handbook of Sports Medicine
Sherry E, Wilson S (Editor)
Oxford University Press, Incorporated 1998.

Oxford Textbook of Sports Medicine
Harries M, Williams C, Stanish WD, Micheli
LJ
Oxford University Press, Incorporated 1995.

Pediatric Sports Medicine
Stricker PR, Landry GL, Micheli LJ
American Academy of Pediatrics 1998.

**Pharmacology for Athletic Trainers:
Performance Enhancement & Social Drugs**
Human Kinetics Staff
Human Kinetics Publishers 1997.

Physical Rehabilitation of the Injured Athlete
Andrews JR, Harrelson GL
Saunders, W.B. Company 1997.

Physical Therapy for Sports
Kuprian W
Saunders, W.B. Company 1995.

Preparticipation Physical Evaluation
American Academy of Family Phys,
Preparticipation Physical Evaluation Task
Force
McGraw-Hill Companies, The 1996.

**Principles & Practices of Isokinetics in Sports
Medicine & Rehabilitation**
Chan KM, Maffuli N, Korkia P, Li R
Human Kinetics 2000.

**Proprioception and Neuromuscular Control
in Joint Stability**
Lephart, SM
Human Kinetics 2000.

**Psychological Approaches to Sports Injury
Rehabilitation**
Taylor J, Taylor S
Aspen Publishers 1997.

Radiological Imaging of Sports Injuries
Masciocchi C, Barile A
Springer-Verlag New York, Incorporated 1997.

Radiology of Sports Injuries
Anderson IF, Steinweg J, Read J
McGraw-Hill Professional Book Group 1999.

Rehabilitation in Sports Medicine
Canavan PK (Editor)
McGraw-Hill Companies, The 1997.

Review of Sports Medicine & Arthroscopy
Miller MD, Cooper DE (Editors)
Saunders, W.B. Company 1995.

Revision of Failed Arthroscopic & Ligament Surgery
Zarins B, Marder RA
Blackwell Science, Incorporated 1998.

Running Injuries
Guten GN
Saunders, W.B. Company 1997.

Science & Medicine in Sport (2nd ed.)
Bloomfield J (Editor)
Human Kinetics 1996.

Shoulder Injuries in Sport Evaluation, Treatment, & Rehabilitation
Ciullo JV
Human Kinetics Publishers 1996.

Shoulder Injuries in the Athlete Surgical Repair & Rehabilitation
Hawkins RJ, Misamore GW (Editors)
Churchill Livingstone, Incorporated 1995.

Shoulder Pathophysiology Rehabilitaiton & Treatment
Haig SV
Aspen Publishers 1995.

Soft Tissue Injuries in Sports Medicine
Almekinders LC
Blackwell Science, Incorporated 1995.

Spiral Manual of Sports Medicine
Safran MR, McKeag D, Van Camp SP
Lippincott-Williams & Wilkins 1998.

Sports Chiropractic & Rehabilitation
Mootz RD, McCarthy KA
Aspen Publishers 1999.

Sports Encyclopedia: Index & Reference Books of New Information, Vol. 3

Sports, Drugs & Doping
Bronsen HH
ABBE Publishers Association of Washington, D.C. 1996.

Sports Encyclopedia: Index & Reference Books of New Information, Vol. 9

Sports, Prevention & Control of Athletic Injuries Vol. 9
Bronsen HH
ABBE Publishers Association of Washington, D.C. 1996.

Sports Gynecology
Warren M, Shagold MM
Blackwell Science, Incorporated 1996.

Sports Injuries Diagnosis & Treatment
Garrick
Harcourt Brace & Company 1999.

Sports Injuries & Illnesses
O'Connor R, Budgett R, Wells C, Lewis J
Crowood Press, Limited, The 1998.

Sports Injuries of the Ankle & Foot
Lian GJ, Marder RA
Springer-Verlag New York, Incorporated 1996.

Sports Injuries of the Lower Extremity
McNerney
Saunders, W.B. Company 1996.

Sports Injuries Sourcebook
Aldred H (Editor)
Omnigraphics, Incorporated 1999.

Sports Injuries Causes, Diagnosis, Treatment & Prevention
Bird S, Black N, Newton P
Singular Publishing Group, Incorporated 1997.

Sports Injuries Recognition & Management
Hutson MA (Editor)
Oxford University Press, Incorporated 1996.

Sports Injury Assessment & Rehabilitation
Reid DC
Churchill Livingstone, Incorporated 1998.

Sports Injury Management
Anderson MK, Hall SJ
Williams & Wilkins 1995.

Sports Medicine
Irvin, Iversen
Prentice Hall 1998.

Sports Medicine
Prentice Hall 1995.

Sports Medicine
Sobell
Wiley, John & Sons, Incorporated 1999.

Sports Medicine Ethics & the Law
Grayson E, Bond C
Butterworth-Heinemann 1999.

Sports Medicine Practical Guidelines for General Practice
MacAuley D
Butterworth-Heinemann 1999.

Sports Medicine for Primary Care
Richmond JC, Shahady EJ
Blackwell Science, Incorporated 1995.

Sports Medicine in Primary Care
Johnson
Saunders, W.B. Company 2000.

Sports Medicine Roles & Responsibilities for High School Team Physicians & Athletic Trainers
Ohio State Medical Association, Ohio High School Athletic Association, Ohio Athletic Trainers Association
PRC Publishing 1997.

Sports Medicine Primary Care & Rehabilitation
Scuderi GR, McCann PD (Editors)
Mosby-Year Book, Incorporated 1996.

Sports Medicine The School Age Athlete
Reuder B
Saunders, W.B. Company 1996.

Sports Neurology
Jordan BD, Tsairis P, Warren RF (Editors)
Lippincott-Williams & Wilkins 1998.

Sports Ophthalmology
Zagelbaum BM
Blackwell Science, Incorporated 1996.

Sports Therapy
Hudson M
Thornes, Stanley Publishers, Incorporated 1998.

Sudden Cardiac Death in the Athlete
Wang, Salem, Estes NA (Editors)
Futura Publishing Company, Incorporated 1998.

Surgical Atlas of Sports Medicine
Miller
Saunders, W.B. Company 1999.

Taping Techniques Principles & Practice
MacDonald R (Editor)
Butterworth-Heinemann 1999.

Textbook of Hyperbaric Medicine
Jain, KK
Hogrefe & Huber Publishers 1999.

The Athlete & Heart Disease
Williams RA
Lippincott-Williams & Wilkins 1998.

The Child & Adolescent Athlete
Bar-Or O, IOC Medical Commission Staff, International Federation of Sport (Editors)
Blackwell Science, Incorporated 1995.

The Clinical Pharmacology of Sport & Exercise: Proceedings of the Esteve Foundation
Symposium VII, Sitges, Spain, 2-5 October 1996
Fundacion AE, Reilly T, Orme M
Elsevier Science 1997.

The Elbow in Sport Injury, Treatment, & Rehabilitation
Ellenbecker TS, Mattalino A
Human Kinetics Publishers 1996.

The Female Athlete
Teitz C (Editor)
American Academy of Orthopaedic Surgeons
1996.

The Hughston Clinic Sports Medicine Field Manual
Baker CL, Flandry F, Henderson JM (Editors)
Williams & Wilkins 1996.

The Hughston Clinic Sports Medicine Book
Baker CL (Editor)
Williams & Wilkins 1995.

The Injured Athlete
Perrin D
Lippincott-Williams & Wilkins 1998.

The Problem Knee
Macnicol MF
Butterworth-Heinemann 1995.

The Role of Dietary Supplements for Physically Active People: Current Bibliographies in Medicine: January 1966 Through April 1996 Current Bibliographies in Medicine: January 1966 Through April 1996
Scannell KM, Marriott BM
DIANE Publishing Company 1996.

The Role of Protein & Amino Acids in Sustaining & Enhancing Performance
Institute of Medicine Staff
National Academy Press 1999.

The Spine in Sports
Watkins RG
Mosby-Year Book, Incorporated 1995.

The Sports Medicine Bible Prevent, Detect, & Treat Your Sports Injuries Through the Latest Medical Techniques
Micheli LJ, Jenkins M
HarperCollins Publishers, Incorporated 1995.

The Steroids Game
Yesalis CE, Cowart VS
Human Kinetics Publishers 1998.

The Team Physician's Handbook
Mellion MB, Walsh M, Shelton GL (Editors)
Hanley & Belfus, Incorporated 1996.

The USSF Sports Medicine Book of Soccer
Garrett WE Jr, Contiguglia SR, Kirkendall DT (Editors)
Williams & Wilkins 1996.

Therapeutic Medications in Sports Medicine
Martin M, Yates WN Jr
Williams & Wilkins 1997.

Therapeutic Modalities in Sports Medicine
Prentice WE
McGraw-Hill Companies, The 1999.

Topics in Sports Physical Therapy
Brown S (Compiler)
Book Tech, Incorporated 1996.

Treatment & Rehabilitation of Fractures
Hoppenfeld S
Lippincott-Williams & Wilkins 1999.

Upper Extremity in Sports Injuries
Jobe FW
Mosby-Year Book, Incorporated 1995.

CHAPTER 13
Sports Medicine Journals

Advances in Sports Medicine and Fitness
ISSN: 08893977
Publisher: Mosby-Year Book, Inc. (Chicago)
Frequency: annual

American Journal of Knee Surgery
ISSN: 08997403
Publisher: Slack, Inc.
Frequency: quarterly
www.slackinc.com

American Journal of Medicine and Sports
Publisher: LeJacq Communications, Inc.
Frequency: bimonthly

American Journal of Sports Medicine
ISSN: 03635465
Sponsor: American Orthopaedic Society for
Sports Medicine
Frequency: bimonthly
www.sportsmed.org

Annals of Sports Medicine
ISSN: 07341997
Publisher: Raven Press
Frequency: quarterly

Athletic Therapy Today
ISSN: 10787895
Publisher: Human Kinetics Publishers, Inc.
Frequency: bimonthly
www.humankinetics.com/products/journals/
journal.cfm?id=ATT

British Journal of Sports Medicine
ISSN: 03063674
Sponsor: British Association of Sport and
Medicine
Publisher: B M J Publishing Group
Frequency: quarterly
www.bjsportmed.com

Canadian Journal of Applied Physiology
ISSN: 10667814
Sponsor: Canadian Society for Exercise
Physiology
Publisher: Human Kinetics Publishers, Inc.
Frequency: bimonthly
www.humankinetics.com/products/journals/
journal.cfm?id=CJAP

Canadian Journal of Sports Medicine
Publisher: Rodar Publishing Inc.
Frequency: quarterly

Clinical Journal of Sport Medicine
ISSN: 1050642X
Sponsor: Canadian Academy of Sport
Medicine
Publisher: Lippincott-Raven Publishers
Frequency: quarterly
www.lww.com

Clinical Sports Medicine
ISSN: 09539875
Sponsor: International Association of
Olympic Medical Officers

Publisher: Chapman & Hall, Journals
Department
Frequency: quarterly

Clinics in Sports Medicine
ISSN: 02785919
Publisher: W.B. Saunders Co.
Frequency: quarterly
http://wbsaunders.com

Foot & Ankle International
ISSN: 10711007
Sponsor: American Orthopaedic Foot and
Ankle Society Inc.
Publisher: Williams & Wilkins
Frequency: monthly
www.wwilkins.com

International Journal of Sport Nutrition
ISSN: 10501606
Publisher: Human Kinetics Publishers, Inc.
Frequency: quarterly
www.humankinetics.com/products/journals/
journal.cfm?id=IJSN

International Journal of Sports Medicine
ISSN: 01724622
Publisher: Georg Thieme Verlag
Frequency: 8 times a year
www.thieme.de

International Journal of Sports Vision
ISSN: 10714235
Sponsor: International Academy of Sports
Vision
Frequency: annual

**Japanese Journal of Physical Fitness and
Sports Medicine**
ISSN: 0039906X
Sponsor: Japanese Society of Physcial
Fitness and Sports Medicine
Frequency: bimonthly

Journal of Applied Sport Psychology
ISSN: 10413200
Sponsor: Association for the Advancement
of Applied Sport Psychology
Frequency: semiannually
www.allenpress.com

Journal of Athletic Training
ISSN: 10626050

Sponsor: National Athletic Trainers
Association, Inc.
Frequency: quarterly
www.nata.org

**Journal of Back and Musculoskeletal
Rehabilitation**
ISSN: 10538127
Publisher: I O S Press
Frequency: bimonthly
www.iospress.nl

**Journal of Orthopaedic and Sports Physical
Therapy**
ISSN: 01906011
Sponsor: American Physical Therapy
Association
Publisher: Allen Press Inc.
Frequency: monthly
www.allenpress.com

Journal of Osteopathic Sports Medicine
ISSN: 08933871
Sponsor: American Osteopathic Academy of
Sports Medicine
Frequency: 5 times a year

Journal of Science and Medicine in Sport
ISSN: 14402440
Sponsor: Australian Council for Health,
Physical Education, and Recreation
Publisher: Sports Medicine Australia
Frequency: quarterly
www.sportsmedicine.com.au
www.humankinetics.com

Journal of Sport Rehabilitation
ISSN: 10566716
Publisher: Human Kinetics Publishers, Inc.
Frequency: quarterly
www.humankinetics.com/products/journals/
journal.cfm?id=JSR

**Journal of Sports Chiropractic and
Rehabilitation**
ISSN: 10841288
Publisher: Williams & Wilkins
Frequency: quarterly
www.wwilkins.com/csm

**Journal of Sports Traumatology and Related
Research**
ISSN: 11203137

Publisher: Editrice Kurtis s.r.l.
Frequency: quarterly

Journal of the American Podiatric Medical Association

ISSN: 00030538
Sponsor: American Academy of Podiatric Sports Medicine
Publisher: Allen Press, Inc.
Frequency: 10 times a year
www.apma.org/www.allenpress.com

Knee Surgery, Sports Traumatology, Arthroscopy

ISSN: 09422056
Sponsor: European Society of Sports Traumatology, Knee Surgery and Arthroscopy
Publisher: Springer-Verlag
Frequency: quarterly
http://link.springer.de/link/service/journals/00167/index.hm

Medicine and Science in Sports and Exercise

ISSN: 01959131
Sponsor: American College of Sports Medicine
Frequency: monthly
www.acsm.org/igrpurp.htm

Medscape Orthopedics & Sports Medicine

Publisher: Medscape, Inc.
Frequency: 6 times a year
www.medscape.com

Musculoskeletal Medicine

ISSN: 09658408
Sponsor: Primary Care Rheumatology Society
Publisher: Imprint Services
Frequency: quarterly

New Zealand Journal of Sports Medicine

ISSN: 01106384
Sponsor: Sports Medicine New Zealand
Frequency: quarterly

Operative Techniques in Sports Medicine

ISSN: 10601872
Publisher: W.B. Saunders Co.
Frequency: quarterly
www.wbsaunders.com

Orthopaedic and Traumatic Surgery

ISSN: 03874095
Publisher: Kanehara Shuppan Ltd.
Frequency: monthly

Scandinavian Journal of Medicine & Science in Sports

ISSN: 09057188
Sponsor: Scandinavian Foundation of Medical Science in Sports
Publisher: Munksgaard International Publishers Ltd.
Frequency: bimonthly
www.munkgaard.dk

South African Journal of Sports Medicine

Publisher: In House Publication
Frequency: quarterly

Sport Health

ISSN: 1032562
Publisher: Sports Medicine Australia
Frequency: quarterly
www.sportsmedicine.com.au

Sportcare

ISSN: 13532693
Sponsor: National Sports Medicine Institute of the United Kingdom
Publisher: Medical College of St. Barts Hospital
Frequency: bimonthly

Sports Injury Management

ISSN: 10489304
Publisher: Williams & Wilkins
Frequency: quarterly

Sports Medicine

ISSN: 01121642
Publisher: Adis International Limited
Frequency: monthly
www.adis.com/biomednet.com/library/jspm

Sports Medicine

Sponsor: Indian Association of Sports Medicine
Publisher: Netaji Subhas National Institute of Sports
Frequency: semiannually

Sports Medicine Alert

ISSN: 15218333

Publisher: Mountainview Publishing, L.L.C.
Frequency: monthly

Sports Medicine and Arthroscopy Review
ISSN: 10628592
Publisher: Lippincott Williams & Wilkins (Philadelphia)
Frequency: quarterly
www.lww.com

Sports Medicine Bulletin
ISSN: 09524630
Sponsor: National Sports Medicine Institute of the United Kingdom
Publisher: Medical College of St. Bartholomew's Hospital
Frequency: monthly
www.nsmi.org.uk

Sports Medicine Reports
Publisher: Mountainview Publishing, L.L.C.
Frequency: quarterly

Sports Medicine Research Today
ISSN: 08979340
Publisher: BIOSIS
Frequency: monthly

Sports Medicine Standards & Malpractice Reporter
ISSN: 1041696X
Publisher: PRC Publishing, Inc.
Frequency: quarterly

Sports Medicine, Training and Rehabilitation
ISSN: 10578315
Publisher: Gordon and Breach - Harwood Academic
Frequency: quarterly
www.gbhap.com/Sports—Medicine

Sports Mediscope
Sponsor: United States Olympic Committee
Frequency: quarterly

Sports Physiology and Medicine
ISSN: 09677755
Sponsor: SUBIS
Frequency: monthly
www.shef-ac-press.co.uk

Sports Trainers Digest
ISSN: 10325506
Publisher: Sports Medicine Australia
Frequency: quarterly
www.sportsmedicine.com.au

Sports, Exercise and Injury
ISSN: 13510029
Sponsor: European Federation of Orthopaedic Sports Traumatology
Publisher: Churchill Livingstone
Frequency: quarterly
www.churchillmed.com

SportsVision Quarterly
Publisher: Miller Freeman Inc. (New York)
Frequency: quarterly

The Journal of Musculoskeletal Medicine
ISSN: 08992517
Publisher: Cliggott Publishing Co.
Frequency: monthly

The Journal of Sports Medicine and Physical Fitness
ISSN: 00224707
Publisher: Alberto Oliaro
Frequency: quarterly

The Physician and Sportsmedicine
ISSN: 00913847
Publisher: McGraw-Hill Companies (Minneapolis)
Frequency: monthly
www.physsportsmed.com

The Year Book of Sports Medicine
ISSN: 01620908
Sponsor: American College of Sports Medicine
Publisher: Mosby, Inc., Continuity Division
Frequency: annual

Wilderness and Environmental Medicine
ISSN: 10806032
Sponsor: Wilderness Medical Society
Publisher: Allen Press, Inc., Division of Alliance Communications Group
Frequency: quarterly
www.allenpress.com